Ethical Issues in Drug Testing, Approval, and Pricing

ETHICAL ISSUES IN DRUG TESTING, APPROVAL, AND PRICING

The Clot-Dissolving Drugs

Baruch A. Brody, Ph.D.

New York   Oxford
OXFORD UNIVERSITY PRESS
1995

Oxford University Press

Oxford   New York   Toronto
Delhi   Bombay   Calcutta   Madras   Karachi
Kuala Lumpur   Singapore   Hong Kong   Tokyo
Nairobi   Dar es Salaam   Cape Town
Melbourne   Auckland   Madrid

and associated companies in
Berlin   Ibadan

Published by Oxford University Press, Inc.
200 Madison Avenue, New York, New York 10016

Oxford is a registered trademark of Oxford University Press

Library of Congress Cataloging-in-Publication Data
Brody, Baruch A.
    Ethical issues in drug testing, approval, and pricing :
  the clot-dissolving drugs /
Baruch A. Brody.
        p. cm.
    Includes bibliographical references and index.
    ISBN 0-19-508831-X
    1. Fibrinolytic agents.
  2. Drugs—Testing—Moral and ethical aspects.
  3. Drugs—Prices—Moral and ethical aspects.
  I. Title.
  RM340.B76   1995   174'.2—dc20   94-4479

9 8 7 6 5 4 3 2 1

Printed in the United States of America
on acid-free paper

To
Ellen and Todd
Rocky and Jeremy
Myles

Preface

This book combines bioethical concerns about clinical issues with philosophical concerns about the policies of a liberal, pluralistic society. The clinical concerns are about the testing, approval, and adoption of new drugs; the philosophical concerns are about people's different rankings of goods, about society's need to respect those rankings, and about the need to be sensitive to the difference between people's expressed rankings of goods and their actual ranking of goods.

I have been fortunate that my academic position has enabled me to explore the interrelationship between these concerns. I am thankful to Baylor College of Medicine, The Institute of Religion, and Rice University for jointly sponsoring the Center for Ethics, Medicine, and Public Issues, a center which I have headed since it was founded in 1982. This arrangement has greatly facilitated my interdisciplinary work; without it, this book would not have been possible.

Because the book focuses on one clinical example to illustrate certain problems and to propose certain solutions, some readers may be tempted to see this book as an exposé of certain blocs within the community of cardiologists. Such a reading would be a great mistake, and I caution against it throughout the book. Even when I conclude that particular groups made faulty decisions (in some cases, tragic errors), I always remind the reader that this shows much more about the need for society to deal with certain issues than it shows about anyone's personal failings. I want to reinforce those reminders in this preface. This is a work of scholarship about issues rather than a journalistic exposé of people.

There are a number of people that I must thank. Bob Arnold, Bob Levine, Allen Matusow, Janet Wittes, Jim Young, and Salim Yusuf read portions of the manuscript and helped me both with their useful suggestions and with their encouragement and support. Audiences at Baylor College of Medicine, the University of Pittsburgh, Prairie Cardiovascular Research Center, a PRIMR conference, the Society for Clinical Trials, The University of Texas at Galveston, and the University of Utah stimulated my continued work on this project with their helpful questions and comments. I am thankful to all of them. Special thanks are due to Sarah

Brakman for her help with the initial gathering of material and for her many suggestions, and to Maureen Kelley for her help in the final production of the book and the index. Finally, in dedicating this book to our sons and our daughters-in-law, I am thanking all of them for the joy and satisfaction that they have given to Dena and me.

Houston   B. A. B.
February 1994

Contents

Ethical Issues in Drug Testing, Approval, and Pricing

Introduction

In the United States, as in most industrialized countries, the process by which drugs are tested, approved, and adopted is heavily regulated. The many regulations attempt to address important ethical and social questions related to protecting research subject safety, to ensuring that approved drugs are safe and efficacious, and to overseeing the marketing process. They constitute an impressive attempt to balance the goals of promoting scientific and medical advances with those of protecting other societal interests.

In this book, however, I argue that this attempt, as impressive as it has been, has failed to adequately address important issues in each stage of the process. In the drug development and testing stage, important issues that have not been adequately addressed include giving some subjects placebos (dummy pills) as a control when testing new life-saving drugs, obtaining informed consent to be enrolled in a trial from research subjects facing emergency life-threatening situations, and avoiding conflicts of interest that inappropriately influence the ways in which drugs are tested. In the drug approval stage, important issues that have not been adequately addressed include how to balance our desire for the best possible evidence with our desire to speed the drug approval process and how to weigh the relative importance of safety and efficacy in approving drugs. In the drug adoption stage, important issues that have not been adequately addressed include how clinicians should take prices into account when prescribing drugs and how new drugs should be priced so as to adequately reimburse companies for the cost of developing expensive new drugs while not excessively burdening consumers.

Some of these issues have been discussed extensively by ethicists; many—particularly those surrounding drug approval and drug adoption—have been glossed over. To my mind, this is part of a general failure of ethicists to pay enough attention to the institutional framework in which health care is practiced. For example, it is not enough to worry about how doctors and patients should deal with the costs of drugs in making clinical decisions, a question that has been scrutinized by ethicists. Ethicists also need to worry about why drugs cost so much, and whether institutional changes resulting in changed prices wouldn't make the clinical decisions easier. This book attempts to deal with these and other institutional issues.

The opening chapter presents a case study (the testing, approval, and adoption of clot-dissolving drugs for patients with heart attacks) that illustrates each of these problems. In the remaining chapters, I will argue that the case study illustrates how the problems in question have not yet been resolved, although much has been said about each one, and I will examine alternative approaches to dealing with each of these problems.

This case study played a very important role in the development of my own understanding of these problems. In the spring of 1984, I was a member of the Baylor College of Medicine Institutional Review Board, the committee charged with the responsibility for protecting human subjects in research at our medical school. We received a research protocol for a series of studies called the TIMI (Thrombolysis in Myocardial Infarction) studies. These studies, to be funded by the National Institutes of Health, were designed to test clot-dissolving drugs in patients who were in the midst of a heart attack. Some of the proposed studies involved testing these drugs against placebos (dummy pills). I was concerned about the plan since I remembered reading that these drugs had recently been shown to save lives in patients who were having a heart attack. Was it ethical to withhold them from some patients? Moreover, could patients make a meaningful choice to participate or not to participate in these studies given their condition in the midst of having a heart attack? If not, would it be ethical to enroll these patients in a research study? The Baylor Institutional Review Board gave approval to the first part of these proposed studies, which did not involve the use of placebos, and reserved its judgment about the rest. I decided to follow these trials, and I opened a file on thrombolytic therapy. Little did I know then how large this file would soon become. As time progressed, more and more material was added to the file (which now occupies a very full file cabinet drawer) as more and more questions arose about thrombolytic therapy. In this book, the case study is presented to illustrate the problems and to evaluate possible solutions. In my professional life, the case study actually taught me what the ethical problems are regarding how drugs are developed, approved, and adopted. Rarely does service on committees in academic institutions yield this type of intellectual reward.

One final observation. There are many points in the book at which it becomes necessary to examine in some detail medical, economic, and legal points, and the treatment may seem too technical for some readers. Unfortunately, understanding these technical points is essential for a responsible treatment of the issues. If medical ethics is to make a difference in the real world in which issues often involve complex technical points, ethicists and others interested in ethics will have to learn to work with them. I write this not to apologize to the reader but to offer an advanced warning and explanation. The story I will tell and the issues it will illustrate are fascinating but not easy.

1

The Development
of Thrombolytic Therapy

This opening chapter presents the history of one of the most important recent developments in modern medicine: a new way of saving the lives of many patients who would otherwise die from a heart attack. Although the history is itself very interesting, since my goal is not just to tell the story but to use it to illustrate the ethical issues we will be discussing throughout the rest of the book, I will be injecting these issues as the history unfolds.

The first section presents the medical developments which serve as the background for the rest of the history. For those who are familiar with the medical background, the history of its development may be of interest. For those unfamiliar with the medical background, the opening sections should provide the needed understanding of that background as well as surveying how that background knowledge developed.

The Medical Background

All stories must begin somewhere, but it's often hard for the storyteller to know where to begin. People have suffered from chest pain and died from heart attacks for as long as there have been people, and it would be of great value for other purposes to trace the history of human reflection on these phenomena. But for our purpose, which is to trace the development of thrombolytic therapy, we can begin with a paper published by James Herrick in 1912. This paper played a central role in the development of modern medicine's emphasis on the obstruction of the coronary arteries—the arteries supplying the heart—as the cause of heart attacks.

James Herrick and the Coronary Thrombosis Hypothesis

Herrick was born in Illinois in 1861, graduated from Rush Medical College in 1886, and served on its faculty for the whole of his teaching career.[1] His main work was in the areas of cardiology and hematology, and his paper of 1912 is widely recognized as a great classic.[2] But even those who give it that recognition often fail to explain why it was such an important paper and how it contributed to further work in the field. We begin our story by trying to better understand Herrick's contribution.

Part of his contribution was reemphasizing the idea that narrowed and eventually obstructed coronary arteries were responsible for chest pain (angina pectoris) and sudden death. William Heberdeen (1710–1801) had first described in 1768 this chest pain and its progression over time; Edward Jenner (1749–1823) and Caleb Parry (1755–1822) had suggested that the reduction of blood flow through narrowed coronary arteries was responsible for the pain.[3] Other authors whose work is described by Herrick had shown that the sudden total blockage of these arteries by a clot could cause death. Herrick's paper supported this view by presenting several cases, the most important of which was a detailed history of a patient who died 52 hours after suffering severe chest pain followed by chills, nausea, and a rapid pulse. Upon autopsy, one could see the severely narrowed and hardened arteries and a red clot (thrombus) which completely blocked the left coronary artery at a point at which it was severely narrowed.

Another part of Herrick's contribution was to emphasize the possibility of people surviving at least for some time after their arteries were completely blocked. In a famous passage, Herrick divided patients into four categories, those who died instantaneously and painlessly, those who died after a few minutes of pain and shock, those who suffered chest pain without ever suffering an acute crisis, and those who survived the type of acute attack which killed the first two types of patients.[4] Herrick emphasized the last group, whose existence had not been adequately noted earlier, since he felt that proper medical care designed to restore the functional integrity of the heart "may occasionally in such cases save life."[5]

Herrick himself said that his paper initially attracted little attention:

> The publication aroused no interest. It fell like a dud. Recognizing the radical nature of the view I held . . . I doggedly kept at the subject, doing what I called "missionary work." . . . I hammered away at the topic. When in 1918 I showed lantern slides and electrocardiograms [of coronary obstruction], physicians in America and later Europe woke up [to the diagnosis which was] later to become a household word translated by the layman into "heart attack."[6]

What Herrick was alluding to in that quote was a paper published in 1919 in which he described the electrocardiogram (ECG) of a patient who had suffered a heart attack.[7] By contemporary standards, the evidence offered in the paper is hardly overwhelming. Herrick persuaded a colleague, Dr. Fred Smith, to do a study in which he compared the electrocardiogram of dogs before and after different coronary arteries were ligated. Following the ligation, various irregularities were noted in the electrocardiograms. Similar irregularities were noted in the electrocardiogram of one patient whose clinical course is described, although the exact similarities are not carefully described in the paper. Herrick admitted that further work was obviously required, and the most he could suggest is that abnormal electrocardiograms might provide helpful confirmation of the existence of blockages in the coronary arteries.

This is the first occurrence of a phenomenon that will be common in our story, namely, that one medical development is influenced in a major way by other initially unrelated developments. In this case, improved understanding of clots and chest disease was made possible by the development by W. Einthoven (1860–1927) of a practical and reliable way to measure electrical activity of the heart.[8] Herrick was able to strengthen the hypothesis that the cause of acute attacks was blockage by clots (the coronary thrombosis hypothesis) by suggesting that patients suffering an acute attack had an ECG that was very similar to animals whose coronary arteries were clearly blocked.

In a recent article, J. E. Muller emphasized that others had put forward the coronary thrombosis hypothesis before Herrick and that they had supported that hypothesis by similar autopsy studies.[9] All of that is correct, but I believe that it misses the point. I believe that Herrick's major contributions were to vigorously advocate the hypothesis, put forward the new ECG evidence for its truth, and suggest for the first time that at least some patients might be saved if a blood supply could be provided. Moreover, and even more fundamentally, Herrick's work combined a physiological interest in the functioning of the heart (as measured by the ECG readings) with an anatomical interest in what was happening to the heart muscle because of the blockage of the coronary artery. As C. Lawrence has argued, it is only this combination of perspectives which led Herrick to begin the modern understanding of a heart attack.[10]

There is a widespread perception of science as a cumulative series of advances, each one building on the previous advances. This picture has been criticized by many modern scholars,[11] and we need not repeat their general observations here. What should be pointed out here is that Herrick's coronary thrombosis hypothesis did *not* serve in the years that followed as the basis for continued progress. Rather, it underwent a series of critiques, some less radical and some more so, which led to considerable doubt about the ultimate truth of the coronary thrombosis hypothesis.

The less radical critiques arose from pathologic studies which showed that many acute episodes did not involve the blockage of a coronary artery by a clot and that some clot blockages did not result in death after an acute crisis. Typical of such studies were those by Friedberg and Horn in 1939[12] and by Blumgart, Schlesinger, and Davis in 1940.[13] The former study expanded on many earlier observations that death of the heart muscle tissue can occur without blockage of a coronary artery by a clot but that the electrocardiogram reading could be the same because it is due to the death of the tissue (the infarction) rather than to the clot. Friedberg and Horn systematically reviewed 2,000 autopsies performed over 4 years at Mount Sinai Hospital. They found 153 deaths involving the death of the myocardium and identified 34 of those as *not* involving a coronary thrombosis. These deaths were due to inadequate blood flow to meet the demands of the heart; they suggested, but this could occur without the formation of a clot which blocked the artery. They proposed that the accurate term for this form of crisis was "myocardial infarction" (death of the tissue of the heart muscle because of inadequate blood flow), and they concluded that many myocardial infarctions were unrelated to coronary thromboses. Blumgart and his colleagues examined 125 autopsies and discovered that coronary thromboses which result in totally blocked arteries do not necessarily produce any clinical manifestations, much less a myocardial infarction. This is due to the fact that during the years in which the arteries were progressively becoming narrower, the patients were developing widened connections between the different coronary arteries so that blood could flow into the area beyond the blockage (collateral circulation) and provide a constant blood flow to that part of the heart's muscle.

The relation between myocardial infarctions and coronary thromboses was further clarified by a pathologic study published in 1951 by Miller, Burchell, and Edwards.[14] They studied 143 cases of myocardial infarctions and found coronary thromboses present in 94 (66 percent) of these cases but absent in 49 (34 percent) cases. Their more crucial finding was an associated difference in the location of the infarcts in the wall of the heart. Some 89 percent of the patients with coronary thromboses had tissue death involving the full thickness of the wall of the ventricle (transmural infarcts) while 82 percent of the patients without coronary thromboses had tissue death only in part of the wall (subendocardial infarcts).

All of these less radical critiques accepted Herrick's basic concept that coronary thromboses caused myocardial infarctions and death. They disagreed only with his emphasis on thromboses as the sole cause, postulating (especially in subendocardial infarcts) other causes and postulating (especially if collateral circulation had developed) the real possibility of survival even after a total blockage of a major coronary artery.

Other critics emerged in the 1950s who were far more skeptical about Herrick's claim. They argued that Herrick had the causal relations backwards; thromboses, they claimed, were the result of the myocardial infarctions, not their cause.

An early version of this alternative is a 1956 article by Branwood and Montgomery arguing that thrombus formation cannot be the cause of myocardial infarctions (but must rather be an effect) in part because thrombi are often not present but even more because the thrombi, even when present, seem to be more recent than the infarctions.[15] Their argument depended heavily on certain assumptions about occlusion thrombi, and they admitted that these assumption were far from established. A few years later, Spain and Bradess argued that since the frequency of thrombi increases progressively with the duration of the acute fatal episode, the thrombi must result from some time-consuming process following the onset of the acute episode of myocardial infarction and cannot be the cause of that acute episode.[16] This view, reinforced by further evidence from other studies, was supported by Dr. William Roberts of the NIH in an influential editorial published 14 years later[17] and by many (but by no means all) of the participants at a 1973 workshop sponsored by the NIH.[18]

By the late 1970s, Herrick's original hypothesis, even when suitably modified, remained a matter of considerable controversy. In a crucial conference sponsored by the National Institutes of Health in 1981 (to which we shall return later) one participant could say, "The controversy as to which comes first, the thrombosis or the myocardial infarct, is still not satisfactorily answered."[19] How that controversy was resolved is an important part of our story, but we need to look first at other developments which provided the background for the resolution.

The Emergence of Streptokinase as a Thrombolytic Agent

The next part of our story is more complicated, because it involves tracing some concepts which developed in the basic sciences and which were to ultimately interact fruitfully with Herrick's hypothesis. We must begin, however, not with that clinical interaction but with the background basic science.

This part of the story starts[20] with another classic article, Tillett and Garner's 1933 article[21] on the peculiar capacity of cultures of organisms drawn from patients suffering from various manifestations of acute streptococcus infections to dissolve clots (composed of fibrin) which had been formed from human plasma by coagulation. The results described in the paper are quite surprising: (1) these streptococci are unique among the species of bacteria which are pathogenic for human beings in that they have the capacity to rapidly transform the solid clotted fibrin into a thin fluid state; (2) normal rabbit fibrin clots formed by mixing calcium chloride with rabbit blood are totally resistant to dissolution by these bacteria under these same conditions; (3) however, when rabbit plasma is clotted by use of human thrombin rather than by use of calcium chloride, the dissolution of the fibrin clots (fibrinolysis) is possible. These results didn't make a lot of sense, and Tillett and Garner didn't even pretend to understand what was happening. The most they could suggest was that the role of human thrombin in making rabbit fibrin susceptible to fibrinolysis might suggest some approaches to discovering the underlying mechanism of fibrinolysis. In short, Tillett and Garner's paper in 1933 looked like a peculiar but interesting result found by bacteriologists, with no suggestion that this might be the first step toward the development of a promising drug to treat heart attacks.

Tillett set up a laboratory at New York University to which he attracted a group of young investigators (in the early years, Haskell Milstone, L. Royal Christensen, Colin MacLeod, and Sol Sherry; in the later years, Alan Johnson and W. Ross McCarthy), and in a series of brilliant papers, Tillett and this group elucidated the mechanism of fibrinolysis. Their results can be summarized very briefly as follows: Milstone showed in 1941 that the fibrinolytic agent in the cultures worked only if there was some agent present in human blood (he called it a lytic factor); pure fibrin was not dissolved by the fibrinolytic agent.[22] Rabbit fibrin will be dissolved by the fibrinolytic agent when some human plasma containing the lytic factor is present. Christensen and MacLeod, four years later, completed the account of how fibrinolysis worked. They showed that the lytic factor normally present in blood (which they called plasminogen) is activated by the fibrinolytic agent derived from the streptococcal culture (which they called streptokinase, or SK) to produce an enzyme (which they called plasmin) that dissolves clots and other proteins.[23] This process can be represented schematically as follows:

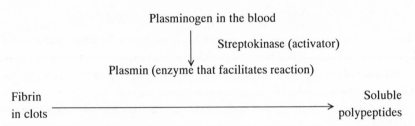

Plasminogen in the blood

Streptokinase (activator)

Plasmin (enzyme that facilitates reaction)

Fibrin in clots ⟶ Soluble polypeptides

By the early 1950s, interest had clearly shifted from understanding the basic biochemistry of dissolving clots (thrombolysis) to the possible clinical use of streptokinase. While various possible clinical uses of streptokinase were investigated, greatest interest lay in the possible use of this drug in breaking up clots in the vascular system since they seemed to be involved in at least some disease processes in that system (especially if Herrick was right). In 1952, Johnson and Tillett showed that clots artificially induced in the ear veins of rabbits could be dissolved by the intravenous administration of streptokinase.[24] Unfortunately, 8 of the 25 rabbits died, so the drug's toxicity would have to be reduced before it could be clinically useful.

By 1957 and 1958, Lederle Laboratory had produced a sufficiently high-quality streptokinase to avoid many of these toxicities.[25] Studies by a St. Louis group (headed by Sol Sherry, who had left New York University), among others, showed that clot dissolution is most effective when streptokinase acts directly on the plasminogen in the clot, rather than when it produces a lot of plasmin circulating in the blood.[26] This led them to a research strategy of infusing high dosages of streptokinase to ensure that streptokinase (rather than plasmin) reached the clot. A year later, the same group reported what they took to be some success in using this therapeutic strategy to deal with patients suffering from myocardial infarction.[27]

By 1960, an atmosphere of great excitement about the clinical use of streptokinase existed. Published symposia, such as one sponsored by Sloan-Kettering in March 1960,[28] evidenced the excitement in the therapeutic community. It seemed that basic scientific research on the dissolution of clots would combine with deeper cardiologic insight into myocardial infarctions to produce a clinical breakthrough of great significance. Plans for clinical trials to prove the benefits of streptokinase were being formed. Sherry and his group, however, had some reservations, which were published in an editorial in the *American Heart Journal*.[29] The reservations centered around possible problems with the proposed clinical trials. Streptokinase, they felt, was not sufficiently pure, very sick patients might react badly with the impurities, and the resulting deaths might outweigh the benefit of thrombolytic therapy. Moreover, they argued, there were too many details of the administration of the drugs (dosage and duration, for example) that had to be worked out before any trials could answer the important clinical questions. They understood the significance of starting trials of promising agents when patient needs were so great, and they themselves ran such trials, but they wanted to express their concerns that the scientific basis for these trials was not firm enough. They argued, moreover, that good science was required to answer the clinical questions, and bad trials wouldn't do the job. This tension between clinical needs and scientific needs is, of course, very real, and we shall return to it again and again. It is important to note its explicit presence so early in our story.

The Initial Failure

The promise that seemed so clear in 1960 that streptokinase would become a major tool in preventing death from heart attacks was unfulfilled 20 years later. In fact, in 1979, an article appeared in the *New England Journal of Medicine* providing guidelines for the use of streptokinase, which had recently been approved by the Food and Drug Administration (FDA).[30] The FDA at that time had approved streptokinase for use only in treatment of massive obstructions in the pulmonary arteries or marked blockages of the veins of the extremities. The authors recommended that this drug, which has potentially serious side effects, not be used for other indications, where its efficacy remained to be proven. Among these other indications were myocardial infarctions. What went wrong? Why was the promise of streptokinase unfulfilled?

The answer is certainly not to be found in a failure of the medical community to explore the use of streptokinase for the treatment of myocardial infarctions. As we will discuss later, all the relevant trials, starting with a trial by the St. Louis group in 1959, have been reviewed,[31] and no less than 18 trials of streptokinase and 4 of urokinase (another thrombolytic agent) were conducted in the period 1959–1979. Of the 22 trials, 13 showed less mortality in the group receiving one of the thrombolytic agents (the treatment group), 3 showed no difference between the group receiving one of the agents and the group not receiving either (the control group), and 6 trials showed less mortality in the untreated group. So a quick look at the 22 trials shows no clear answer to the question of whether thrombolytic therapy actually results in fewer deaths.

There is, however, a second major reason why the trials didn't settle the question of the usefulness of thrombolytic agents. The trials were simply too small to produce significant results. This point needs some explanation. There is a common convention in biomedical research that trials should be analyzed as tests of the null hypothesis. In this case, the null hypothesis is that there is no difference in mortality between the treatment group and the control group. Another convention is that the null hypothesis should not be rejected in light of the evidence unless the evidence is so strong for a positive difference that the likelihood (in light of the evidence) of the null hypothesis being rejected when it is actually true is less than 5 percent.[32] When the evidence is not that strong, the trial is treated as inconclusive and the results are said to be statistically nonsignificant. This stringent convention is a way of avoiding the error of accepting insufficiently supported claims about therapeutic efficacy that turn out to be false. This puts a considerable demand on trials. In order to get statistically significant results, one must enroll enough patients so that the likelihood of rejecting the null hypothesis when it is true is less than 5 percent. Most of the trials were not well-designed because they did not involve enough patients. Only recently have clinicians paid adequate attention to questions of trial design (especially of the size required), and the failure of these trials is further evidence that such questions must be kept in mind if trials of new therapeutic agents are to be of any value.

In short, progress was slowed in the period 1960–1979 because of the failure of the trials which were run to unambiguously indicate that thrombolytic agents administered after myocardial infarctions saved lives. In retrospect, it can be shown that all the significant studies revealed a reduction in mortality in the treatment group, and that combining all the studies shows a highly significant reduction in mortality from 19.1 to 15.6 percent by use of thrombolytic agents. But "Dr. Retrospect" is always wiser than "Dr. Prospect," and part of the problem was that none of the many clinical trials succeeded in making an unambiguous case for thrombolytic therapy.

Historical phenomena rarely have only one cause, and our case is no exception to this generalization. Several other factors contributed to the failure of researchers in the 1960s and 1970s to settle the question of the clinical value of streptokinase after myocardial infarctions. One was the continued controversy over Herrick's coronary thrombosis hypothesis. A second was the controversy, to be explained later, about anticoagulant therapy. A final factor was the emergence of other modalities of treatment for myocardial infarctions, with the suggestion that if they were employed, thrombolytic therapy would be of little significance. Let us examine each of these factors separately.

We have already reviewed the controversy which continued through the 1960s and 1970s concerning the extent to which coronary thromboses were associated with myocardial infarctions and the extent to which, even when associated, they were the causes of the myocardial infarctions. The more unsure people were about those questions, the less likely they were to be convinced that the use of thrombolytic agents was of value. After all, the rationale for the use of thrombolytic agents was that they broke up the clots that caused heart attacks and the resulting death to the myocardium. Doubt about these causal claims created doubt about the use of thrombolytic agents such as streptokinase.

Connected to all of this is the complicated issue of the use, after myocardial infarctions, of anticoagulant drugs such as heparin, which prevent further clot formation.[33] There was originally much enthusiasm for this form of treatment, especially after a 1948 American Heart Association study which concluded that anticoagulation therapy markedly lowered mortality and morbidity when used for 6 weeks after a heart attack. This enthusiasm waned after a critical article by Grifford and Feinstein in 1969 reviewed the many trials which had been run and showed that most of them suffered from fundamental methodological flaws.[34] By the mid-1970s, a much discussed and controversial survey showed that very few American and British teaching hospitals, unlike most West European teaching hospitals, were routinely using anticoagulant drugs for patients who had undergone a myocardial infarction,[35] although there is some evidence that the trend was changing just around that time. Admittedly, the question of the use of drugs (anticoagulants such as heparin) to prevent clotting after myocardial infarctions is very different from the question of using thrombolytic drugs (such as streptokinase) to break up clots which had already formed. But I cannot help but suspect that these issues were linked in the minds of many, and that the decline in the use of heparin was connected—rightly or wrongly—with a decline in the belief in Herrick's coronary thrombosis hypothesis and with increasing hesitation about streptokinase.

Another important factor is that other major medical advances in the management of myocardial infarctions attracted more attention in the 1960s and 1970s. Perhaps the most important of these[36] was the development of coronary care units (CCUs), with their emphasis on the careful monitoring of a patient's cardiac rhythm and on a quick response to those arrhythmias which were so often responsible for the death of patients who had suffered from a myocardial infarction but who arrived in the hospital alive. It seemed to many that reliance on CCUs, rather than thrombolytic agents, was the way to save lives. Now all of these medical developments were perfectly compatible with the continued use of thrombolytic agents, and analyses[37] show that the benefits of thrombolytic therapy continue even for patients in a coronary care unit, but all of this is more retrospective wisdom.

In short, then, the failure of the 1960s and the 1970s to settle the question of the utility of thrombolytic agents after myocardial infarctions was due to many factors. Trials that were run were widely viewed as inconclusive, Herrick's coronary thrombosis hypothesis was challenged by many, and the attention of cardiologists shifted to other therapeutic modalities.

All of this was to change rapidly. A series of interrelated developments was to lead in a few short years to a total reevaluation of thrombolytic therapy and to the emergence of a new era in the management of patients with myocardial infarctions. Some of these developments related to Herrick's hypothesis, while others related to new data about the value of streptokinase. The next section will examine each of these developments.

The Years of Promise

New Evidence for Herrick's Hypothesis

In October 1980 a major study transformed our understanding of the role of thrombi in myocardial infarctions. Dr. Marcus DeWood and his colleagues argued that a new approach provided answers that earlier studies had not been able to provide.[38] Because of the centrality of this study to the coronary thrombosis hypothesis, we will examine it very carefully.

All of the earlier studies were based upon findings of the presence or absence of a clot in the coronary arteries when they were examined on autopsies. There are many reasons why such results may be distorted. To begin with, some of the clots (if present) could spontaneously dissolve, leading to an underestimation of the role of thrombi. Alternatively, a low flow of blood associated with the falling circulation of a sick patient might contribute to thrombus formation, thereby leading to an overestimation of the role of thrombi. Finally, all of the data may be confounded by events associated with the dying process.

DeWood's group decided to study these questions by use of a new technique which enabled one to examine the coronary arteries of live patients during the early stages of their myocardial infarctions. The new technique, coronary angiography, involves introducing a flexible tube (catheter) into a vein or artery and guiding it to the heart or to the arteries. There, dye can be injected and x-rays can be taken so that one can see the blockages.

Because of concerns about its safety, this technique was initially confined to use in patients with chronic stable angina. Starting in 1971, DeWood and his group began using it in patients who presented within 24 hours of the onset of symptoms of a transmural myocardial infarction. By December 1978, when they began analyzing their data for their first publication, they had evaluated 322 of 1,210 eligible patients. An additional 195 patients were studied in 1979, 1980, and the early part of 1981.

There were three major findings of DeWood's study: (1) angiography is relatively safe; (2) findings of angiographic studies are reliable; and (3) the central role of coronary thrombosis in the development of a myocardial infarction is supported by powerful evidence. Because of the importance of each of these findings, we shall examine them separately.

Of the 517 patients DeWood studied, 4 died during the procedure. Three of these four were already in shock (profound depression of the vital processes of the body) at the time of the procedure. DeWood's view was that these deaths could not be associated with the procedure. Forty-four other patients who did not die suffered ventricular fibrillation (rapid, random, and ineffectual contractions of the heart, a very dangerous heart rhythm). The problem was resolved, however, and its incidence was lessened by administering the drug lidocaine before inserting the catheter. Finally, four patients suffered a variety of other problems. Clearly, DeWood's invasive studies were not without risk, but that is perfectly compatible with angiography being relatively safe so long as it sufficiently facilitates therapeutic decisions for the patients. If in our later examination we find these benefits sufficient, then DeWood's first claim will certainly be established.

The second issue is more complex. The problem DeWood was addressing was whether his findings concerning the presence of thrombi were reliable. Two problems were possible. Those examining the films might not see existing thrombi (false-negative findings), or they might "see" a thrombus that wasn't really there (false-positive findings). DeWood tested for these possibilities by examining the 96 patients who underwent emergency surgery. Angiographic results reported that 73 had a thrombus, and the thrombus was found in 65 cases, so there were 8 (11 percent) possibly false-positive claims. They were not certainly false because the thrombus might have been present at the time of angiography but spontaneously lysed before the surgery. Angiographic results reported that 23 did not have a thrombus, but a thrombus was recovered in 6 cases, so there was a 26 percent rate of false-negative cases. DeWood's procedure was then reasonably reliable, although certainly not perfect.

The most important of the findings was, of course, that Herrick was right. DeWood's analysis of this point was very careful. He began by pointing out that his study was confined to transmural infarctions because of Miller's crucial 1951 paper on transmural versus subendocardial infarcts. The total frequency of coronary thrombosis was 379 of the 517 patients with a transmural infarction (73 percent), although 419 (81 percent) had totally occluded arteries. Of equal importance was the fact that thrombi were present to a greater extent in the early hours. The frequency of thrombosis was 80 percent (294 of 368) in the patients studied in the first 6 hours after symptoms appeared, 59 percent (50 of 85) of those studied in the next 6 hours, and 54 percent (35 of 64) of those studied in the next 12 hours. These data supported the view that thrombi were the causes (because they were present early on) of the majority of transmural infarcts, even if there were some caused by other factors producing an occluded artery and there were others where the arteries weren't totally blocked. So Herrick was more or less right. To quote DeWood:

> Nevertheless, our data suggest that coronary thrombosis is associated with the majority of transmural infarctions and may be the final common pathway leading to coronary occlusion in a dynamic interaction between coronary spasm, platelet aggregations and atherosclerotic plaque. These data further suggest that coronary thrombosis is a fundamental mechanism by which chronic ischemic heart disease is converted to acute transmural myocardial infarction in man.[39]

In the years that followed, DeWood's study was cited repeatedly by many investigators; these citations strongly suggest that it is a turning point in our story. Much as Herrick's original proposal was supported by his new ECG findings, new angiographic findings reestablished it as a successful hypothesis.

The Intracoronary Administration of Streptokinase

The use of coronary angiography did more than just provide new evidence for Herrick's hypothesis. It also led to a new approach to the use of streptokinase. This use was ultimately superseded, but it is still very important for our story.

This particular segment of the story began in June 1978 in Göttingen, Germany. A patient with a previous history of a myocardial infarction and unstable angina was admitted to the hospital because of worsening chest pain and was scheduled for coronary angiography. In the midst of the examination, he began to exhibit classical signs of another infarction. His physicians were able to see by angiography that his right coronary artery, which had been partially opened, was now totally blocked. Since he didn't respond to medical treatment, his physicians decided to try something different. The catheter was maneuvered into the right coronary artery just before the site of the obstruction, and its guide wire was advanced through the obstruction. Shortly, blood flow was reestablished through the artery and the patient was free of symptoms.

The physicians who treated this patient, headed by P. Rentrop, published a case report describing what had occurred.[40] They pointed out that others had used special catheters to open up narrowed coronary arteries, but that this was the first time that someone had tried the technique with a total blocked artery in the midst of a myocardial infarction. They concluded that such an approach might be helpful in the future, but that general use would require further study and properly designed equipment (in particular, the guide wire needed to be stiff enough to perforate fresh thrombotic material but flexible enough to decrease danger of injury to the coronary artery itself).

Through the summer and fall of 1978, but particularly after August when a better guide wire became available, Rentrop and his group tried the technique on five additional patients, with further promising results.[41] But in July 1979, for reasons that were not made clear in the published report, they switched strategies.[42] In a patient who had already had some of the blockage opened by the guide wire, they infused streptokinase directly into that artery through the catheter (intracoronary administration of streptokinase). The result was a striking improvement in the amount of blood flow. Encouraged by this success, they followed with several cases in which direct administration of streptokinase into the coronary arteries was tried without any use of a guide wire to break up the blockage. The most impressive result they obtained was on August 30, 1979, when a patient with a totally blocked left anterior descending artery had normal blood flow restored by intracoronary administration of streptokinase. With this case, Rentrop and his group opened up a new chapter in the history of thrombolytic therapy.

At the end of the report on the use of streptokinase, Rentrop drew several conclusions. (1) Since the reopening of the artery produced a marked improvement in symptoms, it is reasonable to suppose that Herrick was right and that the obstruction of the arteries was the cause of the myocardial infarction and its accompanying symptoms. (2) In each of the cases, they had used nitroglycerine first in the hope that it would resolve any spasm in the coronary artery. This was done because spasm was the favorite alternative view of the cause of myocardial infarctions. Rentrop and his group found that nitroglycerine had little positive impact, which of course challenged the alternative account and reinforced Herrick's view. (3) All of their results suggested that intracoronary administration of streptokinase might be a valuable therapeutic modality.

Encouraged by Rentrop's work, Mathey and his group in Hamburg treated 41 patients with the intracoronary administration of streptokinase preceded by use of nitroglycerine to relieve spasm and by an attempt to reopen the blocked vessel by use of a flexible guide wire.[43] Nitroglycerine worked in only one case, but a total of 30 patients (73 percent) had their arteries reopened within 1 hour, with the largest group (18 patients) receiving this benefit from the streptokinase alone. The age of intracoronary streptokinase was clearly beginning. Leinbach and Gold, in an accompany editorial to the Mathey article, expressed their excitement as follows:

> Regional streptokinase treatment requires specially trained teams and available catheter laboratories and they require surgical intervention before therapy is complete. It could prevent major myocardial infarctions, and therefore, shock. In patients who present very early, it may prevent infarction almost entirely. Investigations in this area may change the responsibilities of the angiographer from the recording of coronary events to a participatory role in their reversal. It will be fascinating to see this form of therapy take its place in the management of the acute coronary patient.[44]

It is interesting to note that the editorial suggested a new role for physicians. Cardiologists had traditionally been medical specialists whose work was of a noninvasive nature, and it was they who treated myocardial infarctions. In the 1960s, with the emergence of bypass surgery as a modality of therapy for those who survived their myocardial infarction, invasive treatment began to be more important. Now, Leinbach and Gold were suggesting, cardiologists who were willing to treat patients with invasive techniques, such as catheterization and intracoronary administration of thrombolytic agents, could join their surgical colleagues in playing a more important role than the noninvasive cardiologists in treating myocardial infarctions.[45]

The work by Rentrop and by Mathey in 1979 and 1980 did suggest a new major therapeutic modality, the intracoronary use of thrombolytic agents. In 1981, three controlled trials, designed to test the efficacy and safety of this modality, began. In these trials, some patients—the active group—got the new treatment. They were compared to another group—the control group—who did not. These were randomized trials, with the patients randomly assigned to the active or the control group. Randomized controlled trials have emerged since the 1950s as the paradigm of modern scientific medicine,[46] and their scientific advantages are obvious. But not all new therapeutic modalities have been tested by such trials. It is important for our purposes to understand why the intracoronary use of streptokinase did undergo such trials. Two important factors which deserve consideration, intellectual considerations and governmental regulations, shall each be examined separately.

The intellectual argument was set out in a very impressive and influential article in the *New England Journal of Medicine*.[47] The authors began by pointing out that important medical advances have sometimes been introduced without careful trials designed to test for when they are indicated. The example they gave was coronary artery bypass surgery. They then argued that although the initial evidence documented the potential value of intracoronary thrombolytic therapy, there are important questions that need to be answered: Does it make a difference to long-term survival? Are there any hazards not yet noted? Which patients will benefit and which will not? How does intracoronary administration compare to intravenous administration? What other treatments should accompany this therapy? They concluded that properly conducted randomized trials were needed.

In a very interesting concluding section, the authors raised an important ethical question: Would it be legitimate to submit all patients to coronary arteriography when only half will actually get intracoronary streptokinase (since the members of the control group will not)? They suggested as an alternative randomizing patients before arteriography and getting consent to perform arteriography only from those assigned by the randomization to the treatment group.

While these intellectual considerations were important, governmental regulations might seem to have been even more important. New drugs must be approved for use by the Food and Drug Administration, and its regulations call for controlled trials demonstrating safety and efficacy before approval can be granted. These regulations and their implications will be the focus of Chapter 3. But they suggest that another reason for the clinical trials would be to secure FDA approval. This suggestion is reinforced by the fact that the three trials in question were cited in the *FDA Drug Bulletin* in the explanation of the eventual FDA approval of intracoronary streptokinase.[48] In fact, however, the trials in question were not for the most part completed and analyzed until after FDA approval. That approval was based therefore on other data. So these institutional considerations were of less importance than an initial look might suggest.

Of the three trials of thrombolytic therapy which began in 1981,[49] the most important was the Western Washington trial headed by J. Ward Kennedy. It was the largest trial, enrolling 250 patients, and it was the only one of the three to actually study survival rates as opposed to other measures of the efficacy of streptokinase (for example, opening up of the clogged artery). Interestingly enough, it catheterized all patients before randomization, arguing that it was safe to do so and that the information derived was of great benefit to the patient even if the patient did not receive streptokinase. Its results were very impressive. Of the 134 patients randomly assigned to streptokinase therapy, only 5 (3.7 percent) died within 30 days; on the other hand, of the 116 patients assigned to the control group, 13 died (11.2 percent). In short, the intracoronary administration of streptokinase reduced short-term mortality by nearly two-thirds. While not answering every question raised by Muller and his colleagues, the Western Washington randomized controlled trial provided powerful evidence for the beneficial impact of the intracoronary administration of streptokinase. Herrick's original hope that proper medical care, designed to break up clots and restore the functional integrity of the heart, might save lives seemed finally to be realized.

1982: A Year of Consolidation and Further Initiatives

The rapid changes sketched in the previous section led to a renewal of interest in thrombolytic therapy and to major developments in 1982. Among the most important were the approval by the Food and Drug Administration of intracoronary thrombolytic therapy, the decision by the National Institutes of Health to fund major studies of thrombolytic therapy, and the sudden emergence of new alternatives to streptokinase. Together, those developments made 1982 a crucial year in our study. This section will examine each of these developments separately.

FDA Approval of Intracoronary Streptokinase

Since 1962, drugs can be introduced into interstate commerce only after the Food and Drug Administration certifies, on the basis of adequate and well-controlled investigations, that the drug is safe in use *and* effective in use.[50] On May 7, 1982, the Food and Drug Administration approved streptokinase (as manufactured by Hoechst-Roussel under the name Streptase) as a safe and efficacious intracoronary thrombolytic agent for patients having a myocardial infarction. This approval consolidated the results of all the positive work of the preceding few years.

Since questions of FDA approval are very important in this book, it is of some interest to study the data the FDA used in this case. The best source for these data is an article by Jerome Weinstein, published in 1983, describing the Hoechst-Roussel Streptokinase Registry.[51] The registry was created in response to a meeting held in November 1980 at the Bureau of Biologics of the Food and Drug Administration to discuss assessing the safety and efficacy of this new use of streptokinase. Three questions were raised at that meeting: Are most acute myocardial infarctions the results of a recent blockage of an artery by a thrombus? Can intracoronary streptokinase lyse the thrombus and open up the occluded artery for blood flow? If that occurs, does it produce clinically meaningful benefits? The goal of the registry was to answer these questions.

The registry consisted of patients treated at three clinical centers in Germany and four in the United States that had extensive experience with intracoronary streptokinase. Two-thirds of the patients were from Germany, since it had the longer experience. Intracoronary streptokinase was administered to 224 patients, while 178 received only standard therapy. Weinstein noted very clearly that these patients were not assigned randomly to these two groups. The 178 patients were those who refused to sign consent forms or who could not receive streptokinase because of either contraindications or logistic problems.

Twenty-nine of the patients achieved at least a partial reperfusion (blood flow) of the blocked artery by use of a guide wire to perforate the thrombus. One hundred and forty-seven achieved at least a partial reperfusion of the blocked artery after the intracoronary use of streptokinase. Weinstein argued that this proved both that streptokinase worked to dissolve the clot and that the myocardial infarction was due in most cases to the blockage caused by the thrombus. The third question was answered to his satisfaction by the difference in survival rates. Within 28 days after the onset of the myocardial infarction, there were 26 deaths in the standard treatment group (14.6 percent), as opposed to 9 deaths in the 48 patients who received streptokinase which didn't work (18.8 percent), and as opposed to 8 deaths in the 176 who received streptokinase which broke up the clot (4.5 percent). Although the question of safety was not explicitly raised by the FDA, Weinstein argued that the registry showed that the intracoronary use of streptokinase was safe because of the low incidence of adverse reactions.

In an accompanying article, Dr. Eugene Braunwald raised several major problems with this data.[52] First, the patients were not randomly assigned to the treatment or the control group, so we cannot be sure that the worse results in the control group were due to their not getting thrombolytic therapy or to some other difference between the groups. Second, the physicians reporting the data knew whether the patients had or had not received streptokinase and this may have biased their report; in an ideal trial, those not receiving the drug would get a dummy drug (placebo) so that this possibility of bias is eliminated. Third, the treated patients who did not get reperfused did worst of all, and this might suggest that streptokinase is problematic in some cases.

These issues seem very legitimate, but they did not have an impact upon the FDA, which went ahead with the approval anyway. The FDA did not even wait for the results of the Western Washington trial, which was designed to avoid these methodological issues. That trial had begun in July 1981 and had enrolled 107 of the planned 250 patients by March 1982.[53] In light of some of the delays in approval we shall see later, this haste is quite surprising.

The NIH Steps In

In the post–World War II period, American research has been dominated by projects funded by two major federal agencies, the National Institutes of Health and the National Science Foundation. In the fields of biology, biochemistry, and medical sciences, research run or funded by the NIH has been central to many advances. Even with its considerable funding, however, the NIH must make choices about what areas of research should be funded because they hold out the promise of progress. Consequently, conferences sponsored by the NIH are extremely important, because they often lay the foundation for new directions for NIH funding.

In the latter part of 1981, the NIH sponsored a conference on thrombolytic agents held at its headquarters in Bethesda. The conference involved not only many figures we have already encountered but also those who will be very important in the rest of our story. We pause for a moment to see who attended.

Dr. Marcus DeWood, whose angiographic studies had revitalized Herrick's hypothesis, was there, as were Drs. Rentrop and Mathey, the Germans whose work had sparked the excitement about intracoronary administration. The FDA was represented by Dr. David Aronson, the head of the Section of the Bureau of Biologics that was soon to supervise the approval of intracoronary streptokinase, and Dr. Jerome Weinstein from Hoechst-Roussel, the manufacturer of streptokinase, was also present. The NIH was represented by Dr. Eugene Passamani, who was to play a major role in the years to come in NIH activity in this area, by Drs. David DeMets and Curt Furberg, two of the leading advocates and theoreticians of carefully controlled clinical trials, and by Dr. Peter Frommer, the deputy director of the National Heart, Lung, and Blood Institute of the NIH. Dr. J. Ward Kennedy, who was heading the Western Washington trial, was present. Two extremely distinguished cardiologists, Dr. Eugene Braunwald of Harvard and Dr. Burton Sobel of Washington University in St. Louis, were present, and they presented summary comments on the major areas under discussion. Among the others present who will be important for our story were Dr. Desire Collen, from the University of Louvain in Belgium, and Dr. Victor Marder, a hematologist from the University of Rochester (New York). In short, an extremely distinguished group was brought together by the NIH to address the current status of thrombolytic therapy for myocardial infarction and to discuss the need for future studies. Fortunately, most of the presented papers were later published as a symposium edited by Passamani,[54] so we can get a good sense of what happened at the conference.

One theme that emerged very clearly was that the participants were sufficiently encouraged by the most recent developments in thrombolytic therapy, but sufficiently concerned about specified issues, to strongly urge that the NIH fund a major trial to settle many of the outstanding questions. Braunwald ended his comments with the following observation: "Of all of the available interventions to limit acute infarct size and the subsequent morbidity and mortality from acute infarction, the administration of thrombolytic therapy appears to be the most promising. We should now proceed to design prospective, randomized clinical trials that accurately evaluate the efficacy of this intervention."[55] Dr. John Ross, a cardiologist from the University of California at San Diego, made the appeal even more explicit: "Despite technical problems that may make it difficult to design an optimum clinical trial, plans for designing a trial sponsored by the National Institutes of Health should be developed in the near future."[56]

Another major theme was that such trials would have to consider intravenous as well as intracoronary administration of streptokinase. Braunwald noted that some recent trials of intravenous administration had some very positive results, and Ross suggested that a good trial might have both an intravenous treatment group and an intracoronary treatment group.

A third complicating theme was the question of what measurement of success should be employed in such trials. One obvious answer is that such trials should study differences in survival between the treatment group and the control group (and perhaps even the quality of life of those who survive). Such trials would need to be very large because most of the people in the control group survive anyway, and so you would need a very large group to observe statistically significant differences. Another obvious answer is that such trials should simply consider whether clots are broken up and blood flow restored to arteries, but that begs the question as to whether reperfusion is of clinical benefit. In summarizing that part of the discussion, Sobel emphasized the possibility of using intermediate techniques such as assessing the performance of the left ventricle (the part of the heart that pumps blood to most of the body) after treatment. To quote him: "A prospective, controlled clinical trial should of course consider mortality as a critical end point, but the discriminant power of the trial would be enhanced by reliance on several of the measurements discussed."[57] The crucial point is that such assessments measure whether the reperfusion is of clinical benefit to the heart's actual functioning, and they might detect differences between survivors in the treatment group and survivors in the control group. This last theme, as well as the others mentioned before, became very important in the subsequent work of the NIH.

One final point. Even though there were participants from the FDA at the conference, very little was said about any impending approval by the FDA of the intracoronary administration of streptokinase (an approval which came in May 1982), and there was no discussion (at least in the published papers) about what impact that might have on the possibility and ethics of randomized controlled trials. We have here, I believe, the beginning of a problem (lack of clear coordination between the FDA and the NIH) that became more important as time passed.

The Advisory Council of the National Heart, Lung, and Blood Institute (NHLBI) of the NIH held a meeting on Thursday, May 20, 1982, in Bethesda, Maryland. Among the items on its agenda was a report by Passamani on a proposed new initiative from the NIH entitled "Thrombolysis in Myocardial Infarction." Since this trial became a very important part of further developments, we need to look carefully at its beginning.

The minutes of the council meeting are very sparse.[58] They refer to an April 4–5 meeting of the Cardiology Advisory Committee and to descriptive material sent out in advance, but I have unfortunately not been able to obtain that material. The minutes refer to the proposed study as follows:

> At present there is a controversy regarding the relative efficacies of intra-coronary versus intravenous administration of thrombolytic agents. The TIMI study will be undertaken to determine if fibrinolytic agents are useful in the treatment of acute myocardial infarction. The end points proposed for this study will be cardiac ejection fraction which is roughly inversely proportional to infarct size and seems to be correlated with long-term mortality and mortality rate itself.

The proposed study was approved, with funding of the postplanning phase to be contingent on further council approval.

Fortunately, this rather brief account of the original NIH decision can be supplemented by two additional documents, an observer report and an August 20 document from the NIH requesting proposals from clinical units wishing to participate in the trial.[59] From these documents, we can learn the following additional information. (1) The proposed study was to have two major subtrials. One, TIMI-A (sample size 200), would randomize patients with an angiographically confirmed complete occlusion of the infarct-related artery to receive either intracoronary administration of a thrombolytic agent, intravenous administration of such an agent, or intravenous administration of a placebo. The other, TIMI-B (sample size 1,000), would randomize noncatheterized patients to receive either intravenous thrombolytic therapy or an intravenous placebo. (2) The primary trial end point to be studied was mortality during the follow-up period, but emphasis was also to be placed on intermediate measures of the functioning of the left ventricle such as the left ventricular ejection fraction. (3) Some members of both the Cardiology Advisory Committee and the Advisory Council expressed concerns about the ethics of the trial, in part because of the denial of any thrombolytic therapy to patients in the placebo control group and in part because of doubt about the possibility of getting informed consent from patients in the midst of an evolving myocardial infarction. Although these concerns did not lead to any changes in the proposed protocol for the trials, we will be devoting a considerable amount of attention to them since they affected the actual trial, which was quite different from the proposed protocol.

The influence of the November 1981 meeting at Bethesda on thinking at the NIH was obviously profound. Not only was the NIH moving forward with major funding for a trial of thrombolytic therapy; it was also adopting the suggestions that intravenous as well as intracoronary administration should be studied and that importance should be ascribed to such measures of improvement as left ventricular ejection fraction.

One final observation about the council meeting. The previously mentioned reporter at the council meeting reported that approval had been given for a clinical trial to test the use of streptokinase. The minutes and the request for proposals make reference to thrombolytic agents and to thrombolytic therapy without specifically mentioning streptokinase. This was no accident. By the period May–August 1982, a new competitor to streptokinase was emerging, and thinking at the NHLBI was rapidly shifting from a test of streptokinase to a test of thrombolytic therapy. We turn then to this additional major development in 1982, the emergence of other plasminogen activators as competitors to streptokinase for thrombolytic therapy.

Other Thrombolytic Agents

In order to understand these developments, we need to remind ourselves that by 1945 scientists already understood that streptokinase produced clot dissolution by activating an agent in the blood (plasminogen) so that it became an enzyme (plasmin) which produced the dissolution of the fibrin in clots. Streptokinase does not, of course, occur naturally in human beings; it is produced by streptococci. But some clots in humans do dissolve, so the question arises as to whether there is some substance which naturally occurs in human beings and other animals and which also activates plasminogen to plasmin, thereby beginning the thrombolytic process.

In 1947, two Danish investigators, Tage Astrup and Per Permin, announced that they had identified and prepared such an agent found in animal tissue cells.[60] In 1951, J. R. B. Williams described a similar activator present in human urine, an activator which came to be called urokinase.[61] Both these activators were difficult to study, because they were available only in limited quantities which were also impure.

Things began to improve in the late 1950s, when urokinase was isolated and purified to some degree by a group of Danish investigators associated with Leo Pharmaceutical Products in Copenhagen.[62] However, only modest clinical benefits were found in the earliest clinical studies run by this group. With the help of Abbott Laboratories, the St. Louis group, which had played such a major role in the development of streptokinase, began in 1965 to study the use of highly purified urokinase as a thrombolytic agent.[63] In the years that followed, urokinase had a history quite similar to streptokinase. It underwent various clinical trials, and it was ultimately approved by the FDA for noncoronary use in 1978 and for intracoronary administration for myocardial infarctions in 1982.

Urokinase is not, however, the focus of our attention in this section, because it ultimately attracted little clinical use. Our focus is instead on the activator found in tissue cells. By the late 1970s, it was clear that this activator (called tissue plasminogen activator, or tPA) was different from the activator found in urine and that it had at least one major theoretical advantage over both streptokinase and urokinase. Streptokinase and urokinase both activate plasminogen circulating in the plasma, while tissue plasminogen activator primarily activates plasminogen associated with the thrombus itself.[64] This relative selectivity offers the possibility of two major benefits for tPA. To begin with, it might reduce the risk of bleeding by patients who have received thrombolytic therapy. If circulating plasminogen is activated into plasmin, the resulting plasmin will dissolve not only the fibrin in clots but also other proteins in the blood which defend against systemic bleeding. If, on the other hand, primarily plasminogen associated with the clot is activated to plasmin, it might dissolve the clot but much less of these other proteins in the blood, leaving the patient protected against systemic bleeding. Moreover, it might also increase the lysing of the clots because it produces the plasmin where needed at the clot site.

Whatever its possible theoretical advantages, tissue plasminogen activator was very hard to produce in sufficient quantities and in a purified fashion. The credit for producing purified tissue plasminogen activator in quantities sufficient for simple pilot clinical studies is to be given to a group working in Belgium at the University of Louvain, and particularly to one of its central investigators, Desire Collen.[65] It had been known for some time that tumor cells produced an unusually large amount of plasminogen activators, but they are often urokinaselike activators. Using an established human melanoma cell line (the Bowes cell line) obtained from D. B. Rifkin at Rockefeller University, the Louvain group isolated and purified the tissue plasminogen activator and showed that it could serve as a clot-selective thrombolytic agent.

Rijken and Collen ended their 1981 report with the observation that they now had enough purified tissue plasminogen activator to initiate studies on the thrombolytic properties of this activator in animal and human models. The Louvain group soon joined with a group in St. Louis at Washington University Medical School (headed by Dr. Burton Sobel) to study the effects of this activator in dogs and in humans. The studies were small pilot studies, but they indicated that clot-selective coronary thrombolysis without concomitant systemic effects could be induced in patients with evolving myocardial infarctions.[66]

All of this seemed very exciting, and it no doubt played a major role in the thinking of some at the NHLBI that streptokinase might not be the thrombolytic agent to study. But even the Louvain invention was not sufficient to produce enough tissue plasminogen activator for use in the real world if the studies proved that tPA was safe and efficacious. To quote the end of the report of the pilot study:

> Widespread use of tissue-type plasminogen activator or any activator requires a ready supply of active material. Isolation and purification of protein from tissue-culture supernatant fractions, as in this study, are not likely to meet the need for large-scale availability of preparations. Recent reports of successful cloning and expression of the human tissue-type plasminogen activator gene in *Escherichia coli* suggest that large-scale production can be accomplished with recombinant-DNA technology.[67]

In fact, that new technology would be used to produce the desired tissue plasminogen activator. To understand how that happened, we need to go back in time to the emergence of biotechnology as an industry and to the emergence of a particular company, Genentech.

Biotechnology, Genentech, and tPA

In the mid-1970s a major scientific breakthrough occurred, one which transformed the capacities of biology and created at the same time the foundations of a new industry, the biotechnology industry. Collaborative research carried out by Herbert Boyer at the University of California at San Francisco and Stanley Cohen at Stanford University resulted in a process by which genes could be altered to affect the production by cells of fundamental proteins. Boyer had been studying restriction enzymes that sliced the DNA strands, which are the chemical basis of genes. Cohen had been working with plasmids, tiny rings of DNA that float outside the main chromosomes in bacteria. In their collaborative work, Boyer and Cohen showed that one could use Boyer's enzymes to cut a piece of Cohen's plasmids and insert some foreign DNA, that the plasmid would carry that foreign DNA into the bacteria, and that the resulting altered gene would order the bacteria to produce the desired protein. In this way, bacteria could be turned into factories for producing useful proteins which they normally did not produce. The Boyer-Cohen recombinant DNA technology revolution had begun.

The Government Patent Policy Act of 1980 permitted nonprofit organizations to retain title to inventions and to secure the benefits of commercialization even if the research producing the invention had been done with federal funds. Stanford and the University of California patented both the process invented by Boyer and Cohen and the resulting product, although there was some delay in getting the patent. No company has been granted an exclusive license, since the process is needed by all who would work in genetic engineering. Instead, companies that agree to follow NIH guidelines for use of genetically altered material can get a license in return for royalty payments. Estimates of the value of the Cohen-Boyer patent range from $250 million to $750 million. Thus commercial biotechnology was born. One of its first progeny was Genentech.[68]

The story of the founding of Genentech, the first major biotechnology company, has been told many times, but it is worth retelling at least in outline to see where it fits into our story about thrombolytic therapy. The formation of the company was due to two individuals, Herbert Boyer, whose scientific work it was to use in its activities, and Robert Swanson, a young expert in venture capital.

The venture capital industry had come into its own in the 1970s as people rushed to put their funds into companies which promised to apply the latest technological advances to produce new commercially viable products. Computers and electronics were industries that benefited heavily from the infusion of cash from venture capitalists. In 1976, Swanson was 27 years old and was working for Kleiner Perkins, a California venture capital firm. Swanson telephoned Boyer and asked for a personal meeting. A planned Friday afternoon chat turned into the formation of Genentech. Four years later, Genentech was to go public, selling one million shares at $35 a share. If this is not incredible enough, consider what happened on October 14, 1980, the opening day. Within an hour, Genentech's stock had risen to $89 a share, and even if it was to close at $70 a share later that day, such an opening was unprecedented. What had Genentech done during those first four years? What was responsible for its success?

Genentech's early work, apparently carried on in Boyer's laboratory, involved inducing bacteria to produce a human brain hormone, somatostatin. This was carried out successfully, and even though this success did not lead to any direct commercial exploitation, it did give the new company considerable credibility.[69] In January 1978, Genentech moved into leased facilities of its own and entered into an important agreement with Eli Lilly. Under this agreement, Genentech would do the research to produce insulin bacterially, Eli Lilly would pay for the testing and approval process, and Lilly would also produce and market this insulin. Genentech would receive a royalty on the sales. Genentech soon entered into an arrangement with A. B. Kabi, a Swedish company. Kabi funded the research for the bacterial production of human growth hormone and received in return exclusive manufacturing and marketing rights outside the United States. Most crucially, Genentech retained the right to manufacture and sell this bacterially produced hormone in the United States and Canada, providing it could receive FDA approval. This meant that Genentech would be more than just a research corporation. It would seek to eventually become a fully integrated pharmaceutical corporation, carrying on the entire process of drug development from initial research to manufacturing and marketing. Other agreements were entered into with other corporations.[70] In short, by 1980 Genentech had begun to build a record as a successful innovator in the science and financing of biotechnology, so it is not surprising that it was able to launch a major stock offering which was received with great enthusiasm by the investment community.

In January 1983, in an article in *Nature*, a group of scientists from Genentech along with Collen from Louvain announced that they not only had isolated and characterized the entire genetic coding sequence of human tissue plasminogen activator but also had constructed a plasmid which directed bacteria to produce human tissue plasminogen activator.[71] Some of these results had already been presented in Lausanne in July 1982, and the actual work had been completed slightly earlier. It is not so surprising then that the NIH was no longer committed to streptokinase by summer 1982, when it was planning its trial of thrombolytic agents. Thanks to biotechnology and the efforts of the Genentech group, a real alternative was available.

The Great Clinical Trials

In the years immediately following 1982, physicians increasingly used thrombolytic therapy. They sometimes administered it by the intracoronary route, as approved by the FDA, but more often they administered it intravenously, even though this route lacked FDA approval, because intravenous administration is a far easier way to administer the drug.[72] Nevertheless, the focus in these years was less on actual clinical employment and more on a series of large clinical trials designed to establish the usefulness of thrombolytic therapy administered intravenously. In this section, we will examine the major clinical trials, beginning first with the TIMI trial at the NIH, and then looking at trials of streptokinase, tPA, and still a third thrombolytic agent, APSAC.

We should note, however, that the period 1983–1987 was marked by a real ambiguity, one which gives rise to important ethical questions that we shall examine later. On the one hand, thrombolytic therapy in the form of intracoronary streptokinase was an approved nonexperimental therapy. On the other hand, thrombolytic therapy in the form of the newer thrombolytic agents and/or administered intravenously was clearly experimental. What should physicians say to patients in the experimental trials about the established therapy? Could there be ethically acceptable trials in which the control group received a placebo (inactive substance), given the existence of approved therapies of proven value? As we saw, these questions had already been raised when the NIH voted to conduct the TIMI trial. Throughout this section, we shall see how the various trials dealt with these issues, which we consider further in Chapter 2.

The TIMI Trial and Its European Cooperative Counterpart

As noted previously, the National Heart, Lung and Blood Advisory Council approved on May 20, 1982, a major national trial of thrombolytic therapy. As late as summer 1982, when the NIH requested proposals from clinical units wishing to participate in the trial, the TIMI trial was supposed to be a three-pronged trial of intracoronary and intravenous therapy against a placebo control group. By the time the trial began in 1984, its structure had changed considerably. It had become at least in part a trial of streptokinase against tPA. The process by which this came about was to engender great controversy. We need therefore to carefully review it.

The study chairman for the TIMI trial was Dr. Eugene Braunwald of Harvard

University. The NHLBI, which funded the study, was represented by Dr. Eugene Passamani. The coordinating center, which administered the day-by-day activities of the trial, was the Maryland Medical Research Institute, represented by Dr. Genell Knatterud. These individuals, together with the principal investigators from the thirteen clinical centers and the five core laboratories, formed the steering committee. In addition, there was a Policy Advisory and Data Monitoring Board, chaired by Dr. William Hood. This rather complex structure is typical of multicenter trials sponsored by the NIH.

The crucial decisions to make the changes in the trial were made in the later half of 1983 by the investigators and were approved by Hood's committee in its meeting on January 31, 1984.[73] The new plan was to have an initial trial (TIMI-I) to determine which of two agents (streptokinase or tPA) administered intravenously was more effective in lysing a coronary thrombus within 90 minutes of administration in patients with angiographically proven total occlusion of the infarct-related artery. A later trial (TIMI-II) would be based upon the results of the TIMI-I trial, but no firm plans were made. To quote the minutes:

> The investigators should maintain a flexible approach to TIMI phase II which was not reviewed or approved. The design of phase II should include reconsideration of these (i.e., streptokinase and r-tPA) and other agents, dose and timing based on TIMI phase I and other available studies of thrombolytic agents.

Notice the many changes that had taken place. First, all consideration of the issue of intracoronary versus intravenous administration was dropped. The only concern of the study would be the efficacy and safety of intravenous therapy. Second, heavy emphasis would be placed upon an initial comparison of the two major thrombolytic agents. Third, the primary end point of the study, by which efficacy of the drugs would be studied, would be lysis within 90 minutes, rather than mortality or even the functioning of the left ventricle of the heart. The following reasonable arguments can be offered in justification for each of these decisions. Given the difficulties of intracoronary administration, especially in hospitals without active coronary catheterization facilities, intravenous administration is more practical, so a study of its efficacy is very important. Given the emergence of tPA, it would be foolish to run a trial which left it out. Given that the purpose of the initial trial was to provide data to plan a useful follow-up trial, it needed to be quick, and the use of a simple determinant of efficacy such as reperfusion of the occluded artery was perfect for that purpose. Nevertheless, these rapid changes in trial design, combined with other events to be described later, would become matters of considerable controversy.

One final observation before we turn to the actual conduct of TIMI-I. The design of TIMI-I raised no ethical issues about the use of a placebo control group, since none was involved. All patients in this trial received either tPA or streptokinase intravenously. That is why the Baylor Institutional Review Board, as noted in the introduction, approved TIMI-I while reserving judgment about TIMI-II. If there was any ethical question about this trial, it had to do with the issue of informed consent. Were patients made aware that, as an alternative to participating in this trial of intravenous administration, they could just receive the proven benefit of the intracoronary administration of streptokinase? And if not, did they truly give informed consent? We shall return to these issues.

After some preliminary small studies, TIMI began enrolling patients on August 20, 1984. All of the patients were 75 or younger and had experienced the onset of chest pain within 7 hours. They underwent coronary arteriography and were randomized to one of the two arms of the trial (tPA and streptokinase) if intracoronary nitroglycerin was not effective. The primary study end point was patency of the infarct-related artery 90 minutes after infusion of the thrombolytic agent (30 minutes after the end of the infusion of streptokinase, which took only 1 hour, but only halfway into the infusion of tPA, which took 3 hours).[74]

The original plan was to enroll 340 patients; it was estimated that 272 would have total occlusions of the artery and 68 would have partial occlusions. A plan was also developed to do two interim reviews, one after 50 percent of the patients had been treated and one after 75 percent had been treated. It was agreed that the trial would be stopped if the interim analysis showed such an extreme difference that the probability of its being reversed by the collection of the rest of the data was less than one in a thousand. Such planned interim reviews and stopping plans are now built into many well-designed clinical trials. They are based upon the recognition that a balance must be achieved between the need to stop trials earlier than planned if the data are overwhelming and the statistical concern that stopping too early will lead to incorrect conclusions. A whole science of how to design interim reviews and stopping plans has emerged.[75]

On February 5, 1985, the NIH, following the recommendation of Hood's Policy Advisory and Data Monitoring Board, stopped the TIMI-I trial after 316 patients were randomized because of the substantial differences in patency rates between the tPA patients and the streptokinase patients. A preliminary report on the results was published in April of that year in the *New England Journal of Medicine*, although the final reports (published as three separate papers) did not appear for several years.

There are some differences between the initial report and the final reports, because the former used angiographic results from individual centers while the latter used results from the common core laboratory, but whichever report is followed, the difference in patency rates at 90 minutes is very striking. We shall present here the final data. Seventy percent of those treated with tPA (100 of 143) but only 43 percent of those treated with streptokinase (63 of 147) had partial or complete perfusion at 90 minutes. These figures become even more impressive when one considers only those 232 patients with no real perfusion before administration of the drug. After 30 minutes of therapy, 24 percent of those treated with tPA (27 of 113) but only 8 percent of those treated with streptokinase (9 of 119) had achieved reperfusion. After 60 minutes of therapy, 48 percent of those treated with tPA (54 of 113) but only 23 percent of those treated with streptokinase (27 of 119) had achieved reperfusion. And after 90 minutes, 62 percent of those treated with tPA (70 of 113) but only 31 percent of those treated with streptokinase (37 of 119) had achieved reperfusion. With such differences, it is not surprising that the trial was stopped, given that its end point for study was patency of the infarct-related artery.

This last caveat is, however, very important. Is the difference between patency rates at 90 minutes clinically significant? To be sure, the study also showed that there remained a greater patency at discharge, but is even that very significant clinically? What happens to the results of TIMI-I when you examine other end points?

The quick answer to this question is that the superiority of tPA over streptokinase disappears. One of the three final reports explicitly addressed the issue of left ventricular functioning.[76] As was pointed out earlier, this is a useful end point to study because it measures how well the heart is pumping blood to most of the body, and, as the TIMI investigators pointed out in their report on left ventricular functioning, it "has consistently proven to be a powerful predictor of survival after myocardial infarction." Of the 290 treated patients, 145 had a successful predischarge as well as a successful pretreatment cardiac catheterization, enabling one to study the improvement in the functioning of the left ventricle. Of these, 68 had received streptokinase and 77 had received tPA, and the tPA patients in this subgroup had better reperfusion. Nevertheless, there was no difference between the two treatment groups either in the magnitude of improvement in ventricular function or in the level of functioning measured before discharge. The superiority of tPA over streptokinase disappears when left ventricular function is studied.

All of this raises many questions. Was the NIH right in choosing reperfusion as the primary end point, especially when the 1981 conference had emphasized the importance of studying other end points? Should the initial report in 1985, which attracted so much attention, have focused on the positive benefit of tPA over streptokinase in achieving reperfusion, even if that clearly was the primary end point, or should it have indicated, as did the final reports, that this led to no major difference in ventricular functioning? In fairness, the initial report was based upon data from the local centers while all the final reports used later data from the core laboratory, and it is not clear when the local centers reported initial ejection fraction data. This may help explain why only reperfusion data were presented in the initial report. But despite this logistical explanation, the question still remains as to whether it would not have been better to wait to present a more balanced picture.

And, finally, should the NIH have designed TIMI-II to center around tPA, in light of the different results using different end points? We shall return to all of these questions in Chapters 2 and 3, since they are central both to some of the conflict-of-interest charges that were raised and to some of the issues about drug approval based on these surrogate end points. For now, we will return to the details of the TIMI trial.

We have already noted that the issue of how the results of TIMI-I would shape the TIMI-II trial had been raised but not settled at the January 31, 1984, meeting of Hood's committee. Given the two-phase design, it was natural to suppose that the plan would be to test the "winner" of TIMI-I against a placebo in a trial with mortality as the end point. Apparently, just that was suggested by Braunwald at the fall 1984 meeting of the American Heart Association in Miami. He was certainly interpreted that way by one of the members of Hood's committee, Dr. Victor Marder. On November 26, Marder wrote Hood challenging the statement on the grounds that the issue had not been settled and suggesting that a three-way trial (involving, presumably, a placebo group, a streptokinase group, and a tPA group) would be best since "it is not a foregone conclusion that an agent with a lower reperfusion rate will necessarily have a lesser effect on mortality."[77] Hood responded cautiously, suggesting a conference call, but reminding Marder that "the results are quite impressive."[78] The events of the next few months are less clear, but two points should be noted: the study group was planning a trial involving tPA against a placebo with 10-day mortality as the outcome; and a decision was made to confine Hood's committee to overseeing two other clinical trials being run by Rentrop and Kennedy, and a new board (*not* including Marder, even though he volunteered to be part of it) would be constituted to supervise the rest of the TIMI trial.[79]

In fact, however, none of these trials was carried out. By late 1985, the investigators had decided on ethical grounds not to run any placebo-controlled trial of tPA but to focus instead on other issues associated with the use of tPA. This decision was announced publicly on February 16, 1986, at the meeting of the American College of Cardiology. Braunwald, in an interview with the *Wall Street Journal*, had the following to say: "I would be happier if the evidence on tPA were buttoned up a little firmer. . . . I wavered for three or four months and didn't come lightly to the decision."[80] In the same article, Marder expressed his concern that the NIH was neglecting other new thrombolytic agents (such as APSAC, a drug we will discuss shortly).

There are two aspects of the decision that need discussion. One, on which Marder focused, was whether it was a good idea to limit study to tPA. The other was whether a placebo-controlled trial was ethically unjustified, as the NIH now seemed to be saying. The second is clearly the more crucial question, for as we shall see later, many other groups continued to run placebo-controlled trials of thrombolytic agents to see whether reperfusion actually reduced mortality. The public record unfortunately provided little evidence as to what led to this decision, but several events can be suggested. Oddly enough, these events are connected with streptokinase, but they indirectly affected the NIH's views about legitimate tPA trials.

The first was the publication in mid-1985 of a review article by a group headed by Dr. Salim Yusuf of the NIH.[81] Although not the first article of its type, it was certainly the most comprehensive. It reviewed all the trials of thrombolytic therapy and concluded that there was powerful evidence for a reduction of mortality by intravenously administered streptokinase. To quote the abstract:

> Because all of these IV [intravenous] and IC [intracoronary] trials were small (the largest including only 747 patients), their separate results appear contradictory and unreliable. But, an overview of the data from these trials indicates that IV treatment produces a highly significant (22 percent ± 5 percent, $p < 0.001$) reduction in the odds of death, an even larger reduction in the odds of reinfarction, and an absolute frequency of serious adverse effects to set against this that is much smaller than the absolute mortality reduction.

One might well argue as follows. Even granted all the problems involved in pooling data from many studies, the Yusuf review certainly provided powerful evidence that IV streptokinase saved many lives. Given that tPA had been shown to be better than streptokinase in producing reperfusion, it would surely reduce mortality by at least that same percentage (22 percent), if not more. One cannot therefore justify a trial of tPA in which half the patients will get a placebo and in which many additional patients in that group will needlessly die.[82] This line of reasoning was surely reinforced by data becoming available in late 1985 and early 1986 from a very large trial of intravenous streptokinase (the GISSI trial, to be discussed later) which showed an 18 percent reduction in mortality. Such data would surely reinforce the view that a placebo-controlled trial would be inappropriate.

To say that these data would reinforce the view that placebo-controlled trials would be inappropriate is not to say that all investigators would draw that conclusion. In fact, that conclusion was *not* drawn by another group, the European Cooperative study group, whose early research (and some of whose post-1986 research) paralleled the research of the TIMI group. Let us turn then to their activities.[83]

In early 1984, Genentech entered into an agreement with Boehringer Ingelheim to supply tPA for clinical trials in Europe, which would be funded by Boehringer Ingelheim. Boehringer then entered into a sponsorship relationship with a European Cooperative study group, set up under the chairmanship of Dr. M. Verstraete of Louvain (where Collen had done his work on tPA). The clinical centers for the trials were in Belgium, France, Germany, and the Netherlands. Their earliest studies, paralleling the NIH TIMI-I trial, studied patency of the infarct-related artery, comparing both tPA against streptokinase and tPA against a placebo-controlled group. As in the TIMI trial, this group found that tPA produced a greater percentage of patency than streptokinase. Their results were published in 1985.[84] Like TIMI, they also began in 1986 to study other issues associated with the use of tPA. But unlike the TIMI investigators, they found it ethical to start in May 1986 a trial of tPA against placebo to study the impact on left ventricular function and on survival; this trial continued until November 1987 and the impressive positive results for tPA were published in 1988.[85]

This raises two very important questions. Can we attribute the difference in the decision made by these two groups to the fact that the TIMI investigators were funded by a public agency and the European Cooperative investigators were funded by a drug company which might need the data from a placebo-controlled trial of mortality to secure approval for its drug? In any case, whose decision was ethically more appropriate?

Returning to TIMI, we need to note that the group continued its activities, even if there was to be no placebo-controlled trial with mortality as its end point, focusing on various questions related to the use of tPA. Their activities in the next few years are of lesser significance for now, although we will return to them when they become important during the FDA approval process, so we can temporarily summarize them briefly as follows:[86]

1. During the period August 1985 to March 1986, the group studied a new form of tPA with single-chain molecules that Genentech said would be relatively easy to produce in large-scale production. (Note the close collaboration with Genentech at this point.) The new form seemed less efficacious, so 100 mg had to be used to get the same results as with 80 mg of the old type of tPA. Even higher rates of reperfusion were obtained with a 150-mg dose of the new tPA.

2. The TIMI group then began its new TIMI-II trial designed to find out whether the use of coronary angioplasty (the opening up of a coronary artery by passing a catheter to the diseased area and inflating it to compress the plaque obstructing the artery) and of a class of drugs called beta blockers after the use of tPA would produce even better results. Early on in that trial, they had to reduce the dosage of the new tPA back to 100 mg because of an unexpected increase in intracerebral hemorrhages.

3. Angioplasty used routinely offered no advantages, but early intravenous beta blockage appeared to be of benefit in reducing recurrent infarctions and ischemic episodes.

Thus the TIMI trial never settled the question it was originally perceived as settling: Did thrombolytic therapy actually save many lives? It did, however, establish that on at least one measure (reperfusion), tPA was better than streptokinase, and it also established a great deal of information about how tPA should be used in conjunction with other therapeutic modalities.

The Trials of Streptokinase: GISSI, ISIS-2, and Others

The TIMI group was not the only group to study the efficacy of thrombolytic therapy. Many other groups were extremely active in that process (they are listed in Appendix A of this chapter). In this section, we will examine the activity of those groups which conducted trials of intravenous streptokinase against a placebo control group. There were at least five such groups: an Italian group, the Gruppo Italiano per lo Studio della Streptochinasi nell'infarto Miocardico (GISSI), whose research was supported in part by a variety of Italian foundations and governmental agencies; a multinational group, centered at the Radcliffe Infirmary at Oxford, which conducted the second international study of infarct survival (ISIS-2), that was supported predominantly by Behringwerke, a subsidiary of Hoechst, one of the manufacturers of streptokinase; a German group, whose work was funded by the German Federal Ministry for Research and Technology, which conducted the Intravenous Streptokinase in Acute Myocardial Infarction (ISAM) study; the Western Washington group, which had conducted a very important study of intracoronary streptokinase, and which turned its attention to the use of intravenous streptokinase and conducted a trial funded in part by the NIH; and a group from New Zealand, led by Dr. Harvey White, which conducted a trial of intravenous streptokinase funded by the National Heart Foundation of New Zealand and the New Zealand Medical Research Council.

Of all these trials, the GISSI trial and the ISIS-2 trial were to attract the most attention. These trials were in many ways different from American trials such as TIMI. First, they were extremely large trials. GISSI enrolled 12,000 patients while ISIS-2 enrolled 20,000 patients. These numbers are required if you want to be able to detect differences in mortality when the base mortality rate in the control group is low. Second, these trials were less rigorous in design, allowing different trial centers and/or different physicians to treat their patients in different ways. Thus, for example, the GISSI study explicitly allowed some centers to use heparin while other did not. ISIS-2 did not even impose a policy of uniformity within a center on the use of heparin. Finally, there were few restrictions on enrollment, thereby producing a patient population which is closer to the actual patient population seen in normal clinical practice.

The GISSI trial was planned in the fall of 1983 (at the same time as the planning of TIMI-I) and was conducted from February 1984 to June 1985.[87] A crucial component of its design, in addition to those already mentioned, is that informed consent was not obtained from the patients before they were enrolled in the trial.

Those conducting the trial were aware that this seemed to breach the standard principles of ethics governing research trials, but they argued for the breach in the following passage: "The research protocol, approved by the ethics committee of the regional health authority, did not require informed consent—mainly because the patients' predicament was judged too acute for acceptable application of the procedure. Medical staff were ready to provide explanations to the patients upon request."[88] The argument can be interpreted in several ways. The benefit of thrombolytic therapy is greater when it is administered as soon as possible. Any realistic and meaningful process of informed consent would slow the process too much and is therefore too risky for the patients. Moreover, in light of the acute anxiety and stress suffered by the patient, and in light of the further possible impairment of the patient's mental processes by medications, it is not meaningful to talk in this setting of obtaining competent informed consent. Finally, it would be disturbing and cruel to the patient in this setting, where his or her life is acutely threatened, to have to explain all the uncertainties which have given rise to the trial.

A total of 11,806 patients were randomized into the GISSI trial and full data were available for 11,712. The results in terms of lessening in-hospital mortality were impressive. The 21-day overall mortality rate was 10.7 percent in the streptokinase group (628 of 5,860) as opposed to 13 percent in the placebo group (758 of 5,852), a relative reduction of 18 percent in the number of deaths and an absolute 2.3 percent lowering of the death rate.[89] The results were particularly impressive for patients presenting within 6 hours of the onset of chest pain. Moreover, the major feared side effects (serious bleeding, allergic reactions, and hypotension) were found in only a small number of patients. Naturally, there were more deaths in both groups when the patients were followed for a full year. Even then, however, the survival rate was impressively better in the streptokinase group. Only 17.2 percent of the streptokinase group (1,005 of 5,851) died, as compared to 19 percent (1,113 of 5,846) of the placebo group. This difference in long-term mortality was entirely due to the difference in the in-hospital mortality; there was no extra long-term benefit.

Similar striking results were found in the ISIS-2 trial.[90] It was a somewhat more complicated trial than GISSI since it was interested in studying both the effects of streptokinase and the effects of aspirin (as an antiplatelet agent) on patients with acute myocardial infarction. Patients were divided into four groups: a group which received streptokinase alone, a group which received aspirin alone, a group which received both, and a group which received neither. Different centers involved in these trials adopted a variety of approaches to informed consent, ranging from not obtaining consent to having the patients sign a detailed consent form.

The ISIS-2 group began enrolling patients in March 1985 and continued enrolling them through the end of December 1987. This meant that half the patients in the years 1986 and 1987 received no thrombolytic therapy (only a placebo) even though the GISSI results were available and even though the NHLBI was no longer willing to run placebo controlled trials. In this respect, the ISIS group agreed with the European Cooperative investigators. But another episode which occurred in the midst of the ISIS trial raised even more serious ethical issues. This had to do with the ethics of continuing to randomize patients who presented within the early hours (less than 4 hours) after the onset of chest pain in light of the trial's own initial data about efficacy of treatment. Let me elaborate upon this point.

In January 1987, the Data Monitoring Committee of the ISIS-2 trial (chaired by Sir Richard Doll) informed the ISIS-2 investigators that there was proof beyond reasonable doubt that streptokinase reduced mortality among these early patients (from about 12 percent to about 8 percent). Despite that finding, the steering committee conducting the trial felt that it would be appropriate to allow the responsible physician to continue to enroll patients even in the early hours after onset of chest pain if that physician remained uncertain as to whether streptokinase is indicated. To quote Sir Richard Doll:

> We did in fact report at an intermediate stage that, in our view, it was beyond reasonable doubt that one particular treatment was more beneficial than another. *We were, however, not responsible for conducting the trial*, and the steering committee that was conducting it preferred to pass our information onto the participating doctors and to allow them to stop or continue to admit patients as they thought wise.[91]

In fact, many additional early onset patients were enrolled after the interim data on the nearly 4,000 early onset patients were analyzed by the monitoring committee, and half of them continued to receive a placebo. Was this appropriate in light of the interim data? What is the purpose of collecting interim data? What is the role of the monitoring committee as opposed to the study steering committee in making these decisions?

Putting aside these issues for now, let us return to the results of the ISIS-2 trial. Both streptokinase alone and aspirin alone produced a highly significant reduction in 5-week cardiovascular mortality. Even more exciting was the fact that the reduction produced by these two agents was additive, producing a 42 percent relative reduction and a 5.2 percent absolute reduction in cardiovascular mortality (from 13.2 percent to 8 percent) in patients allocated both agents as opposed to patients receiving neither. All of this was accomplished with a very low percentage of side effects. Not surprisingly, then, the ISIS-2 investigators concluded that the use of streptokinase and aspirin could avoid several tens of thousands of deaths each year.

Given the results of these two major trials, far less attention has been paid to the others, but it seems to be worth noticing at least the following:

1. At least one of the placebo-controlled trials, the Western Washington trial,[92] was stopped before it had enrolled as many patients as planned (368 out of 660) because it was deemed inappropriate, in light of the GISSI data and other similar data, to continue to enroll further patients in the placebo control group.

2. The appropriateness of informed consent was controversial in many of these studies. The Western Washington group attempted to involve a family member in the process. A Dutch group, which began studying intracoronary streptokinase but ended up studying intravenous streptokinase, decided to get informed consent only from patients who were assigned to the streptokinase group.[93]

3. Several of these smaller trials, such as ISAM,[94] found a trend toward reduced mortality only at 21 days, although the New Zealand study[95] did find a significant improvement in 30-day survival (from 12.9 percent to 2.5 percent) in what was a very small study.

As noted in the previous section, the NIH never ran a trial which many thought in 1982 that it should run, a trial of streptokinase against a placebo to see whether the intravenous administration of streptokinase would save lives. In the period 1983–1987 such trials, run primarily in Europe, established beyond any doubt that the intravenous administration of streptokinase could save a significant number of lives. As we have seen, many ethical questions were raised in the course of these trials, and the design of these studies was not as tight as the NIH design. They did, however, provide a definitive answer to a very important question. What does this mean for the future of clinical trials? Can important results be obtained in scientifically and ethically unquestionable trials?

The Trials of tPA: ASSET and Others

While the trials of streptokinase were being conducted, other groups turned their attention to placebo-controlled trials of tPA. The major trial was another very large European trial, involving 5,011 patients, called the ASSET (Anglo-Scandinavian Study of Early Thrombolysis) trial.[96] It was funded by Boehringer Ingelheim, the European company to which Genentech had licensed distribution rights in Europe of tPA. The study was coordinated from Nottingham University, and it involved patients from England, Norway, Sweden, and Denmark. This largest and most important trial of tPA against a placebo with mortality as the end point will be the major focus of this section, but we begin by briefly reviewing some other trials.

One such trial was the European Cooperative Group trial mentioned earlier. At least three others should be mentioned. One was a trial headed by Dr. Alan Guerci, at Johns Hopkins Hospital, funded by a grant from the NHLBI and by Genentech. After enrolling 138 patients, the trial was stopped in March 1987 when the publication of the preliminary ISIS-2 data following the GISSI data led the investigators to conclude, "We did not consider it ethical to continue a placebo-controlled trial in the light of these data."[97] The study took ejection fraction as its end point (it was too small to study mortality) and concluded that the use of tPA produced a significantly better ejection fraction. The second study also examined ejection fraction, comparing tPA with a placebo. It was conducted by the TICO group (Group for the Study of Thrombolysis in Acute Coronary Occlusion) in Australia and was funded by Boehringer Ingelheim. It also showed a significantly better ejection fraction in the tPA group, and it was stopped in June 1987 because an interim analysis of the first 119 patients showed that the results were so impressive that a continuation was unjustified.[98] The last of these trials was the National Heart Foundation of Australia study of ejection fraction in a tPA-treated group as compared to a placebo control group, a study in which Boehringer Ingelheim had a representative on the study management committee. It too showed a significant improvement in the 103 patients who had usable ventriculograms. Finally, it too struggled with the question of the placebo control group. To quote its report: "In December, 1986, the management committee decided that random allocation to placebo administration in patients admitted under 2 hours was no longer ethically tenable because of the findings of the GISSI trial, and from January 1, 1987, only patients in the 2–4 hours time period were admitted to the trial."[99]

Several points should be noted about these small trials. To begin with, by using as a measure of heart performance left ventricular ejection fraction rather than mortality as the end point, these groups were able to run small trials with statistically significant results. The contrast between the numbers of patients they enrolled and the number of patients in such large trials as GISSI, ISIS-2, and ASSET, which used mortality as their end point, is very striking. Second, each of these trials struggled with the question of how long placebo-controlled trials could be justified in light of positive data coming either from other trials or from the trial in question.

Having looked briefly at these other trials, we return to the ASSET trial. The trial randomized 5,011 patients within the first 5 hours of the onset of symptoms of myocardial infarction (MI) to receive either tPA or a placebo. All received heparin, but they did not receive anticoagulants or antiplatelets after discharge. In this way, the ASSET trial was more carefully structured than the GISSI trial and the ISIS-2 trial. As mentioned previously, ASSET took 1-month mortality as its end point, and data were available for nearly all the 5,011 patients. Of 2,515 patients getting tPA, 182 (7.2 percent) died, whereas 245 of 2,494 patients getting a placebo died (9.8 percent). This represents a highly significant 26 percent relative reduction of mortality and a 2.6 percent actual lowering of the death rate by using tPA. While there were more complications (especially bleeding complications) among the patients receiving thrombolytic therapy, these were clearly outweighed by the tremendous reduction in mortality. ASSET then joins GISSI and ISIS-2 in showing that lives are saved by using thrombolytic therapy, although none of these trials show which agent saves more lives, since they were not designed as comparative trials.

The ASSET trial first enrolled patients in November 1986, nine months after the GISSI data had been published, and continued enrolling patients until February 29, 1988, one year after the preliminary data from ISIS-2 were published. We have already seen that some of the other placebo-controlled trials of tPA found this unacceptable. The Johns Hopkins trial, for example, stopped after the ISIS-2 data became available. The National Heart Foundation of Australia partially stopped enrolling patients because of GISSI. What was the stance of the ASSET group on this issue? They had the following to say:

> The trial results were monitored by an independent ethical committee who would have advised premature termination of the study if predetermined differences between the treatment group has been observed. These "stopping rules" were not needed. The ethical committee did advise, on the basis of the published results of other studies of thrombolysis, that it was no longer reasonable to include patients in a placebo-controlled study, but this advice coincided with the inclusion of the intended total of 5000 patients.[100]

This is a very interesting passage, for it raises the question of what study led the committee to make its decision in February 1988 as opposed to earlier, when other impressive data were already available. What was the relation between this delay and the fact that they made the decision when they had all the patients they needed? Were there any special considerations causing the trial to continue?

One final observation about these trials and their corporate sponsorship. TIMI and GISSI were publicly funded trials. ISIS-2 was funded by Boehringer, but the study made a point of insisting that it was designed, conducted, analyzed, and interpreted independently of the companies funding it. ASSET let sponsoring company personnel attend meetings as observers, and the National Heart Foundation of Australia had sponsoring company personnel on the management committee of the trial. Since the companies in question had significant economic interests in the outcomes of these trials, it is worth considering how closely they should have been involved in the conduct of the trials.

Putting aside these ethical questions for the moment, we can say that ASSET as a trial of mortality (supported by the smaller trials of left ejection fraction) laid the foundation for the claim that tPA was a safe and efficacious drug, a claim that would become very important when approval was to be sought for use of the drug in regular clinical practice. But before turning to that question, we need to look at trials of one more thrombolytic agent.

Trials of APSAC

This last thrombolytic agent, anisoylated plasminogen streptokinase activator complex (APSAC), does not occur naturally but was produced in 1979–1980 in the laboratories of Beecham Pharmaceuticals, a British pharmaceutical company. Beecham was attempting to design a thrombolytic agent with certain very specific properties (giving, perhaps, a newer and nicer meaning to the phrase "designer drug").[101] The investigators wanted to produce an agent better than streptokinase in at least three respects. It should produce more fibrinolytic activity at the site of the clot and less elsewhere (thereby reducing the threat of bleeding), it should have a longer period of activity, and it should be protected from destruction by inhibitors circulating in the blood. The molecule they created, one of several experimented with, is a complex of plasminogen and streptokinase with an inactivated center. When injected into the body, the complex binds to fibrin and begins to be activated to produce fibrinolysis. Because the activation takes a fair amount of time, the complex can produce fibrinolytic activity for a longer period of time. Moreover, because it is activated slowly, it can be administered very quickly without fear of excessive activity. When APSAC was announced in 1981, it looked extremely promising. But it did not get picked up by the NIH, although Marder, while still on the Data Safety Board, had urged the NIH to study it. Nevertheless, by 1985 it had been studied sufficiently so that clinical trials of its efficacy could begin.

Two approaches were adopted in these clinical trials. The first, comparing APSAC to other thrombolytic therapies, was adopted for the trials in the United States. In a series of trials headed by Dr. Jeffrey Anderson, begun in 1985 and continuing into 1990, APSAC was compared first to intracoronary streptokinase, then to intravenous streptokinase, and finally (in a trial continuing into 1990) to tPA.[102] The end points were angiographically confirmed reperfusion and patency of the infarct-related artery. The second, comparing APSAC to a placebo, was adopted in a large trial in Europe called AIMS (APSAC Intervention Mortality Study).[103] In it, APSAC was compared to a placebo control group with mortality as the end point.

Why did the first group adopt its approach of avoiding placebo control groups? We must remember that this decision was made at the beginning of 1985, before any results were in from the GISSI and ISIS-2 trials, and even before the publication of Yusuf's article about pooled data. Consequently, this group could not have been influenced by the factors that led the NIH (1 year later, after GISSI) to stop the originally planned placebo-controlled TIMI-II trials, or the factors that led others (2 years later, after the preliminary report of ISIS-2) to stop other placebo-controlled trials. The reasoning of Anderson's group, based upon their understanding—whether correct, we shall see in Chapter 3—of FDA policy, is best stated in the following passage from the report of their first trial, which compared APSAC with intracoronary streptokinase (which had, of course, already been approved by the FDA in 1982 for use in patients with an MI):

> The selection of intracoronary streptokinase as the control arm and its dose and duration of administration deserve comment. During initial new drug development, federal (FDA) policy required controlled comparisons with placebo or with an *approved* standard therapy. Comparison with placebo was considered unethical at the time of this study, and intravenous thrombolytic therapies (streptokinase, tPA) were not approved until November, 1987.[104]

The argument is that it would be unethical to deny treatment to a control group because there exists an approved standard therapy. Therefore, the only trial that could be run was APSAC against intracoronary streptokinase (intravenous streptokinase had not yet been approved). The argument seems to have force, unless alternative forms of trials are available, in light of the life-threatening nature of the condition and the demonstrated benefit of intracoronary streptokinase. No doubt Anderson was particularly sensitive to this point because he had run one of the studies demonstrating the benefit of intracoronary streptokinase.

The European AIMS trial began more than a year later, and these investigators had available the data from the Yusuf article and from the GISSI trial. Moreover, Anderson's argument about the existence of an approved therapy was certainly still valid. So how did the AIMS investigators respond to the question of the legitimacy of a placebo-controlled trial? They responded by going ahead with the trial but they added provisions for stopping it earlier if their own data proved significant. To quote their preliminary report:

> However, in the light of other trials showing highly significant mortality reductions after thrombolytic therapy, the data monitoring committee redefined the plans for interim analyses as follows. Such redefinition was done after patient entry had begun but before any survival results were known. Analysis would be undertaken of the accumulating data after each consecutive 500 patients had been followed for at least 30 days, and would use a logrank analysis of survival up to 30 days as the primary test statistic. Statistical guidelines for stopping were based on an O'Brien and Fleming rule with a maximum of four analyses and an overall two-sided type I error = 0.05.[105]

In fact, this led them to stop the trial after an interim analysis of 1,004 patients showed a 47 percent reduction in 30-day mortality in the APSAC-treated group as opposed to the placebo group. Whether this provision for interim analyses was an adequate resolution of the ethical issues will be discussed in Chapter 2.

Let us turn now to an analysis of the results of the various APSAC studies. The multicenter APSAC trial headed by Anderson took angiographically demonstrated reperfusion as its study end point and compared the use of APSAC with the use of intracoronary streptokinase. Reperfusion was studied for the first 90 minutes after thrombolytic therapy commenced, although APSAC, because of its long duration of action, was administered for only 2–4 minutes while streptokinase was administered for 60 minutes. After the 90-minute time frame, physicians were allowed (because of "ethical considerations") to treat the patient at their discretion.

For patients treated within 4 hours of the onset of symptoms, there were no differences between APSAC and intracoronary streptokinase. APSAC was successful in 60 percent (47 of 79) of patients treated in that time frame, while intracoronary streptokinase was also successful in 60 percent (50 of 83) of those patients. For patients treated after 4 hours of the onset of symptoms, APSAC did not do as well as intracoronary streptokinase. Anderson pointed out that these results compare favorably to intravenous streptokinase in the TIMI-I trials and are as good as the results of tPA in that trial. Anderson and his colleagues concluded that, given the ease of administration of APSAC, thereby facilitating early thrombolytic therapy, APSAC's further development should be encouraged.

Given the limited end point in the Anderson study, it did not attract as much attention as the European AIMS trial, which involved a larger number of patients and had mortality as its end point. As indicated earlier, the AIMS trial was designed to compare APSAC to a placebo-controlled group. Initial statistical considerations suggested a need to study 2,000 patients, but, for reasons stated previously, that plan was enlarged to allow for interim analysis after each 500 patients were enrolled. In fact, the trial was stopped because of the impressive results in the first 1,004 patients, but by the time the analysis of the data was completed, 1,258 patients had been randomized.

What were the impressive results? To begin with, if administered within 6 hours of the onset of symptoms, APSAC produced a 50 percent relative reduction and a 6 percent absolute reduction of 30-day mortality, from 77 of 634 patients on placebo (12 percent) to 40 of 624 on APSAC (6 percent). Even on long-term survival data, APSAC did very well. On 1-year follow-up, 69 of the APSAC patients (11 percent) had died, compared to 113 of the placebo patients (18 percent). What makes these results particularly striking is the comparison of the 30-day mortality data in the APSAC group with similar data from trials of streptokinase and tPA. Table 1.1 illustrates the comparison. Even given the need for great caution in comparing data across different trials (because of different entry criteria, forms of concomitant therapy, and so on), this difference is quite striking and it attracted

Table 1.1 Comparison of Mortality Data

	Mortality rate in treatment group (%)	*Reduction in mortality (%)*
GISSI (SK)	10.7	22.6
ISIS-2 (SK)	9.2	29.4
ASSET (tPA)	7.2	28.4
AIMS (APSAC)	6.0	50.0

Source: Data from AIMS Trial Study Group, "Long-Term Effects of Intravenous Anistreplase in Acute Myocardial Infarction: Final Report of the AIMS Study," *Lancet*, February 24, 1990, pp. 427–31.

a lot of attention. With the conclusion of the AIMS trial, APSAC had progressed very quickly from design to demonstration of great clinical benefit.

1987: The Year of FDA Approval

The many clinical trials we examined in the last section illustrate the power of clinical investigations to settle important issues. GISSI, ISIS-2, ASSET, and AIMS demonstrated beyond a doubt that thrombolytic therapy administered after an acute MI would save many lives, and TIMI began the process of evaluating the respective merits of different thrombolytic agents. But these trials were not designed just to advance the state of clinical knowledge; they were also intended to influence actual clinical practice.

In the United States, as in other countries, clinical trials of new drugs can influence actual clinical practice only if they result in government approval of the use of the tested drugs. With that approval, the drug companies can begin the commercial distribution of the drug; without that approval, the drug's use is severely limited. In this respect, new drugs differ from other new therapeutic interventions such as new forms of surgery. As the results of the major trials came in, attention turned to the FDA to see how quickly it would approve the new agents, tPA and APSAC, and how quickly it would approve the new mode of administration, intravenous injection, for streptokinase.

In November 1987, the FDA approved intravenous streptokinase and tPA for use in the treatment of myocardial infarctions. APSAC, whose application came into the FDA later because its trials began later, was approved in November 1989. Given the fact that the major trials were completed in 1986 and 1987, it might seem as though the process of FDA approval went extremely smoothly and expeditiously. This is, however, a very misleading impression. Few events in the history of thrombolytic therapy were as controversial as the FDA approvals. We turn next to an examination of that process and to the issues which it raises.

The May 29 Meeting of the Cardio-Renal Drugs Advisory Committee

While final decisions about the approval of drugs are in the hands of the FDA staff, normal operating procedure is to review applications submitted by manufacturers internally and to solicit the advice of an advisory panel before any final decision is made. That process was followed in the case of thrombolytic agents, and both the intravenous streptokinase and tPA requests were forwarded to the Cardio-Renal Advisory Committee for discussion at its May 29, 1987, meeting.

There was one crucial change in the process, a change whose significance will emerge as we go along. The Center for Drugs and Biologics is the part of the FDA devoted to approving new pharmaceuticals. Most of that work, especially in the cardiovascular area, is carried out at the Center for Drug Evaluation and Research. Certain pharmaceuticals (large biologic molecules) are, however, under the control of the Center for Biologics Evaluation and Research, and among these are the thrombolytic agents. In particular, the thrombolytic agents are under the supervision of the Division of Blood and Blood Products of the Center for Biologics, headed in 1987 by Dr. Tom Zuck. But there was no advisory committee on cardiovascular drugs, so these agents were assigned to the Center for Drug's Cardio-Renal Advisory Committee, which had greater expertise in this area. Thus in May 1987 the advisory committee was working with a division of the FDA with which it had not interacted before.

Both the formal agenda of the meeting and the transcript are available as public documents.[106] They reveal a very full day, with the morning devoted to examining ten major issues surrounding intravenous streptokinase and the afternoon devoted to examining seven major issues surrounding tPA.

What happened at the meeting? Simply, the committee recommended the approval of intravenous streptokinase but suggested deferring action on tPA. It was the deferral of tPA that led, of course, to the controversy. The immediate reaction of many was extremely negative. Dr. Eugene Braunwald, who led the TIMI trials, said at the meeting: "I think you have to be very careful that you are not rejecting a drug that is twice as effective as a drug that you approved a few hours ago" (p. 547). This reaction, no doubt reflecting Braunwald's position that the TIMI trial had proven the superiority of tPA over streptokinase, was very mild compared to an editorial a few days later in the *Wall Street Journal*. The following excerpts from an unsigned editorial give a good sense of its outrage:

> Last Friday an advisory panel of the Food and Drug Administration decided to sacrifice thousands of American lives on an altar of pedantry . . . the advisory panel decided to approve intravenous use of streptokinase, but not approve the superior thrombolytic tPA. This is absurd. . . . Patients will die who would otherwise live longer. Medical research has allowed statistics to become the supreme judge of its inventions. The FDA, in particular its bureau of drugs under Robert Temple, has

driven that system to its absurd extreme. . . . The advisory panel's suggestion that tPA's sponsor conduct further mortality studies poses grave ethical questions. . . . We'll put it bluntly. Are American doctors going to let people die to satisfy the bureau of drug's chi-square studies?[107]

Naturally, others saw it differently. Among those who did were the members of the committee itself. Writing in *JAMA* almost a year later, they stated their position as follows:

Given our concerns, the committee had no choice but to recommend postponement of approval pending further data analysis and to ask the sponsor to provide the FDA with the results of ongoing trials when they were available. To do otherwise would have been inconsistent with good science and good medicine.[108]

What were the concerns raised by the advisory committee at its May meeting? In its 1988 defense of its actions, the committee identified its concerns as follows:

1. There was inadequate evidence of efficacy at the recommended dose of 100 mg, when efficacy was defined as something more than clot lysis. Improvement in ventricular function would be sufficient; mortality studies would not be required.
2. There was concern about intracerebral bleeding. An unacceptable incidence of bleeding had occurred at the 150-mg dose in the TIMI trial, leading to a dose reduction in that trial to 100 mg, and the committee wanted to know the incidence of that severe complication at 100 mg.
3. All of the data were hard to evaluate because the sponsor had changed the form of the drug, as well as its dosage, during the crucial trials.

Indeed, all of these issues are raised in the transcript of the committee's deliberations. Moreover, when the FDA finally approved tPA in November, in a process to be discussed shortly, it announced its responses to just these questions, arguing that these responses justified the eventual approval.[109] All of the evidence points to these being the major issues. They need to be reviewed one at a time because of their importance for our evaluation of the FDA's standards of drug approval.

Determining the criteria that would demonstrate efficacy of tPA was quite complex. Obviously, a placebo-controlled trial of tPA with mortality as its end point which showed a major reduction in mortality by the use of tPA would be the best evidence. Unlike streptokinase, for which evidence of improved survival was available from GISSI and ISIS-2, evidence from such a trial of tPA was not available in May 1987, since ASSET had just begun enrolling European patients in such a trial and the European Cooperative Group's much smaller trials had not yet finished enrolling patients. Moreover, the NIH (and others) had quite reasonably adopted the view that such placebo-controlled trials were not ethically acceptable once the GISSI data and the Yusuf pooled data became available. Evidence of lysing clots and restoring artery patency derived from placebo-controlled trials of tPA or from trials of tPA versus streptokinase was available (the most important being the results in TIMI-I indicating that tPA was better than streptokinase in restoring patency), but such evidence left open the question of the clinical significance of restoring patency. Would it save lives by improving ventricular functioning? That left the possibility of trying to get from already-run placebo-controlled trials or new streptokinase-controlled trials evidence about ventricular function. But the data about that were unclear in May 1987. So everybody was groping with this issue at the meeting.

Dr. Elliot Grossbard, speaking for Genentech at the May 1987 meeting, began his presentation with a pretty clear statement that tPA should be approved as a thrombolytic agent designed to restore patency to infarct-related arteries. Grossbard clearly appealed to previous decisions which Genentech thought had settled the question:

> In late 1983, we met with the representatives of the Office of Biologics and described a clinical plan which basically suggested that we were going to attempt to demonstrate coronary thrombolysis as a primary efficacy end-point in our trials. There were a number of reasons why we did that. Over the next 2 or 3 years we have sequentially done that in a number of studies, and we have in no way attempted to avoid issues regarding ventricular function and mortality, but we have operated within certain constraints that existed with regard to our participation with the NHLBI TIMI group and with the impact that the GISSI trial had on the ability to conduct certain placebo controlled trials in this country. (p. 372)

Grossbard was making two points. He thought that Genentech had a clear understanding with the Biologics Division that evidence of thrombolysis would be sufficient. Here, the sudden switch to an advisory committee of the Drug Division may have been crucial, and it has been widely speculated that Genentech felt that the rules of the game had been unfairly changed at the last minute.[110] Equally important, Grossbard felt that the evidence required was determined by the NIH when it had taken (in TIMI-I) patency of arteries as the appropriate end point and when it had canceled (in 1986) further placebo-controlled trials. These points have validity, and they certainly indicate the need, which we have alluded to on several occasions, for collaboration between the relevant government agencies.

Independent of these procedural points, however, the question still remains as to what should be taken as adequate evidence of efficacy. Many would argue that evidence of patency should be sufficient. After all, they would say, heart attacks cause death because myocardium is destroyed by a lack of blood due to clots in the relevant arteries. If you can break up those clots and restore blood flow, that should save lives. GISSI, available to the committee, shows that lives are saved by streptokinase. As shown in TIMI-I, tPA produces patency in more cases, so it must save more lives. But the committee saw it differently. The clearest statement of their position is found in the remarks of one of the members, Dr. Giardina:

> The major difference really is that there were thousands of patients to draw upon in the streptokinase data, and streptokinase, the mechanism of action by which streptokinase improves mortality or improves reperfusion may, in fact, be different than what we are seeing here. There may, in fact, be other mechanisms that come into play with streptokinase but haven't been evaluated or worked out or presented here with tPA, and so, I don't think we can completely extrapolate. . . . I think that what we need is more numbers, more studies, and again, I say that intuitively I want to believe that it will improve mortality. (p. 530)

Other mechanisms that had been suggested include the lowering of blood viscosity (allowing blood to reach heart muscle through unblocked collateral vessels) and the lowering of blood pressure (which may decrease both the strain on the heart and the loss of myocardium) by streptokinase. So the committee felt that the evidence of tPA's efficacy was suggestive but not conclusive. Is that enough to justify approving the drug as efficacious? Just how much evidence should be required?

Two final points on this question of efficacy. First, Genentech presented as evidence of efficacy the positive results of the recently stopped Guerci trial at Johns Hopkins, which (we now clearly know) showed evidence of improved left ventricular functioning in a placebo-controlled trial. And it also presented as evidence of efficacy the TIMI-I results showing that tPA and streptokinase produced equivalent left ventricular functioning. The former data looked impressive, but the committee members, who had not seen them in advance, were noncommittal. It was late on Friday, and several members had to leave before the end of the meeting, so the Guerci data may have fallen prey to a too lengthy agenda for one day. The latter data raised all of the usual issues about active-controlled trials, to which we shall return. Second, at the very end of the meeting, at least two people—Dr. Borer, the chair of the committee, and Dr. Zuck, from the Biologics Division—wondered what to tell sponsors about what evidence was required for approval. By the time they asked this question, much of the committee had left, but the answers they got, especially those from Dr. Raymond Lipicky and Dr. Robert Temple of the FDA, are particularly interesting. Lipicky expressed the hope that placebo-controlled data might yet be coming in (pp. 545–46, 550–51 of the transcript). Temple's response was more complex. He suggested that once additional lysing agents, which didn't lower viscosity or blood pressure, had been shown to be effective, then further placebo-controlled trials might not be required, although such trials might be required until then (pp. 548–51 of the transcript). Neither specifically said that mortality data would be needed, and at least Lipicky suggested that ventricular functioning data would be enough. Still, the message to be drawn from the end of the meeting was very unclear.

The safety of tPA with respect to intracerebral bleeding was the second issue raised by the advisory committee. To understand the issue, one needs to remember certain facts about the history of the TIMI trials discussed earlier. After the ending of TIMI-I, the TIMI group adopted a new single-chain-molecule form of tPA, compared to an earlier double-chain form. Studies conducted in late 1985 and early 1986 (the open-label studies) suggested that the new tPA required a higher dose (either 100 or 150 mg) than the older tPA (80 mg), but that it was as safe.[111] TIMI-II was therefore planned using 150 mg of the new tPA. In March and April 1986, TIMI-II and another open-label pilot trial began using 150 mg. By October 20, 1986, it was clear that this had been a mistake. A total of 326 patients in the open-label trial had received the higher dosage, as had 581 patients in TIMI-II. In these 907 patients, there were 16 intracranial hemorrhages (1.76 percent). Even if you add the 107 patients who had received the higher dosages in the 1985–1986 trials and none of whom had suffered a hemorrhage, you get 16 hemorrhages in 1,014 patients (1.6 percent). Given the seriousness of this problem, the investigators returned to the 100-mg dosage of the new single-chain molecule. By May 1987, when the hearing was held, over 1,400 patients had received the lower dosage with a hemorrhage rate of only 0.6 percent, clearly a much more acceptable rate.[112] These are the facts that need to be kept in mind as one looks at the discussion at the advisory committee meeting.

Were these facts understood at the meeting? It is clear from the transcript that they were not. One immediate question is why Genentech did not present these data. Early in his discussion, Grossbard's own frustration about this issue is clear:

> I think to a certain extent I am a little bit constrained by what I can say about the TIMI trial, and I hope that Dr. Braunwald will elaborate on the results of the TIMI trial because it has been our practice not to make public statements about the TIMI trial that have not been disclosed. (pp. 422–23)

Because NIH procedures dictated that unpublished data from ongoing trials could not be revealed, Genentech put together a lot of other data that left people thoroughly confused.

Things got worse a little later in the hearing when Lipicky from the FDA introduced the claim that only 350 patients had received 150 mg and that they had suffered 16 intracranial hemorrhages (p. 435). He was right about the numerator of 16, but very wrong about the denominator, as Grossbard tried to point out (p. 436)—with little success. Grossbard again referred to the frustrations of not being able to talk clearly about the TIMI unpublished data, especially the data showing the low rate in the patients who got only 100 mg. Unfortunately, things did not get better when Braunwald made his presentation. Part of the problem was that he felt unable to present data from the blinded ongoing trial (p. 469), although in fact he presented at one point or another all the information. In general, moreover, too much attention was devoted to the incidence rate at 150 mg and not enough to the incidence rate at 100 mg, the dosage for which approval was sought.

Many speculations have appeared about what caused this total failure of communication.[113] I think that they are not as important as the obvious point to be drawn from this story. It is absurd for one agency of the government (the FDA) to be making decisions about a drug while having available only some of the relevant data available at other agencies (the NIH), especially when people who have access to complete data are testifying. At one point in the hearing, Grossbard found himself saying:

> We have tried within keeping, as I said, with our commitment to the NHLBI not to divulge their information in our presentation, we have collected everything we could that was public and given you what I think reflects a 1.2 percent [at 150 mg] versus 0.4 percent [at 100 mg] relative incidence *which I think is essentially the same as has been observed in another 1500 patients in the TIMI trial.* (p. 436; italics added)

Witnesses should not have to present information in such a confusing manner because of commitments to other agencies. Surely, clearances can be obtained in advance, even if this must be done in a way that minimizes interference with ongoing trials (especially because of the unblinding involved).

There are important issues about what level of intracranial hemorrhaging is safe enough. But these issues never were seriously discussed at the meeting, because the available data were not presented in a straightforward fashion and because members of the committee may have been influenced by reports of individual cases.

What shall we conclude about the meeting and its decision to postpone recommending the approval of tPA? As a meeting, it was a disaster. The crucial Guerci data about efficacy were not made available sufficiently in advance, leaving the committee, which was clearly rushed, no chance to study them carefully. The withholding of the TIMI data about safety, combined with some related misinformation presented at the meeting, only made things worse. It is not necessary for our purposes to settle the question of whether the blame lies with Genentech for making a bad presentation or the FDA for running a bad meeting. It is sufficient to note that, as a matter of policy, important decisions should not be made in such a manner.

But what about the specific decision to defer approval? As we shall see, the FDA, when it later approved tPA, made it clear that it felt the Guerci data, supplemented by another small trial, and the TIMI safety data, properly understood, would justify the approval of tPA. Apparently the FDA felt that the data were available at the meeting but unfortunately not understood.

Final Approval of the Thrombolytic Agent

Despite all the fuss surrounding the recommendations made at the May 29 meeting, final approval of both streptokinase and tPA came in the same week in November 1987. There are two ways of looking at this. The first is that the FDA worked with real dispatch to clear up all the issues left unresolved at that meeting, and this expeditious effort is evidence of the FDA's capacity to move forward without undue delay. The second is that the FDA gave in to the tremendous public outcry following the May 29 meeting, and this episode is evidence of the agency's inability to hold firm under inappropriate pressures. Because of the importance of this process for our understanding of standards for approval of drugs, we need to review the record of this period of time carefully.

The critics of the FDA were quick to state their case. On June 2 the *Wall Street Journal*, which was to take a major role in leading the critics, published the editorial quoted earlier, called "Human Sacrifices."[114] The thrust of its claims was that the committee was sacrificing lives by insisting on pedantic statistical points. It called upon Dr. Frank Young, the commissioner of the FDA, to repudiate the panel, and on Dr. Otis Bowen, the secretary of Health and Human Services, to support Young in fixing the FDA. This attitude reflected the *Journal*'s general support of less bureaucratic regulation of the economy as well as the unhappiness of the investment community, which had backed Genentech as a big winner and which now saw the stock drop from a high of $64.50 in March 1987 to $36.35 on the Monday following the committee's meeting (with a drop of $11.75 on that Monday alone).[115]

But unhappy members of the investment community did not stand alone; distinguished members of the community of cardiologists who had been associated with the testing of tPA were also unhappy. Dr. Eugene Braunwald described himself as "flabbergasted, just shocked," while Dr. Eric Topol of Michigan said, "I think everyone just went into shock."[116]

The FDA was clearly very sensitive to the criticisms that were being raised. It issued a document on June 5, 1987, discussing the concerns which had been raised, and this was followed by a trade press briefing by FDA Commissioner Young on June 17.[117] The very opening portion of the June 5 document shows the FDA as distancing itself from the committee while not explicitly repudiating it:

> There is room for honest disagreement with the advisory committee's recommendation on tPA. . . . Nonetheless, the advisory committee reached a clearly reasoned decision which deserves careful consideration. The following discussion, prepared by FDA staff, is intended neither to support nor rebut the advisory committee's recommendation, but simply to explain the basis for it.[118]

The FDA went on to say that the crucial questions would be the effect of tPA on mortality or cardiac function (efficacy) and the proper dose of the drug (safety).

Commissioner Young stated that the FDA expected to resolve remaining questions expeditiously.

The nature of that expeditious review can be reconstructed from a variety of sources. The review was put under the control of the Center for Biologics, with the review being headed by its director for research, Dr. Elaine Esber. A special tPA licensing committee was formed to review the data. It met on September 2 and was not satisfied with the revised data, but it was satisfied with the final data submitted at the end of September.[119]

Before looking at the data, it is worth spending a little time carefully examining this process. That the review was put in the hands of the Center for Biologics is not surprising since thrombolytic agents had always been under their control. What was more surprising was the formation of the licensing committee rather than a return to the Cardio-Renal Advisory Committee, even if that committee was an advisory committee to the Center for Drugs and even if some of its members were invited to be consultants to the new licensing committee. In the June 17 briefing, Young was still talking about repolling the Cardio-Renal Advisory Committee if a further data analysis showed that there was enough evidence to justify approval. He even said, "They probably should have knocked off at five o'clock and reconvened Monday morning," suggesting, as I did above, that the whole problem was due to a late-running Friday meeting.[120] But sometime later all of this was dropped, and a new licensing committee was formed; by whom and why are open to speculation. Suggestions might range all the way from the idea that this was an attempt to get a more pliable committee to the thought that the FDA had decided that the old committee was excessively demanding. We just don't know.

What data led the new committee to recommend approval in late September? The best sources to answer that question are Dr. Young's November press conference to announce tPA's approval and the FDA's Summary Basis of Approval.[121] The safety issue was settled by TIMI data about bleeding at the 100-mg dose. To quote from a document handed out at the press conference: "Safety data from more than 2,000 patients at a dose of 100 mg. from TIMI-II and other studies *not available at the advisory committee meeting* have convinced FDA scientists that there is not an undue risk of intracranial bleeding using tPA." In fact, of course, most of the data had been known by both Grossbard and Braunwald, but they felt they could not reveal them because of promises of the NIH. Other sources[122] make it clear that Braunwald had persuaded the NIH to let him reveal the safety data. He is quoted as saying, "We decided the hurt of the trial was minor but the enlightenment of the FDA was major." The efficacy data were supplied by the Guerci study from Johns Hopkins (which had been available to the committee, but only at the last minute) and some additional Australian studies which were stopped before originally planned. To quote once more from the FDA handout: "The question [of whether clot lysis is sufficient evidence of efficacy] is no longer relevant because new data were made available from the Johns Hopkins and Australian studies showing that tPA clearly improves heart function in patients treated."[123]

In short, data on record in September clearly were or could have been available to the advisory committee at its May meeting, reinforcing the view that poor coordination between the FDA and Genentech and between the FDA and the NIH was responsible for the mess at the May meeting. But all of this still leaves open the fundamental question: Should the FDA have demanded from the sponsors of tPA evidence—analogous to the GISSI data for streptokinase—of improvement in mortality, should it have been satisfied with clot lysis data of the sort initially presented, or should it have insisted on what it finally got—ventricular function data? This issue of what type of evidence of efficacy should be required by the FDA is an extremely important issue deserving further attention, and we will return to it in Chapter 3.

Two final observations. The first is that it is interesting that streptokinase was approved early in the week while tPA was approved later that week. Symbolically, this is very appropriate: the FDA accepted the advisory committee's recommendations approving streptokinase first but it acknowledged all the criticisms by approving tPA almost immediately. The second is that there was much less controversy two years later when APSAC was approved on November 27, 1989. In part this was because APSAC was the third thrombolytic agent to be approved, and later agents of the same type are usually approved quickly. In part, however, this was due to the fact that the APSAC sponsors had the results of AIMS, which showed a marked reduction in mortality with the use of APSAC as compared to a placebo control group. According to a report in *Business Week*, Genentech slowed the process of approval by using political influence to ensure that the approval was reviewed by an advisory committee.[124] Moreover, one of Genentech's representatives appeared before that committee to raise questions about immunologic sequelae of APSAC.[125] But approval was forthcoming anyway, and by the end of 1989 three major thrombolytic agents were approved for use in the United States.

Our story has focused on the controversy surrounding the FDA examination of tPA in May 1987, and it has raised many issues about that particular approval process. But it is important to remember that the fundamental question is what degree of evidence of safety and efficacy should be demanded before drugs are approved for general use. That will be one of the central issues discussed in Chapter 3.

Money Issues

With the November 1987 approval by the FDA of streptokinase and tPA, American clinicians were free to use thrombolytic therapy on a routine basis to treat patients with myocardial infarctions. The existence of this freedom did not mean, however, that such patients routinely began to receive thrombolytic therapy. The process by which drugs actually are adopted for routine use, as opposed to merely being approved for use, is important and deserves further study. In this part of our story, we will examine one aspect of that process, the impact of financial considerations on the adoption of the newly approved thrombolytic agents. We are focusing on that aspect because it was crucial in the adoption of the thrombolytic agents.

Financial considerations have, in fact, plagued the recent history of the thrombolytic agents, particularly tPA. Patent conflicts, with tremendous amounts of money involved, have emerged, as have charges that financial conflicts of interest undercut the validity of the studies supporting thrombolytic therapy. In this section, we will examine these issues as well, thereby enabling us to form a picture of the interaction between economics and medicine in the process of the development, approval, and adoption of the thrombolytic agents.

Medicare Reimbursement for tPA

American hospitals have traditionally been reimbursed by third-party insurance payers for each service they provide to their patients. Thus when a new drug was approved for use, hospitals that used it would bill the insurance companies for the drug. This approach certainly encouraged and facilitated the introduction of new therapies, but it did little to control the resulting costs, since hospitals had no incentive to limit in any way the introduction of new technologies. In response to these concerns, Congress introduced in the fall of 1983 a new way of reimbursing hospitals for Medicare patients. Under this new form of reimbursement, prospective payment, the hospital receives a flat payment fixed in advance for the care of each patient, a payment determined by the Diagnostic Related Group (DRG) into which the patient falls. If the hospital introduces additional forms of therapy for such patients, it does not receive any additional payment. This scheme was designed to provide an incentive for hospitals to limit the introduction of new technologies as part of their plan for introducing cost controls.

The approval of tPA dramatically illustrates the nature of these issues.[126] In early 1988, hospitals were receiving from $3,579 to $4,200 to treat a Medicare patient who had an uncomplicated myocardial infarction and were receiving from $5,449 to $6,007 to treat a Medicare patient who had a myocardial infarction with complications. The initial cost of tPA was $2,200, although streptokinase cost less than $200. Therefore, hospitals administering tPA to Medicare patients were adding tremendously to their costs without receiving any additional reimbursement. The financial implications of this could be very staggering. A sense of the dimension of this concern can be found in a letter (dated January 1988) from the executive vice president of the American Society of Hospital Pharmacists, Joseph A. Oddis, writing to Congressman Henry Waxman:

> As a result of these new drugs, our members, responsible for drug costs and thera-
> peutics, have found themselves in a dilemma. On the one hand is the need to pro-
> vide optimum patient care. On the other is the unfortunate reality that the current
> reimbursement mechanism for Medicare and Medicaid . . . has not accounted for
> these new products in its payment rates. In a preliminary survey on the matter our
> members have reported, for example, that a hospital will lose between $225,000–
> $655,000 per year when TPA is administered to patients covered by the DRG mecha-
> nism.[127]

At the end of his letter, Dr. Oddis proposed that Congress create a new mechanism for dealing with the problem posed by the sudden introduction of expensive
new technologies.

In fact, two such mechanisms were already in place. The 1983 legislation creating the prospective payment system had mandated that the DRG system should
periodically be adjusted by the Health Care Financing Agency (HCFA) to "reflect changes in treatment patterns, technology, and other factors that may change
the relative use of hospital resources."[128] In other words, as experience shows
unusually high increases in expenditures under a given DRG, HCFA is supposed
to pay more for such patients. Moreover, it created an independent body of experts, the Prospective Payment Assessment Commission (PROPAC), to advise
HCFA on a variety of factors, including the cost of technological advances, when
setting annual payment increases, as opposed to periodic adjustments.[129] So those
wanting increased reimbursement for myocardial infarction patients could turn
to PROPAC and ask it to advise HCFA to increase the payment for myocardial
infarctions in the next annual budget or it could wait for HCFA to recalibrate the
DRGs for myocardial infarctions in its next periodic adjustment of the levels of
reimbursement for each DRG. The latter approach would obviously take longer,
since it would require waiting until hospitals actually spent the extra money and
until HCFA did one of its periodic recalibrations, so it is not surprising that those
wanting an increase turned to PROPAC. The only thing that is surprising is how
quickly they did so. PROPAC considered the issue in its January 13, 1988, meeting, just two months after the FDA approval of tPA.

The minutes of the January 13 meeting make it clear that this was the most
controversial issue discussed that day.[130] It was the only issue which attracted
testimony of outside experts, and eleven individuals made comments, including
two representatives of Genentech and two representative of Hoechst-Roussell (the
distributors of streptokinase). Among the options considered were creating a special DRG for thrombolytic therapy; increasing in one way or another the payment
for current DRGs in which patients got thrombolytic therapy; and adding the
estimated cost of tPA to the total amount that hospitals would get under the DRG

system and waiting for the recalibration to ensure that the money actually went to hospitals caring for patients by using thrombolytic therapy. Oddly enough, it was this last, least-focused option which was actually recommended by PROPAC.

The official explanation of this option and the reasoning behind it are explained in PROPAC's Annual Report and in a letter of its executive director, Donald Young, to Senator Bill Bradley.[131] The commission began by noting that there exists considerable controversy in the literature as to whether tPA is better than streptokinase (which is so much cheaper that it hardly required any extra payment). It also noted that thrombolytic therapy is so efficacious that it may sufficiently shorten hospitalization so that hospitals will save more than the cost of the drugs.[132] Both of these considerations would argue not merely against the rejected proposals of directly adding money to the reimbursement of hospitals treating myocardial infarction patients with tPA, but also against any additional funding. But the commission also seemed to feel that it didn't want to stand in the way of those who might want to use tPA, believing that it was superior even if that superiority had not been fully demonstrated, and it didn't want to rely entirely upon the preliminary findings of shorter hospitalization. It calculated that the additional cost of thrombolytic therapy for 1989 would be $44 million (35,000 patients, one-half of whom got tPA for $2,332 while one-half got streptokinase for $186, with no cost savings). It suggested adding that amount to the total amount hospitals received from Medicare. It also suggested waiting for the recalibration in a few years to reassign that money directly to the relevant DRGs in which the extra money was actually expended.

One cannot read this analysis without finding it less than convincing. A closer reading of the discussion suggests that other factors were operative. On the one hand, as the commission itself noted (in a handout at the meeting discussing the options), HCFA had rejected previous suggestions that extra money should be provided to DRGs before historical experience showed that extra costs were incurred. This fact, together perhaps with pressure from those who supported the use of streptokinase, made any suggestion of extra direct reimbursements politically implausible. On the other hand, pressure from Genentech and its supporters in the community of cardiologists (some of which will be discussed later) made it difficult for the commission to recommend that nothing be done. So it came up with the compromise which it actually recommended.

The reaction to PROPAC's recommendation was quite predictable. Supporters of streptokinase found it very appropriate. Dr. Victor J. Bauer, president of the pharmaceutical division of Hoechst-Roussell, said:

> PROPAC's conclusion was reached after the kind of dispassionate examination which we welcome and which is being called for increasingly by physicians in their analysis of different thrombolytic agents. If implemented, this decision will benefit the patient, the taxpayer and the health care system, which will be able to allocate valuable but limited resources to other areas of need.[133]

Others, more sympathetic to the use of tPA, found the decision less satisfactory. Leigh Hopkins, of Thomas Jefferson University Hospital in Philadelphia, put their point as follows:

> There is the potential for TPA to be much better than streptokinase, and on the downside there's little chance that it's worse. Given the choice, a hospital like ours will always err on the side of the potentially more effective medicine, even though it's ten times more expensive. I think you'd want us to do that if you were a patient. That's the crux of the whole thing.[134]

PROPAC is only an advisory committee; everyone was well aware that the final decision would be made by HHS secretary Otis Bowen and by William Roper, the administrator of HCFA. On March 7, 1988, Jack Owen of the American Hospital Association met with Secretary Bowen to express the concern of his association that a failure to increase the reimbursement would lead to hospitals limiting access to high-quality health care because of financial considerations.[135] In an editorial, Owen made it clear that he was more concerned with the general question of government reimbursement for new technology than with the specific issue of tPA reimbursement:

> TPA is today's hot issue, but as technology breaks new ground, others will surface. Government can choose to respond by charting a course of non-involvement, but hospitals don't have that option. Committed to maintaining high-quality care at all costs, some might have to limit access to selected services, particularly expensive treatment options such as TPA.[136]

In short, Owen made it clear that the real issue was how an increasingly cost-conscious government was going to respond to the emergence of controversial and expensive new technologies.

The governmental response came quickly. On March 29, HHS said that there would be no increased payment for myocardial infarction patients receiving tPA, and it quietly rejected even PROPAC's compromise recommendations to add $41 million to total hospital reimbursement.[137] Bowen's decision was made in response to a memo from Roper, which I have not been able to locate. Quotations from the memo in other sources[138] make it clear that at least part of Roper's reasoning was skepticism about the legitimacy of the high cost of tPA. At one point in the memo, Roper wrote: "To recognize the high cost of one manufacturer's product, especially when its price is so far above that of similar drugs, would encourage other companies to follow suit." He also said: "Any special provision for tPA which is based on the price charged could result in a windfall for the manufacturer—i.e., a direct subsidy of Genentech by the Medicare trust fund." This was an important development, for it was the first time in the debate that anyone asked why tPA was priced as high as it was, refusing to simply take the price for granted.

Those using tPA would therefore have to wait at least until the 1991 recalibration before they began getting extra reimbursement. That decision ended the official consideration of the cost issue in 1988, but it did not of course end the cost issue. Each hospital would have to decide for itself whether it would spend the extra money on tPA. We will examine that decision in the next section. But before doing so, we should note two other 1988 developments on the cost issue, both actions on the part of Genentech.

On April 21, 1988, attorneys representing Genentech wrote to HCFA to ask for a clarification as to whether some hospitals in certain situations could get special reimbursement for the use of tPA.[139] It was settled by the HCFA decision that hospitals administering tPA in the emergency room and then admitting the patient would not get extra reimbursement. But what about hospitals administering tPA in the emergency room but then transferring the patient to another hospital for inpatient coverage? In such a case, the second hospital would get the DRG payment. Could the first hospital, asked the Genentech attorneys, bill separately for the cost of administering tPA to an outpatient? HCFA's response was that it could, but HCFA quickly added that this is true only if the transfer was medically appropriate. This response was distributed by Genentech in June 1988. Obviously, HCFA was concerned about this decision being used as a general way of getting special payment. Within a year, a HCFA program memorandum advised Medicare claim processors to "be alert for situations where tPA is approved for payment on an outpatient bill, but your data shows that the patient was admitted to a different hospital shortly after the receipt of the drug. Refer cases to the RO (regional office) for referral to the PRO (peer review organization)."[140] It has not been possible to find out how often this has actually occurred, although one report indicated that in at least seven states, large hospitals had developed networks of smaller referring hospitals to take advantage of this opportunity for increased funding.[141]

Many analysts had predicted that Genentech would have to lower the price of tPA after the HCFA ruling. It did not. What it did do, however, was to introduce a special program for providing free tPA to patients with income less than twice the poverty level who were not covered by private or government insurance (including Medicare or Medicaid).

Many issues were raised by these developments in the early spring of 1988, but two deserve to be highlighted at this point. One is the question which received the largest amount of attention during the HCFA funding debate: Should we adopt reimbursement policies which encourage the introduction of promising technologies or should we adopt policies which promote caution until it is clearly shown that the cost is justified by extra benefits? The other is the question which was not sufficiently discussed, but which seems deserving of attention: How should drug prices be set and what is the appropriate price for new drugs like tPA? We shall return to this fundamental question in Chapter 4.

The Influence of Economics on Usage

By the spring of 1988 America's physicians and hospitals faced conflicting signals about thrombolytic therapy. On the one hand, there was certainly considerable pressure to employ thrombolytic therapy, whose efficacy had been clearly demonstrated, and even to use tPA, although its advantage over streptokinase had not been fully demonstrated. On the other hand, economic forces pressed in the other direction, although the extent of that economic pressure varied from one institution to another. Institutions that were heavily dependent upon Medicare reimbursement and those that operated on fixed budgets (especially derived from public funds) would obviously feel the problems caused by the high cost of tPA more than institutions that could pass on those costs to private third-party payers who were still reimbursing for all services on a fee-for-service basis. How did American physicians and hospitals respond to these varying pressures? Fortunately, data derived from a series of surveys enable us to answer that question in ways that shed much light on the process of drug adoption.

The data come from a variety of sources, beginning with a survey conducted by a group from Duke in January 1987.[142] This survey is very important because it provides us with a profile of the use of thrombolytic therapy before the FDA's approval of intravenous streptokinase and tPA in the fall of 1987. It serves then as baseline data for our analysis. In addition, there is a series of three surveys, one run by commercial sources[143] and two by scientific investigators,[144] which assessed patterns of use of thrombolytic agents in 1988, after FDA approval. From all these sources, we can put together a very detailed picture of patterns of use and of differing responses to economic pressures.

The data from early 1987 are drawn from a questionnaire distributed to a random sampling of American cardiologists, internists, and family practitioners. They are somewhat soft data, based on a 21 percent response rate. Still, the data provide us with some picture of pre-FDA approval use of thrombolytic therapy. About two-thirds of the responding physicians reported using thrombolytic therapy, but most of the users reported using it in less than one-fourth of their patients, primarily because the patients were not presenting in the first 4–6 hours after the onset of chest pain. Nearly all (92 percent) were using streptokinase, and the vast majority were using it intravenously (72 percent). Cardiologists and internists were far more likely to use thrombolytic therapy than were family practitioners.

It is not at all surprising that thrombolytic therapy was beginning to find widespread acceptance by early 1987 given the studies we analyzed earlier. Nor is it surprising that streptokinase was being used by nearly everybody, since tPA was available in early 1987 only on research protocols. What is interesting to note is the predominant use of the intravenous mode of administration, although this had not yet been approved by the FDA. Once a drug is approved and available, physicians are free to use it as they see fit, and America's physicians were certainly doing so in early 1987.

The three other studies looked at patterns of use 1½ years later, in August 1988 (the survey conducted by Shearson Lehman Hutton analysts of hospital pharmacists), in November 1988 (the survey conducted by Grasela and Green of a sample of hospitals pharmacists), and in October 1988–February 1989 (the survey conducted by the author and his colleagues of 2,651 hospital physician-administrators). During these 18 months, tPA and streptokinase had been approved for intravenous use and the Medicare reimbursement decisions had been promulgated. How then did American hospitals and physicians respond in this changed environment?

One pattern which emerges clearly from all the studies is that the use of thrombolytic agents continued to grow in 1988. The Shearson Lehman Hutton group reported that in their 200 responding (of 234 contacted) hospitals, over 90 percent were stocking at least one thrombolytic agent. The Grasela-Green survey reported that in their 164 responding (of 381 surveyed) hospitals, all used at least one thrombolytic agent. Finally, the Brody study reported that in the 2,651 responding (of 5,792 contacted) hospitals, 90 percent were using thrombolytic therapy. In short, a pattern of very widespread use of thrombolytic therapy had emerged. But one needs to be careful about what this means, since even hospitals using thrombolytic therapy were not necessarily using it on all patients with myocardial infarctions. The Grasela-Green hospitals reported using thrombolytic therapy on only 17 percent of their MI patients, while the Shearson Lehman Hutton hospitals reported using thrombolytic therapy in only 12 percent of their MI patients. The primary limiting factor continues to be that patients were not showing up soon enough (within 6 hours).

What about the choice between streptokinase and tPA? APSAC was not yet a serious option since it had not yet received FDA approval. Here, the change from early 1987 is extremely striking, as is evidenced by Table 1.2 from two of the studies (comparable data are not available from the third study). There are differ-

Table 1.2 Streptokinase versus tPA Use

	Primarily tPA	*Primarily SK*	*No clear preference*
Shearson Lehman Hutton	108/194 (56%)	37/194 (19%)	49/194 (25%)
Brody et al.	1,314/2,293 (57%)	886/2,293 (39%)	93/2,293 (04%)

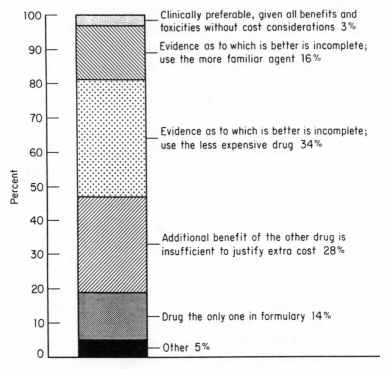

Figure 1. Reason for SK use.

ences between the percentages in the two studies. This is probably due to the fact that the Shearson Lehman Hutton study focused on larger hospitals, while the Brody study included smaller hospitals (which more often used streptokinase). But what is striking is that despite these differences, the picture which emerges is that tPA was more widely adopted than streptokinase.

These two studies examined rather carefully the reasons for this choice. What emerges is a striking difference, as is evidenced by Figures 1 and 2 drawn from the Brody study. The choice of tPA was almost always based upon a judgment of clinical efficacy, while the choice of streptokinase was almost always based upon cost considerations. The same picture emerges from Table 1.3.

The Brody study adds to our understanding of how economic pressures affected the choice of thrombolytic therapy by looking at the association of the type of hospital ownership with the choice of agent. The data are presented in Table 1.4, which presents the responding physician's choice of agent. Other physicians at the hospital might have been using the other agent. Excluded were physicians who said they were users but who failed to indicate a choice or who said they used both agents equally.

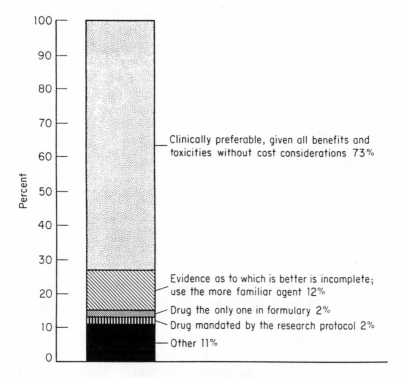

Figure 2. Reason for tPA use.

As can be seen from Table 1.4, publicly owned hospitals with budgets fixed in advance were far more likely to use streptokinase, presumably because the financial constraints they faced made it harder for them to absorb the cost of using tPA. What is surprising, however, is that federal public hospitals were more affected by economic considerations than nonfederal public hospitals; after all, the latter seem particularly prone to fiscal crises. A possible explanation is that the Genentech program for absorbing the cost of providing tPA to uninsured indigent patients had primarily benefited nonfederal public hospitals, because most of the patients treated at federal public hospitals were ineligible for this program.

This information raises many interesting questions. Some, descriptive in nature, relate to the way in which physicians choose among newly available drugs. Others, more normative in nature, relate to the way in which they should choose between newly available drugs. I want to focus on the latter questions, and I shall formulate the crucial question as follows: Given both the difference in cost between tPA and streptokinase and the scientific information available in 1988, should clinicians have chosen to use tPA or streptokinase?

Table 1.3 Most Frequently Cited Reasons for Choosing the Hospital's Future Drug

Prefer tPA(56%)
Clinical effect (28%)—tPA appears to work better than SK or is safer
Publicity (22%)—Doctors and patients are more aware of the benefits of tPA because of medical journals or newspaper articles

Prefer streptokinase (19%)
Cost/benefit (8%)—Doctors feel that SK is as good as tPA and much less expensive
Cost/benefit (7%)—Doctors feel SK should be used whenever possible; use tPA only for special situations

No clear preference (25%)
Awaiting studies (6%)—Doctors are unsure if tPA is better than SK and are awaiting academic studies or their own internal monitoring
Differing opinions (8%)—Some doctors at the hospital are convinced tPA is better while some think SK is just as good
Cost/benefit (6%)—SK should be used whenever possible, and tPA only in special situations

Source: T. Lerner and B. Fradd, *Thrombolytic Therapy: What Users Are Saying* (New York: Shearson Lehman Hutton, September 6, 1988), p. 13.

Opinions on this question obviously varied considerably. The Loran Commission, formed in 1985 by New England's oldest health maintenance organization (HMO), the Harvard Community Health Plan, expressed the following opinion: "There seems to be an unspoken, yet strong, presumption in favor of adopting new procedures, even in the absence of proof that they are better than old ones. The rapid adoption of tissue plasminogen activator (TPA) may prove to be just such a case."[145] Others obviously felt very differently. For example, in a debate at the meeting of the American College of Cardiology, Dr. Eugene Braunwald expressed his view that physicians in 1988 should use tPA:

> I believe that TPA has the edge for efficacy since, in the only three head-to-head comparisons, it resulted in patency of the occluded coronary artery more often than did streptokinase. . . . Both drugs have been shown to improve left ventricular function and to reduce mortality, but there had not yet been a head-to-head comparison insofar as these important end-points are concerned. . . . When we look at adverse effects, TPA again appears to have the edge. . . . I think that price is obviously an important consideration in this era of cost containment, but if the agent is more effective, then it is our job to fight to make it available to our patients.[146]

Table 1.4 Physicians' Choice of Thrombolytic Agent by Hospital Ownership

	Types of ownership			
	Federal public	*Nonfederal public*	*Private nonprofit*	*Investor-owned*
Physician responders, *n*	132	541	1,357	170
SK users, *n* (%)	91 (69)	255 (47)	477 (35)	63 (37)
tPA users, *n* (%)	41 (31)	286 (53)	880 (65)	107 (63)

Two questions emerge here. The first is the question of how to assess efficacy of competing drugs. Braunwald was obviously satisfied with the demonstrated difference in patency while the Loran Commission wanted more evidence of better efficacy of tPA. This is a question we have already discussed. The other question, to my mind the harder question, is this: Assuming that the known difference in patency was ultimately correlated with an improvement in survival, how much of an improvement would justify the use of tPA? Suppose that tPA resulted in a 1 percent absolute improvement in survival rate over streptokinase. With a $2,000 difference in cost, would that justify the use of tPA? You would have to spend $200,000 to produce one more patient who leaves the hospital alive and lives for some indeterminate additional time. Just how much is that worth? And how should society settle that question? As we shall see when we discuss the GUSTO trial, this is not just a theoretical question.

One final observation. As in the Medicare debate, the debate over the choice between tPA and streptokinase took, for the most part, the price difference for granted. But at least one set of commentators did not. Topol and Califf, in an editorial in the *Journal of the American College of Cardiology*, saw the price differential as inappropriate and as the root of the problem: "The 10-fold price differential between rtPA and streptokinase is most unfortunate. Tissue plasminogen activator clearly does not open 10 times as many arteries, save 10 times as much heart muscle or save 10 times as many lives."[147] Whether the argument they offer resolves the question is certainly open to discussion, but there is no doubt they were right in raising the question.

Conflicts over Patents

Many of those involved in the Medicare reimbursement debate and in the tPA–streptokinase debate recognized that at stake were far-ranging issues relating to the pricing, adoption, and reimbursement of the many pharmaceuticals which would result from the biotechnology revolution, rather than issues related to tPA exclusively. That recognition was present as well in the next part of our story, the fight over the tPA patents. Those involved, as we shall see, recognized that the future of biotechnology hinged on the extent to which patent law would reward companies like Genentech by offering them broad protection against infringement of their patent rights. The Genentech patent infringement suits became a forum for a discussion of a broader set of issues our society needs to confront.

To understand why these cases are paradigmatic, it is necessary to remember the central role of the patent law in promoting research. Research in biotechnology is very expensive, and the private companies involved in it can hope to reap sufficient rewards to justify investing their funds only if they can count on the monopoly given them by a patent to fully exploit the results of successful research.

But at the same time, by giving the holder of the patent a monopoly for a period of time, patents can be costly to society. Patent law is an attempt to draw a balance between granting monopolies to promote needed research while withholding monopolies to avoid unnecessary costs on the rest of society. To quote Lord Justice Mustill, who sat on the Court of Appeals in the British Genentech patent case:

> The kind of research which leads to a marketable form of t-PA is very expensive. The success rate is low. The benefits to suffering humanity are great. If a sufficient reward is not given in those instances where the research bears fruit, the industry will not attract the venture capital which it needs for survival, the research will cease, and humanity will continue to suffer. . . . [Yet] the arguments are not all one way. If the criteria for patentability are pitched too low there is a risk that mere hard work or superiority of resources, or simple good luck, will entitle a researcher to a monopoly, the commercial and social justification for which is by no means clear, given the risk of stultifying the development of the industry by open competition.[148]

With this understanding of the issue, we turn to an analysis of how the American and British courts dealt with this problem in very different ways.

The United States Patent Office had issued three patents for tPA. The first (Desire Collen and others, U.S. Patent 4,752,603, June 21, 1988) covered tPA isolated in good amounts from the culture fluid of human melanoma cells. This patent was ultimately rooted in an application filed on September 3, 1980, and it reflected Collen's original work using the Bowes cell line. The other two patents (David Goeddel [assigned to Genentech], U.S. Patents 4,766,075, Aug. 23, 1988, and 4,853,330, Aug. 1, 1989) covered tPA produced free of contaminants in useful quantities using recombinant DNA techniques. These patents were ultimately rooted in an application filed on July 14, 1982, and they reflected the work Genentech did using Collen's melanoma cell tPA. It is worth noting the period of time (more than 6 years) between the initial filings and the issuance of the patents, since a recent General Accounting Office report sharply criticized the Patent Office's slowness in issuing biotechnology patents.[149] TPA was certainly an example of that slowness.

On the basis of these patents, Genentech and its allies filed an American suit in 1988 against Burroughs-Wellcome and its allies. The suit alleged that Burroughs-Wellcome and its allies were developing a modification of tPA for sale in the United States, thereby infringing upon Genentech's patent. In return, Burroughs-Wellcome sued Genentech, claiming that Genentech was attempting to fraudulently monopolize the tPA market and more generally the thrombolytic market.[150]

In March 1990, the United States District Court in Delaware issued a summary judgment that none of the Genentech patents had been literally infringed by any

Burroughs product because of differences between them. The judgment left it to a jury to decide whether the patent had been infringed because the drugs are equivalent in that they "perform substantially the same overall work to achieve substantially the same overall results by substantially the same means."[151] This question of equivalency gets to the heart of the issue of the protection afforded by patents. It is clear that with the resources made available by the new biotechnology, one company can modify a patented product of another company in a variety of ways. If patents in biotechnology are to serve their role without going too far, some doctrine of equivalency will have to be adopted, treating at least some of these modifications as patent infringements. If, of course, one goes too far in extending the protection, the results could be equally bad.

Just a few weeks after this judgment, on April 6, 1990, a jury found on behalf of Genentech. It said in its special verdicts that the modified agents produced by Burroughs-Wellcome and its allies were equivalent to the products protected by the three tPA patents. It did not, however, award any damages, presumably because these new agents were not yet being sold. Finally, it did not find any evidence of attempts to create a monopoly by unfair competition.[152] Because this is only a jury verdict, we do not have any account of the jury's reasoning. We can only guess that it may have felt the need to protect the patent but that it also may have been influenced by the judge's very broad interpretation of the doctrine of equivalents. Burroughs-Wellcome shortly afterward announced its plan to abandon attempts to produce an improved tPA.[153]

Burroughs-Wellcome is the American subsidiary of the Wellcome Foundation, which fared much better in the British courts in the same suits. These suits considered, however, very different questions, and they were therefore not entirely analogous to the American suits. The American suits focused primarily, as we saw before, on the question of whether Burroughs was infringing upon the Genentech patents. The validity of those patents was not central. In the British courts, however, the fundamental claim was that the Genentech patents were invalid.

The British Genentech patent was published in February 1986, and Wellcome immediately sued for a revocation of those patents in order to continue the development of its own drug. Genentech shortly afterward sued Wellcome for infringement. In 1987, Mr. Justice Whitford decided against Genentech, but on grounds that were overturned on appeal. Instead, on October 31, 1988, the Court of Appeals ruled that Genentech's British patent was invalid under the British Patent Act of 1977. It is this ruling that we need to analyze.[154]

The 1977 British Patent Act was designed to make Britain part of the European Patent Convention. That act requires the invention to be new and to involve an inventive step. It is new if it does not form part of the state of the art (all matters made available to the public anywhere before the priority date of the invention).

It is an inventive step if it is not obvious to a person skilled in the art, taking into account any matter that forms part of the state of art. The three judges in the Court of Appeal were called upon to rule whether the Genentech patent met these requirements. This was obviously difficult, given the technical complexity of the issues, and the judges were called upon to employ outside experts (whose report provides the best data about what was going on in many research labs in the crucial period 1980–1982).

Lord Justice Purchas thought that Genentech had clearly produced an inventive step because of all of the efforts required to genetically produce tPA. To quote a portion of his very long decision:

> The numerous and technical steps involved in this process, in my judgment, carry the matter beyond the obvious activities of those skilled in the art, as opposed to the activities of those bent upon research and discovery. . . . I do not think that fairness will be achieved as between the patentee and the rest of those involved in the practice of the art concerned if, through the application of the principles of obviousness, it was to be held that there was no invention step involved in the discovery of the . . . data.[155]

At the end, however, he denied the validity of the patent for other reasons.

The other two justices, Dillon and Mustill saw it very differently. Lord Justice Dillon, while accepting the fact that Genentech had invested a lot of work and money in the production of tPA by genetic technology, argued as follows that the result was not patentable:

> All the steps taken by Genentech in finding out the composition of the sequences and applying that knowledge to produce human tPA, as defined in the specification, by recombinant DNA technology were applications of known technology, and no step was by itself inventive.[156]

A similar point, but supported by a fuller understanding of the policy issues, was made by Lord Justice Mustill, who wrote as follows:

> Dr. Goeddel [the Genentech team leader] seems to have been a first rate team leader. He assembled the right people, the right machinery and the right money, and kept the project moving to a conclusion. . . . The whole enterprise was well run, and it is not surprising that Genentech finished first. Yet it is inventiveness which counts, and I cannot find it here in any degree which exceeds the amount of resource to be expected of a group mustering the skills, remarkable as they seem to a layman, ordinarily to be expected of persons skilled in this most difficult array of arts. It may well be said that the work done by Genentech seems worthy of a reward greater than a few months' start on the road to a marketable product. Yet I am driven to conclude both that the monopoly claim exceeds any legitimate award, however exactly it ought to be formulated; and also that for want of an inventive step Genentech is not entitled to any reward through the medium of a patent monopoly.[157]

All of these discussions raise many important issues: How shall we properly but not excessively reward private research companies for their efforts, even if a full inventive step is not involved? Should a monopoly be granted in the form of a patent, or should some other system be developed? And if a patent is awarded, how far should it extend? Which modifications are so great that the patent should not cover them? Finally, and perhaps most crucially in a world of international biotechnology, can we afford to have different countries using different standards? Because of their technical legal complexity, however, we will not discuss them any further in this book.

Conflict-of-Interest Issues

In September 1987, just as the FDA was completing its work on the approval of thrombolytic agents, another issue emerged that would raise many troubling questions about commercial biotechnology and its relation both to scientific studies and to governmental agencies. Writing in *Newsday*, David Zinman revealed that at least two of the members of the TIMI steering committee, Dr. Harold Dodge (who headed the Radiographic Core Laboratory for the study) and Dr. James Willerson (who was the principal investigator at the University of Texas in Dallas clinical center), owned shares in Genentech.[158] Willerson reported that he had bought the shares only after the decision to stop TIMI-I, so his ownership could not have influenced any crucial decision. Dodge reported that he had bought the shares before the results were in, so his ownership was not based upon trading on insider information.

It turned out that they were not alone. During the TIMI-II trial, 8 of the 34 principal investigators either served as consultants to Genentech or owned shares in Genentech, although none were on the Operations Committee or on the Data Safety and Monitoring Board.[159] Four of the investigators involved in the Guerci trial at Johns Hopkins University (which was crucial for FDA approval), Drs. Bush, Chandra, Healy, and Weisfeldt, were shareholders in Genentech at the time of the trial.[160] One of the most prominent figures in American cardiology, Dr. Burton Sobel (the editor of *Circulation*), was a consultant for Genentech and had an option to purchase 14,000 shares, although he did voluntarily interrupt this consultancy during the crucial TIMI trial comparing tPA and streptokinase.[161]

The initial report in *Newsday* quoted a lot of people expressing differing attitudes toward the revelations. Dodge and Willerson, concerned about possible charges of fraudulent data, pointed out that the trial involved too many investigators to allow any one individual to change the outcome by fudging data. But Dr. Paul Meier, a leading statistician from the University of Chicago, argued otherwise, suggesting that a few fudged data might be just enough to make marginal results statistically significant. Dr. William Raub, of the NIH, was less concerned about fraud and more concerned about potential abuse of inside information for trading purposes on the stock market. But Dodge and Willerson thought that, as private citizens, they were entitled to be free to invest in the stock market. Dr. Claude Lenfant, the director of the Heart Institute at the NIH, was happy to require that NIH officials not own shares in companies manufacturing drugs under their scrutiny but felt that private investigators should be free to own such shares. Dr. Arnold Relman, the editor of the *New England Journal of Medicine*, felt that they should at least be required to disclose their holdings.

These early discussions focused on the questions of fraud and insider trading, and they led to no definite results. However, the issue was picked up and further developed in a series of hearings held by Congressman Ted Weiss in 1988 and 1989. We turn then to an examination of his hearings and of their impact.

Congressman Weiss headed the Human Resources and Intergovernmental Relations Subcommittee of the House's Committee on Government Operations. His subcommittee held three hearings, on April 11, 1988, September 29, 1988, and June 13, 1989. The first of these three hearings, which focused on broad problems of scientific fraud, is of no further significance for our story. But by the time of the second hearing, much of the attention of the committee had turned to the implications of conflicts of interest for fraud in research and in the practice of medicine.[162]

The first witness to be called at the second hearing was Jacques Galin. About two years earlier, his mother had had a heart attack and was admitted to Montefiore Medical Center in New York City. After several hours of being with his mother, Galin was told that the worst was over and left the hospital. When he returned, he found that his mother had had a cerebral hemorrhage subsequent to being given tPA. According to Galin, his aunt, who had remained with his mother, had refused to sign a consent form for her being admitted to TIMI-II (the study under which his mother received tPA), but the doctor had gotten the mother, who was "very dopey," to sign the form. Much of the discussion focused on the adequacy of the consent form and whether a woman in this condition could give informed consent, issues which we have already raised and to which we shall return. It was Galin who raised the crucial question about the conflict of interest faced by the doctor-investigator:

> Later on I found out that it [TIMI-II] was funded by the Federal Government and that it was a very competitive program and that you had to enter a certain amount of patients in it in order to be eligible for the second half of the program. I just question whether a doctor, given a situation and knowing the importance of his research grant and the dollars involved, if that can possibly cloud his judgment. Does he really look out for the benefits of that one particular patient or the possibilities down the road?[163]

This is a crucial remark. It suggests that conflicts of interest may be problematic not only because of fraud or insider trading but because it clouds the clinical judgments of investigator-clinicians who are under pressures to enroll patients and get their studies done.

The second witness who appeared that morning to testify about tPA was Dr. Victor Marder, who had served on the TIMI Data Safety and Monitoring Board until May 15, 1985. Marder never actually discussed the conflict-of-interest issue, but he did focus on several issues about TIMI-I. One was the decision to publish the TIMI-I preliminary report with the emphasis on tPA's better reperfusion result and without mention of the lack of difference in impact upon left ejection fraction or mortality. The other was the decision to drop streptokinase from TIMI-II. We discussed both of these issues earlier, so we need not return to the details now.

Marder's testimony opened up new areas of possible conflicts of interest. Throughout clinical trials, major decisions have to be made about the design of the trial and about the interpretation of the data. Should reperfusion by itself be interpreted as a significant end point or should one insist on evidence of improved left ventricular functioning? Should one drop streptokinase to focus on tPA alone? Whenever these types of questions are discussed, there is the potential for conflicts of interest leading investigators to adopt an answer they might not otherwise adopt. Whether or not conflicts of interest played a role in these particular decisions, their potential to do so is always present. The conflict-of-interest issue goes far beyond the questions of fraudulent data and insider training.

In the afternoon, a number of representatives from the NIH testified before the committee. These included Dr. James Wyngaarden, the director of the NIH, Dr. Charles McCarthy, the director of its Office for Protection from Research Risks, and Dr. Eugene Passamani, from the National Heart, Lung and Blood Institute. Several issues were discussed, especially in response to questions by Congressman Weiss, but it is my impression that the crucial issues were missed. For example, Congressman Weiss and Dr. McCarthy discussed the adequacy of the consent process for TIMI-II, but they focused on the adequacy of the language in the consent form and only once approached the questions of whether such patients could give meaningful consent and whether there were undue pressures on investigators to enroll patients.[164] Again, there was no real discussion of how conflicts of interest might have led people to emphasize reperfusion rather than ventricular functioning as an end point or to drop streptokinase after TIMI-I. The closest they came to those issues is when Dr. Passamani assured Congressman Weiss that Dr. Marder's concern about these issues had nothing to do with the decision to reconstitute the Data Safety and Monitoring Board for the TIMI trials or the decision to leave Dr. Marder off the new board.[165]

Unlike the original *Newsday* article, which attracted very little other news media attention, the hearing of September 29, 1988, led to follow-up articles in such respected journals as the *Washington Post, Barron's*, and the *Wall Street Journal*.[166] Even more important, greater sensitivity began to be evidenced about these issues. For some, this meant more disclosure. Thus when the major article on TIMI-II appeared in March 1989, information was provided about the stockholding and consulting relations between the investigators and Genentech.[167] For others, it meant guidelines limiting potential conflicts of interest. In a much-discussed article appearing in April 1989, the principal investigators in a major NIH trial (including some who had been involved in the tPA conflict-of-interest issue) adopted the following principles governing the behavior of the investigators in the trial (and of their spouses and dependents): (1) they will not buy, sell, or hold stock or options from the companies providing the medications under study and (2) they will not serve as paid consultants to those companies.[168]

Finally, the NIH moved to adopt regulations in this area. As this last development was particularly important, we shall review it in more detail. On January 20, 1989, the NIH issued the following notice:

> Growing expressions of public concerns suggest that N.I.H. act to limit possibilities for actual or apparent financial conflicts of interest by investigators in research and development projects funded by N.I.H. extramural awards. . . . N.I.H. expects that participating investigators and consultants will not have financial interests in organizations or entities that produce drugs, devices, or other interventions, studied in a controlled clinical trial. N.I.H. therefore intends to take steps to develop appropriate guidance for such relationships.[169]

Comments were invited from the public.

In June 1989, at a public forum held at the NIH, various viewpoints were expressed.[170] Some attendees felt that it would be best if each university developed and monitored its own rules. Others (such as Dr. Katherine Bick, from the NIH, who chaired the conference) felt that federal guidelines were needed so that there would be some uniform standards. Still others felt that regulations and not just guidelines were needed. Among the last group was Dr. Diana Zuckerman, an aide to Representative Weiss. She was quoted as saying: "Nobody has to abide by guidelines. Congress is looking to NIH for regulations that can be enforced. If NIH does not provide them, Congress has the power to do it."

On September 15, 1989, the NIH, joined by the Alcohol, Drug Abuse, and Mental Health Administration, issued proposed guidelines for investigators receiving funding from these agencies. The guidelines addressed both the issue of disclosing funding from commercial sources and the issue of prohibiting stock ownership in companies whose products were being tested. Additional provisions covered the sharing of unpublished information among companies, honoraria or fees for services, and the ability of private companies to limit or delay the dissemination of research results. For some, the guidelines were not strict enough. Representative Weiss, for example, thought that enforcement provisions weren't sufficiently clear and there were too many provisions allowing universities to issue waivers and exemptions.[171] For others, the guidelines were too restrictive and threatened to undermine the federal policy encouraging universities and industry to collaborate in research. To quote Robert Weinberg, a researcher at the Whitehead Institute for Biomedical Research: "Had these rules been in effect a decade ago, then the vast majority of biotechnology firms would never have been started. And many of the existing ones, which depend on close ties between university labs and their own scientific advisory boards, would die on the vine."[172] In January 1990, Louis W. Sullivan, the secretary of Health and Human Services, rescinded the proposed guidelines and announced that his department would begin a new process to determine federal policy on this topic. That policy has still (in September 1993) not been issued.

The episode raised many questions. For example, how can we identify all the potential places where conflict of interest could pose problems? Recall that four of the researchers involved in the Guerci trial at Johns Hopkins University had shares in Genentech, yet nobody questioned whether that influenced their decision to stop that trial before its planned termination, when its data were desperately needed for presentation to the FDA to secure approval of tPA. I am certainly not claiming that it did. My claim is only that this sort of influence is possible. Unless we can identify all the possibilities, how can we adopt a policy to protect against them? Another question is, How should we weigh the potential harmful effect of conflict of interest against the potential harmful impact upon the growth of biotechnology which might result from limiting the contact between university investigators and the biotechnology industry? At a time in which the United States is struggling to maintain its strong research position, with the major economic implications of that position, can it afford the bans which have been proposed? Or alternatively, can it take the risk of allowing the bad effects which might be produced by conflicts of interest? We will return to these questions in Chapter 2.

The End of the Story

Events continue to move forward, and tellers of stories must recognize that there is a point at which they must stop their story even as the events continue to progress. We will end our story on September 30, 1993. In this section we review the developments of the final period, developments which showed a new maturity for thrombolytic therapy but which revealed continued questions about the biotechnology industry and its role in the development of new modalities of therapy.

The Coming of Age of Thrombolytic Therapy

We have already seen that FDA approval led to widespread use of thrombolytic therapy (even if in a limited set of patients), though there was considerable variation in the drug actually used. The end of the 1980s saw thrombolytic therapy taken for granted, as researchers turned to issues surrounding the best way to use this form of therapy. Of the many issues discussed, three are of special significance for the future of thrombolytic therapy.

The first is the issue of the role of invasive cardiological interventions after or in place of thrombolytic therapy. As thrombolytic therapy breaks up clots in clogged arteries, a natural suggestion is that it should be followed by invasive procedures (such as balloon angioplasty), which might unclog the affected arteries. As noted previously, the TIMI-II trial ultimately addressed that issue. Its results began to become available at the end of 1988.

There were many publications in 1988 and 1989 of data from TIMI-II, but the most helpful is an early 1990 editorial which summarizes what was learned.[173] The basic idea behind the trial was to compare three *strategies* for using invasive techniques such as coronary arteriography after thrombolytic therapy followed by angioplasty if there was a greater than 60 percent blockage of the infarct-related artery. The first strategy was to use these techniques even while tPA was being administered. The second strategy was to use them between 18 and 48 hours after tPA therapy. The third was to use them only if the patient at a later stage developed spontaneous or exercise-provoked myocardial ischemia. The crucial result is relatively easy to state: there are no advantages to the more invasive strategies whether judged in terms of mortality or in terms of subsequent myocardial infarctions. Interestingly enough, a very similar result was found in a much smaller trial (the SWIFT trial) involving APSAC.[174]

There are many important implications of this study. The first has to do with the relative significance of invasive versus noninvasive cardiology in the management of patients who have suffered myocardial infarction. The 1960s and 1970s were the decades of the invasive cardiologists. One of the morals of TIMI-II is that the 1980s and 1990s may be the decades of the noninvasive cardiologists. The second implication of these findings concerns cost. If thrombolytic therapy is successful without further routine invasive procedures, then it may be cost-saving (in that it replaces the need for these procedures in routine cases) even if the actual medications are quite expensive.

These results, as important as they are, do not resolve all the issues about the use of these invasive techniques. While casting doubt on routine angiography followed by angioplasty after thrombolytic therapy, they leave open such questions as the value of these invasive techniques by themselves in all or some cases and of a more invasive approach to patients in trouble after thrombolytic therapy. These many complicated issues, and the trials designed to settle them, were reviewed in 1991.[175] More recent trials have been even more encouraging.[176] For our purposes, it is sufficient to say that the final evaluation of invasive techniques after or in place of thrombolysis has not yet been completed.

The second of the major clinical issues relates to the early administration of thrombolytic therapy. As early as 1985, some investigators had attempted to increase the impact of thrombolytic therapy either by administering it in the mobile care unit on the way to the hospital or by speeding up the process by which patients were treated once they got to the hospital.[177] Either way, patients had better left ventricular functioning. This study, backed up by the theoretical consideration that earlier therapy is better therapy, led to further studies of both approaches in the late 1980s.

One approach studied delays in the in-hospital administration of thrombolytic therapy.[178] It found that the majority of patients with myocardial infarctions did not arrive by ambulance, so they could not be helped by in-ambulance administration of thrombolytic therapy. It found, moreover, that the largest delays were delays in getting a first ECG to confirm the diagnosis of a myocardial infarction and delays in transferring the patient to the coronary care unit. Consequently, the investigators recommended the following procedures: (1) any patient presenting with symptoms suggesting a myocardial infarction should have an immediate ECG; (2) positive ECG readings should lead to the establishment of intravenous lines *while* the patient is being checked for exclusion criteria; (3) if there are no reasons for exclusion, the emergency room physician should begin therapy immediately, and ancillary drugs (lidocaine, heparin, morphine) should be administered later; (4) the patient should be transported afterward to the CCU. Implementing this approach, they report, significantly reduced delays.

The other approach involved several studies of in-ambulance administration of thrombolytic therapy.[179] Several of the studies involved physician-administered thrombolytic therapy in ambulances transporting patients; at least one, the Myocardial Infarction Triage and Intervention (MITI) study funded by the NIH, involved paramedic-administered thrombolytic therapy in ambulances transporting patients.

The earliest trials of physician-administered in-ambulance thrombolytic therapy were encouraging, but they were not large enough to yield statistically significant results. This defect was to be corrected in the European Myocardial Infarction

(EMIP) study, which randomized patients to prehospital versus in-hospital administration of thrombolytic therapy. Preliminary data, announced in the spring of 1992, showed a reduction of 30-day mortality from 11.1 to 9.7 percent. But the final report made it clear that these encouraging results did not quite reach the level of statistical significance because of enrollment and funding problems.

The MITI trial, which had adequate statistical power, involved paramedics providing in-ambulance thrombolytic therapy. Its first published report simply presented results about the feasibility of prehospital initiation of thrombolytic therapy by paramedics working under base station physician control and transmitting ECG data by cellular telephone. Its final report failed to show statistically significant improvements in the outcome, primarily because the patients in the trial who did not get thrombolytic therapy until they arrived in the hospital got it quicker than normally. One can only conclude, therefore, that part of the coming of age of thrombolytic therapy will be techniques designed to facilitate the early use of thrombolytic therapy, but it is not clear whether the emphasis should be upon the period before the patient arrives at the hospital or upon arrival.

The final, and perhaps most important, clinical issue studied in this period was the respective merits of the various thrombolytic agents. Three major trials were planned, GISSI-2, ISIS-3, and GUSTO, as well as some other smaller studies. These trials were crucial for the future of thrombolytic therapy, for at the time of FDA approval in 1987, little was available from direct trials comparing tPA and streptokinase. Eugene Passamani of the NHLBI was quoted in late 1988: "The bottom line is, nobody knows which is best."[180] Data relevant to that question began to become available in 1989 and have appeared with increasing frequency since then.

The earliest study which attracted a lot of attention was conducted by Dr. Harvey White and his colleagues in New Zealand (under the auspices of the Heart Foundation of New Zealand and the New Zealand Medical Research Council, with support from Boehringer Ingelheim, the international distributor of tPA) and was published in 1989.[181] It looked at 270 patients admitted at an average of 2.5 hours after the onset of chest pain from a first myocardial infarction, and it studied left ventricular functioning 3 weeks after treatment. At 3 weeks, patency of the infarct-related artery and ejection fraction was nearly identical in both groups. There was a trend toward increased survival in the tPA group, but it was far from statistically significant and the number of patients was too small to expect significant results. The accompanying editorial announced that its author used streptokinase in patients admitted within 4 hours and would have no quarrel with those who used it in all patients except those who are hypotensive.[182]

The reaction from Genentech was not surprising.[183] It criticized the study as too small. It also argued that one should use mortality rather than ventricular functioning as the end point; this is somewhat surprising since Genentech had taken the opposite position in the FDA approval debate. The spokesperson added that the true test would come from GISSI-2. The stock market didn't see it that way, and Genentech stock fell from 19⅜ to 17¾ the next day on active trading.

Within a year, the GISSI-2 results became available. Announced in March 1990, they were published in *Lancet* in July.[184] The trial, begun in February 1988 in Italy, was funded in large part by Boehringer Ingelheim. It was expanded in October 1988 to cover other countries and to raise the number of enrollees from 12,000 to 20,000.

Patients were randomized to receive either streptokinase or tPA and to receive heparin (subcutaneously, starting 12 hours after therapy) or no heparin. All patients without contraindicators received beta blockers and aspirin. Originally, the end point was mortality, late heart failure, or late extensive ventricular damage. With the addition of 8,000 subjects, there was a large enough number of patients to run a trial whose only end point was mortality. We will focus on these data since they address the most crucial question: Which drug saves more lives?

The quick answer is that there were no significant differences. The mortality rate for tPA was 8.9 percent (929 of 10,372) and for streptokinase was 8.5 percent (887 of 10,396). When you add heparin, you get mortality rates ranging from 9.2 percent (tPA with heparin and streptokinase by itself) to 8.7 percent (tPA by itself) to 7.9 percent (streptokinase with heparin). For a variety of reasons, the authors conclude that this variation was also not significant. Finally, while there was more bleeding with streptokinase, tPA was associated with a higher incidence of strokes.

This study was clearly very disappointing for Genentech and for the supporters of tPA. What they most feared were reactions like that of Dr. Claude Lenfant, the director of the NHLBI, who was quoted in the *New York Times* as saying, "streptokinase would now appear to be the drug of choice based on factors of cost."[185] Stuart Weisbrod, biotechnology analyst at Prudential-Bache Securities, was quoted as saying, "I think it's terribly negative. . . . I think hospital administrators are going to crack down. I think insurance companies are going to crack down."[186] All of this was particularly troubling for Genentech, because just a year earlier it had dismissed the White study by saying that people should await the results of GISSI-2.

As in the rest of our story, the actual picture is more complicated than this quick answer would suggest. Data had begun to be available in 1989 that indicated that the benefit of tPA, which produced greater earlier patency, was sustained only if heparin was administered concurrently with, or shortly after, the administration of tPA, to prevent new clots from forming. This was not known when GISSI-2 and its International Counterpart were planned and implemented. Consequently, those who believed in the superior efficacy of tPA could, and did, argue that GISSI-2 was not the appropriate trial. Within days of the March announcement, a two-page issue of *Advances in Cardiology*—whose distribution was funded by

Genentech—appeared on the desks of many doctors. In it, these arguments were made. For example, Dr. Ferrari of Italy said:

> It appears that the results of the International Study were not indicative of the optimal efficacy of tPA as was shown by studies employing early IV heparin. Indeed the choice made for administration of heparin subcutaneously starting 12 hours after thrombolysis may well have prevented the previously documented superior patency profile of tPA vs. SK from translating into a greater mortality reduction.[187]

Similar results showing no significant differences in mortality were reported by the ISIS-3 trial in a preliminary fashion in 1991 and in a final format in 1992.[188] This trial involved all three agents, and the mortality rates were 10.6 percent for streptokinase, 10.5 percent for APSAC, and 10.3 percent for tPA. These differences were not statistically significant. The question of whether heparin added to aspirin was more efficacious than heparin alone is more complicated, and we need not consider it here. However, what we do need to note is that in ISIS-3 heparin was first administered 4 hours after thrombolytic therapy commenced (concurrent with the end of the administration of tPA). One final point about ISIS-3: it presented data showing an excess of strokes in the tPA group, which, when combined with the data from GISSI-2, suggested that tPA was more dangerous to use than streptokinase. The death rate in the two trials combined was 10.0 percent for each drug, but there were moderately significant differences in the number of living patients who had suffered a stroke (0.5 percent for SK versus 0.7 percent for tPA).

The reactions to these data were quite predictable. Sherry and Marder wrote an article arguing that all of this showed that the belief that tPA was superior was based upon the mistaken emphasis of TIMI-I on clot lysis at 90 minutes:

> Why then did the TIMI-I data lead to incorrect predictions about the clinical superiority of rt-PA therapy for acute myocardial infarction? . . . In retrospect, the over-emphasis on reperfusion rate or patency at a single time point (90 minutes after treatment onset) as the main determinant of ultimate clinical benefit underlies the flawed predictions of the TIMI-I trial.[189]

In the year following the preliminary report of the ISIS-3 data, tPA market share dropped from 61 percent to 53 percent.[190] Typical of the attitude of those making the change were the remarks of Dr. Donald P. Fischer of the Kaiser-Permanente system in northern California, which saved $1,000,000 annually by making the switch: "We took a look at the data and were impressed."[191] On the other hand, the friends of tPA and Genentech argued that neither GISSI-2 nor ISIS-3 was a good trial, primarily because the delay in the administration of heparin at least until the end of 4 hours (in ISIS-3) or 12 hours (in GISSI-2) meant that tPA's benefits in producing greater patency in 90 minutes were being lost by a failure to use heparin soon enough to prevent reocclusion of the artery.

The last of the major trials planned was the Global Utilization of Streptokinase and TPA for Occluded Coronary Arteries (GUSTO) trial. This trial, funded by Genentech but run totally independent of it, was designed to test the relative efficacy of streptokinase, tPA, and a combination of the two, with the concurrent rather than the delayed use of heparin. The trial involved more than 40,000 patients at a cost of over $55 million. It is clear that GUSTO was crucial for Genentech's claims for tPA. To quote Genentech:

> The GUSTO trial will evaluate the hypothesis that opening closed arteries fast and keeping them open longer will have the most favorable impact on mortality associated with heart attack. The trial was designed to be a definitive comparison between Activase t-PA and streptokinase using the United States–recommended AMI treatment regimen, and the Company believes that the results of this trial may have a significant effect on Activase t-PA market share.[192]

As the day for the release of the GUSTO data approached, there was considerable pessimism expressed about the likelihood of its showing a clinical advantage for tPA over its competitors. An article appearing in the *Wall Street Journal* captured the spirit of many very well:

> The company is hoping against hope that the test will show something previous trials didn't: that a Genentech heart drug costing $2,200 a dose is superior to an older, rival drug that costs only $200 a shot. . . . "My friends in the pharmaceutical industry think that I'm nuts," says Genentech president G. Kirk Raab. But TPA's share of the clot-busting market has been dwindling; this is a long-shot bid to turn it around. Many analysts think that this test will come out like previous ones. . . . Given the price difference, such a draw would be the same as a loss. TPA sales would hemorrhage.[193]

The results were more favorable for tPA than had been expected.[194] Patients receiving tPA with immediate intravenous heparin had the lowest mortality rates (6.3 percent), while patients who received streptokinase had a somewhat higher mortality rate (7.2–7.4 percent, depending upon how the heparin was administered). Genentech's leadership was obviously pleased about the results. Raab said: "It used to be that doctors had to find a reason to use TPA; now they're going to have to find a reason not to use TPA. . . . We could save six lives a day in the U.S.—or 2,000 people a year." Biotechnology stock analyst Weisbrod predicted a major increase in the sales of tPA. The stock market must have agreed, because Genentech shares rose 4¾ points upon the release of the results. But others disagreed. Dr. Richard Peto, the Oxford statistician, argued that the differences disappeared if you combined the data with the data from ISIS-3 and GISSI-2. Dr.

Thomas Graboys, a Harvard cardiologist, argued: "There have been so many prior studies showing no survival difference, and there is such a cost difference, that my recommendation would be to continue with streptokinase." But perhaps the most insightful comment was the observation by Marilyn Chase of the *Wall Street Journal* that the results meant that you had to spend $200,000 ($2,000 extra per patient × 100 patients) to save one additional life by the use of tPA. As she put it, "Health economists and cardiologists now have a sticky issue to consider: Is a human life worth $200,000?"[195] We will return to that issue, both from a social perspective and from a clinical perspective, in Chapter 4.

In summary, then, the final details of how thrombolytic therapy will be used (with or without invasive interventions, in the hospital or in ambulances, as tPA or streptokinase) are far from settled in September 1993. But in the 6 years since they were approved by the FDA, the thrombolytic agents have clearly become standard therapy for patients who have had a myocardial infarction, and the challenge is to ensure that all patients receive at least one of them.[196]

The Fortunes of Genentech

The fate of tPA was obviously very important for the practice of cardiology, but it was also extremely important for Genentech and for the biotechnology industry. Genentech was the first major biotechnology company to have its shares traded publicly on a major stock exchange, and tPA was its most promising product. What happened to Genentech was closely connected to what happened to tPA, and the fate of Genentech was crucial to the attitudes of the financial community toward the biotechnology industry. In this section we examine the history of Genentech in the second half of the 1980s and the early 1990s, the period we have been examining closely, with an eye toward what its fate means for the future of American biotechnology.

As late as 1984, Genentech had derived no revenues from the direct sales of any products. Its recombinant-produced insulin was marketed by Eli Lilly, and Genentech received royalty income from Eli Lilly's sale of that product. It had some other royalty and patent-based income. But most of its income came from research it performed on behalf of research and development limited partnerships that it had sponsored. In 1985, the FDA approved Genentech's new drug Protropin, a growth hormone for the treatment of short stature due to growth hormone deficiency. In 1985, it received its first income from product sales, $5,182,000 out of a total revenue of $89,599,000.[197] But Protropin is a drug with limited indications, although they have grown over time, and Genentech needed a drug with far greater sales potential to become a serious integrated pharmaceutical firm as opposed to a research and development firm. Although it was working on many products, tPA was closest to approval for use, so it became Genentech's major hope.

Genentech entered 1986 with every reason to be confident in the future of tPA.

After all, it had been declared the winner of TIMI-I, and the NIH wasn't even bothering to run a placebo-controlled trial of tPA. Instead, the NIH was moving toward the TIMI-II trials using only tPA. In April 1986, Genentech filed its product licensing application for intravenous tPA with the FDA. Moreover, it made two major moves on the financial front. In June 1986, it entered into an arrangement by which it received $30,000,000 for tPA development costs from Boehringer Ingelheim, which received in return tPA marketing rights in many foreign markets at reduced royalty payments. Moreover, on December 30, 1986, it bought back with 3,385,000 shares the rights to tPA from a limited partnership, Genentech Clinical Partners II, which had financed its development. Clearly, Genentech was using the waiting time for FDA approval to develop an international marketing plan and to position itself to reap the profits from future sales of tPA.

All of this optimism rested, of course, upon the FDA's approval of tPA. That is why the May 29, 1987, meeting of the Cardio-Renal Drug Advisory Committee, with its recommendation to delay approval, came as such a shock to Genentech and to the stock market. Both the management of Genentech and the stock market were reminded of the vulnerability of research and development companies to regulatory delays. It must have come as a great relief to Genentech when FDA approval was finally secured late in 1987. Much of the 1987 Genentech Annual Report was devoted to Activase (Genentech's name for tPA). Some $55.8 million of Activase was sold between November 23 and the end of 1987, in part because a powerful marketing campaign. Genentech had recruited a sales force of 160 who were to call at least twice a month at the 2,800 hospitals that treat the overwhelming majority of heart attack patients. Moreover, it sponsored a 3-hour nationwide video conference, which was broadcast directly to 513 locations and featured such important figures as Burton Sobel and Eric Topol. Things were beginning to shape up for tPA and for Genentech.[198]

Initial sales are not necessarily indicative of continued sales, and 1988 was a challenging year for Genentech. It had lost the fight at HCFA for increased Medicare reimbursement for patients receiving thrombolytic therapy and it was facing an economic challenge from the supporters of streptokinase. Moreover, it had lost its patent battle in England and was connected to conflict-of-interest challenges in Congress. In addition, no new trial data supported the claims of the superiority of tPA, and APSAC was moving forward to approval as a third thrombolytic agent. Finally, sales were not holding up, and in October 1988, Genentech had to stop production of tPA for the rest of the year because distributors had too much stock in their inventory. Net sales for 1988 ended at 151.4 million.[199] This was a disappointment, and the market reacted accordingly.[200] The stock closed in October 1988 as low as 16¾, down 69 percent from its early 1988 high.

Analysts and Genentech officials agreed that the problem was one of excessive expectations. Both had been estimating a $400 million sales figure, and that was certainly a mistake. The problems were manifold, and we have already discussed a number of them. But Genentech felt that all of those problems, including the reimbursement issue and the streptokinase competition issue, could be overcome if it could increase the percentage of myocardial infarction patients who were getting thrombolytic therapy as well as the percentage of patients getting tPA as opposed to streptokinase or APSAC. To do that, Genentech began to stress in its promotion the value of thrombolytic therapy (hoping that once people chose to use it, they would use tPA), rather than pushing tPA directly. Genentech also enlisted the American sales force of Boehringer Ingelheim. Finally, it began trials of the use of tPA for other indications such as pulmonary emboli. The 1989 results were an improvement, with net sales equaling $196.4 million, but they were hardly what had been expected. Still, Genentech could say that its introduction of tPA was a success by all measures except the original hyperbolic Wall Street expectations.[201]

A very balanced report issued in August 1989 neatly summarized the situation.[202] It pointed out that Genentech had been able to reverse some of its sales problems of 1988, and that its aggressive marketing would probably lead to improved sales. It also noted that this might be changed by the introduction of APSAC (with its ease of administration) and by the results of GISSI-2 (which might greatly influence thinking on the question of whether tPA was sufficiently better than streptokinase to justify its much higher costs). Finally, it pointed out that Genentech was still positive about the future of biotechnology and was sacrificing short-term profits in the hope that research and development would lead to important new drugs. In the short term, however, much of Genentech's fate would depend upon the results of trials such as GISSI-2 and ISIS-3 comparing tPA with streptokinase and APSAC.

The first 6 months of 1990 produced startling results, even before the public release of the results of GISSI-2. On February 2, 1990, Genentech announced that Roche Holding Company, a Swiss health products company, would purchase a majority of the outstanding shares of Genentech. Genentech would use the net proceeds for new-product development. Reaction to this announcement varied. Some saw it as a disappointing admission of the failure of America's largest biotechnology company, raising great concerns for the future of American biotechnology. George Rathmann, the chairman of Amgen (America's second largest biotechnology company), was quoted as saying: "I think people will worry about that. . . . It's a little disappointing, if you have to pick a word."[203] Others, including Genentech's leadership and some market analysts, saw it as a wise move enabling Genentech to continue its aggressive approach to research and development without having to worry about Wall Street demands for immediate earnings. Indeed, from their perspective, there was no problem at Genentech; the whole problem was on Wall Street.

The results of both GISSI-2 and ISIS-3 were obviously very disappointing from from the Genentech perspective. As noted, Genentech's 1991 reports showed a decline both in sales and in market share. This was particularly distressing for Genentech, because it had only two other approved products, one of which (Protropin, used for treating growth deficiencies) would shortly lose its Orphan Drug Act protection, and the other of which (Actimmune) was approved for use in a market with only 250–400 patients each year. Although the short-term perspective was not positive, Genentech continued to pursue its long-term program of product development, aided by the $487.3 million it received from Roche. It expanded its facilities, adding at a cost of $75 million a new research facility. It focused its development activities on such drugs as DNase, a mucus-dissolving enzyme for the management of cystic fibrosis and chronic bronchitis; CD4–IgG, a drug aimed at preventing the spread of human immunodeficiency virus (HIV) from pregnant women to their fetuses; HER2, a monoclonal antibody which may be useful in the treatment of breast and ovarian tumors; and relaxin, a naturally occurring hormone which may ease childbirth. Hoffman-Laroche played a major role in financing the development costs for DNase. But, as we have seen, Genentech also committed itself to spending more than $50 million on the GUSTO trial in the hope that it would reactivate enthusiasm for tPA.[204] Only time will tell whether this aggressive long-term strategy has worked, even given the help of the results of the GUSTO trial. The answer to that question may say a lot about the future of the biotechnology industry in the United States.

Final Considerations

The story of thrombolytic therapy is a fascinating combination of scientific-technological advances and social-ethical problems. My purpose in retelling the story was to illustrate the social and ethical problems that arise in the development, approval, and adoption of new drugs. I have tried to call attention to these problems as the story progressed, but it seems worthwhile in conclusion to enumerate them here.

We have seen how the process of drug trials is structured by several federal regulations and is oriented toward meeting the requirements for FDA approval. But this leaves open such ethical issues as when placebo-controlled trials are no longer appropriate and what type of informed consent is adequate when doing emergency research. Moreover, these regulations may not have appropriately structured the research environment to avoid decisions about the design and conduct of trials that are flawed because of conflicts of interests. All of these ethical issues will be carefully analyzed in Chapter 2.

The FDA approval process raises other questions. The fundamental value issue is how to balance the goals of efficacy and safety and how to balance the desire for the best possible evidence with the need for speedy approval. Has the FDA properly balanced these goals and needs, both in the initial approval process and in the later process of approving drugs for additional indications? Are there better alternatives to the current scheme? These questions have been amply illustrated by our story, and they will be fully analyzed in Chapter 3.

Ethical issues arise even after drugs are approved. Most of them are related to financial questions. How are the prices of new drugs set and can that process be improved? What role should cost play both in social reimbursement decisions and in individual clinical decision making? We will turn to these questions in Chapter 4.

The development of thrombolytic therapy has illustrated a full agenda of important issues; they deserve the careful attention they will receive in the rest of this book.

Appendix A. Timetable of Initial Clinical Trials of Thrombolytic Agents

	1982	1983	1984	1985	1986	1987	1988
AIMS					Summer: Begin	Mar.: Interim analysis Aug.: Interim analysis Nov.: End early	Mar.: Report
ASSET					Nov.: Begin in England and Norway	Apr.: Begin in Sweden Fall: Begin in Denmark	Feb.: End Sept.: Report
European cooperative group[a]							
A			July: Begin Dec.: End	Apr.: Report			
B			July: Begin	May: End Nov.: Report			
C					May: Begin	Nov.: End	Nov.: Report
GISSI			Feb.: Begin	June: End	Feb.: Report	Oct.: Follow-up report	
Guerci			Dec.: Begin			Mar.: End due to ISIS-2 Dec.: Report	

[a]Further angioplasty studies are not included.

Timetable of Initial Clinical Trials of Thrombolytic Agents (*continued*)

	1982	1983	1984	1985	1986	1987	1988
ISAM	Mar.: Begin			Mar.: End	June: Report	Jan.: Follow-up report	
ISIS-2				Mar.: Begin		Feb.: Preliminary report Dec.: End	Aug.: Report
Multicenter APSAC				Feb.: Begin		Jan.: End	June: Report
NHF, Australia New Zealand			Aug.: Begin		May: Begin Aug.: End	Aug.: End Oct.: Report	Jan.: Report
TICO			Aug.: Begin	Feb.: End early Apr.: Report	Feb.: Begin	June: End	June: Report
TIMI[a]					Feb.: Decision not to run TIMI-II Apr.: Begin IIA	Sept.: End IIA	Nov.: Report IIA
Western Washington		Sept.: Begin			July: End early		Feb.: Results
Summary Article	Nov.: Stampfer			June: Yussuf			Mar.: *Lancet* June: Marder and Sherry Oct.: 2nd Yusuf

[a]Further angioplasty studies are not included.

Appendix B. Estimates of Additional Short-Term Deaths in Placebo Control Groups

	After FDA approval of intracoronary streptokinase (May 1982), but before GISSI publication (Feb. 1986)	After GISSI publication (Feb. 1986) but before ISIS-2 preliminary publication (Feb. 1987)	After ISIS-2 preliminary publication (after Feb. 1987)
AIMS	N/A	14	15
ASSET	N/A	16	49
European cooperative group			
B	*	*	*
C	N/A	5	5
GISSI	132	N/A	N/A
Guerci	*	*	N/A
ISAM	7	N/A	N/A
ISIS-2	84	84	70
NHF, Australia	N/A	*	*
New Zealand	8	2	N/A
TICO	N/A	*	*
Western Washington	5	1	N/A
Total	236	122	139

Key: N/A = not applicable because trial was not run during that period; * = not a trial of mortality.

Notes: Multiple APSAC, TIMI, and European Cooperative Group A are excluded because they had no placebo control group. Definition of "short-term" varies from study to study. These are estimates because, unless published data indicate otherwise, we assume: that enrollment for each month of the trial was equal; that the types of patients enrolled (e.g., early vs. late presenters) were the same during each month of the trial; and that the percentage of mortality in the placebo control group would have been the same as the actual percentage of mortality in the treatment group if the placebo group had been treated.

Appendix C. Backup Calculations for Estimates of Additional Deaths in Placebo Control Groups

AIMS (patients from prelimary report only):
   61 in control group of 502, or 12.2 percent
   32 in treatment group of 502, or 6.48 percent
   6.4 percent of 502 = 32
   61 – 32 = 29 total additional deaths
   Breakdown:
   Beginning of Mar. 1987 = 502 (after ISIS-2 preliminary) = 14
   They report 502 later = 15
ASSET:
   245 in control group of 2,495, or 9.8 percent
   182 in treatment group of 2,516, or 7.2 percent
   7.2 percent of 2,495 = 180
   245 – 180 = 65 additional deaths
   Breakdown:
   Nov. 1986–Feb. 1987 (4 months before ISIS-2 preliminary) = 16
   Mar. 1987–Feb. 1988 (12 months after ISIS-2 preliminary) = 49
European Cooperative group C:
   29 of 366 in control group, or 7.9 percent
   18 of 355 in treatment group, or 5.1 percent
   5.1 percent of 366 = 19
   29 – 19 = 10 additional deaths
   Breakdown:
   May 1986–Feb. 1987 (10 months before ISIS-2 preliminary) = 5
   Mar. 1987–Nov. 1987 (9 months after ISIS-2 preliminary) = 5
GISSI:
   758 of 5,852 in control group, or 13 percent
   628 of 5,860 in treatment group, or 10.7 percent
   10.7 percent of 5,852 = 626
   758 – 626 = 132 additional deaths all before GISSI publication (Feb. 1986)
ISAM:
   63 of 882 in control group, or 7.1 percent
   54 of 859 in treatment group, or 6.3 percent
   6.3 percent of 882 = 56
   63 – 56 = 7 additional deaths all before GISSI publication (Feb. 1986)
ISIS-2:
   1,029 of 8,595 in control group, or 12 percent
   791 of 8,592 in treatment group, or 9.2 percent
   9.2 percent of 8,595 = 791
   1,029 – 791 = 238 additional deaths
   Breakdown:
   Mar. 1985–Feb. 1986 (12 months before GISSI publication) = 84
   Mar. 1986–Feb. 1987 (12 months after GISSI publication, before ISIS-2 preliminary) = 84
   Mar. 1987–Dec. 1987 (10 months after ISIS-2 preliminary) = 70
New Zealand:
   12 of 93 in control group, or 12.5 percent
   2 of 79 in treatment group, or 2.5 percent
   2.5 percent of 93 = 2
   12 – 2 = 10 additional deaths
   Breakdown:
   Aug. 1984–Feb. 1986 (18 months before GISSI publication) = 7.5 or 8
   Mar.–Aug. 1986 (6 months after GISSI publication and before ISIS-2 preliminary) = 2.5 or 2

Western Washington:
   17 of 177 in control group, or 9.6 percent
   12 of 191 in treatment group, or 6.3 percent
   6.3 percent of 177 = 11
   17 – 11 = 6 additional deaths
   Breakdown:
   Sept. 1983–Feb. 1986 (30 months before GISSI publication) = 5
   Mar. 1986–Aug. 1986 (6 months after GISSI publication but before ISIS-2 preliminary) = 1

Notes

1. A brief biography of Herrick can be found in F. Willius and T. Keys *Cardiac Classics* (St. Louis: Mosby, 1941), pp. 815–16.

2. J. B. Herrick, "Clinical Features of Sudden Obstruction of the Coronary Arteries," *JAMA* 59 (1912): 2015–20.

3. The contribution of these early figures is described in W. L. Proudfit, "Origin of Concept of Ischaemic Heart Disease," *British Heart Journal* 50 (1983): 209–12.

4. Herrick, "Clinical Features," p. 2017.

5. Ibid., p. 2020.

6. J. B. Herrick, *Memories of Eighty Years*, quoted in J. O. Leibowitz, *The History of Coronary Heart Disease* (Berkeley: University of California Press, 1970), p. 150.

7. J. B. Herrick, "Thrombosis of the Coronary Arteries," *JAMA* 72 (1919): 387–90.

8. For a brief account of the history of the development of the ECG, see Leibowitz, *History*, pp. 155–59.

9. J. E. Muller, "Coronary Artery Thrombosis: Historical Aspects," *JACC* 1 (1983): 893–96.

10. C. Lawrence, "Moderns and Ancients: The 'New Cardiology' in Britain 1880–1930," in *Medical History*, Supplement No. 5 (1985): 1–33.

11. The most prominent is T. Kuhn, *The Structure of Scientific Revolutions*, 2nd ed. (Chicago: University of Chicago Press, 1979). A full discussion of these issues is found in L. Laudan, *Progress and Its Problems* (Berkeley: University of California Press, 1977).

12. C. K. Friedberg and H. Horn, "Acute Myocardial Infarction Not Due to Coronary Artery Occlusion," *JAMA* 112 (1939): 1675–79.

13. H. L. Blumgart, M. J. Schlesinger, and D. Davis, "Studies on the Relation of the Clinical Manifestations of Angina Pectoris, Coronary Thrombosis, and Myocardial Infarction to the Pathologic Findings," *American Heart Journal* 19 (1940): 1–91.

14. R. D. Miller, H. B. Burchell, and J. E. Edwards, "Myocardial Infarction with and without Acute Coronary Occlusion," *Archives of Internal Medicine* 88 (1951): 597–604.

15. A. W. Branwood and G. L. Montgomery, "Observations on the Morbid Anatomy of Coronary Artery Disease," *Scottish Medical Journal* 1 (1956): 362–75.

16. D. M. Spain and V. A. Bradess, "The Relation of Coronary Thrombosis to Coronary Atherosclerosis and Ischemic Heart Disease," *American Journal of Medical Science* 240 (1960): 701–10.

17. W. C. Roberts, "Coronary Thrombosis and Fatal Myocardial Ischemia," *Circulation* 49 (1974): 1–3.

18. A. B. Chandler et al., "Coronary Thrombosis in Myocardial Infarction," *American Journal of Cardiology* 34 (1974): 823–33.

19. Donald B. Hackel, "The Coronary Arteries in Acute Myocardial Infarction," *Circulation* 68, suppl. I (1983): I-6–I-7.

20. Following the valuable summary in S. Sherry, "The Origin of Thrombolytic Therapy," *JACC* 14 (1989): 1085–92; others, such as F. Koller, "The Development of Our Knowledge of Fibrinolysis," *American Journal of Cardiology* 6 (1960): 367–70, emphasize the continuity of Tillett and Garner's work with earlier studies.

21. W. S. Tillett, and R. L. Garner, "The Fibrinolytic Activity of Hemolytic Streptococci," *Journal of Experimental Medicine* 58 (1933): 485–502.

22. H. Milstone, "A Factor in Normal Human Blood which Participates in Streptococcal Fibrinolysis," *Journal of Immunology* 42 (1941): 109–16.

23. L. R. Christensen, "Streptococcal Fibrinolysis: A Proteolytic Reaction Due to a Serum Enzyme Activated by Streptococcal Fibrinolysin," *Journal of General Physiology* 28 (1945): 363–83, and L. R. Christensen, and C. M. MacLeod, "A Proteolytic Enzyme of Serum: Characterization, Activation, and Reaction with Inhibitors," *Journal of General Physiology* 28 (1945): 559–83.

24. A. J. Johnson and W. S. Tillett, "The Lysis in Rabbits of Intravascular Blood Clots by the Streptococcal Fibrinolytic System," *Journal of Experimental Medicine* 95 (1952): 449–63.

25. There is an element of irony here. Lederle, unable in the years that followed to produce enough high-quality streptokinase, dropped out in the 1960s to be replaced by Behringwerke in Germany and Kabi in Sweden.

26. S. Sherry, A. Fletcher, N. Alkjaersig, and F. E. Smyrniotis, "An Approach to Intravascular Fibrinolysis in Man," *Transactions of the Association of American Physicians* 70 (1957): 288–96.

27. A. P. Fletcher, N. Alkjaersig, F. E. Smyrniotis, and S. Sherry, "The Treatment of Patients Suffering from Early Myocardial Infarction with Massive and Prolonged Streptokinase Therapy," *Transactions of the Association of American Physicians* 71 (1958): 287–95.

28. "Symposium on Fibrinolysis," *American Journal of Cardiology* 6 (1960): 367–563.

29. S. Sherry and A. Fletcher, "Thrombolytic Therapy," *American Heart Journal* 61 (1961): 575–78.

30. W. R. Bell and A. G. Meek, "Guidelines for the Use of Thrombolytic Agents," *NEJM* 301 (1979): 1266–70.

31. M. J. Stampfer et al., "Effects of Intravenous Streptokinase on Acute Myocardial Infarction," *NEJM* 307 (1982): 1180–82, and S. Yusuf et al., "Intravenous and Intracoronary Fibrinolytic Therapy in Acute Myocardial Infarction," *European Heart Journal* 6 (1985): 556–85.

32. On these matters, see L. Friedman, C. D. Furber, and D. L. Demets, *Fundamentals of Clinical Trials*, 2nd ed. (Littleton, Mass.: PSG Publishing, 1985), Chapter 7.

33. A balanced history and treatment of this issue is found in P. H. Rogers and S. Sherry, "Current Status of Antithrombotic Therapy in Cardiovascular Disease," *Progress in Cardiovascular Diseases* 19 (1976): 235–53.

34. R. H. Grifford and A. R. Feinstein, "A Critique of Methodology in Studies of Anticoagulant Therapy for Acute Myocardial Infarction," *NEJM* 280 (1969): 351–57.

35. S. Rogel and M. Bassan, "Anticoagulants in Ischemic Heart Disease," *Archives of Internal Medicine* 136 (1976): 1229–30.

36. E. Braunwald, ed., *Heart Disease*, 3rd ed. (Philadelphia: Saunders, 1988), Chapter 38.

37. Ibid.

38. M. DeWood et al., "Prevalence of Total Coronary Occlusion During the Early Hours of Transmural Myocardial Infarction," *NEJM* 303 (1980): 897–902, supplemented by M. DeWood et al., "Coronary Arteriographic Findings in Acute Transmural Myocardial Infarction," *Circulation* 68, suppl. I (1983): I-39–I-49.

39. DeWood et al., "Coronary Arteriographic Findings," p. I-48.

40. P. Rentrop et al., "Acute Coronary Occlusion with Impending Infarction as an Angiographic Complication Relieved by a Guide-Wire Recanalization," *Clinical Cardiology* 1 (1978): 101–6.

41. K. P. Rentrop et al., "Initial Experience with Translumimal Recanalization of the Recently Occluded Infarct-Related Coronary Artery in Acute Myocardial Infarction," *Clinical Cardiology* 2 (1979): 92–105.

42. K. P. Rentrop et al., "Acute Myocardial Infarction: Intracoronary Application of Nitroglycerin and Streptokinase," *Clinical Cardiology* 2 (1979): 354–63.

43. D. G. Mathey et al., "Nonsurgical Coronary Artery Recanalization in Acute Transmural Myocardial Infarction," *Circulation* 63 (1981): 489–97.

44. R. C. Leinbach and H. K. Gold, "Editorial: Regional Streptokinase in Myocardial Infarction," *Circulation* 63 (1981): 498–99. Quote, p. 499.

45. Of interest was the fact that cardiologists soon focused just on the use of medications administered noninvasively. There has, however, been a renewed interest in the more invasive interventions analogous to those originally employed by Rentrop. See, for example, C. L. Grines et al., "A Comparison of Immediate Angioplasty with Thrombolytic Therapy for Acute Myocardial Infarction," *NEJM* 328 (1993): 673–79, and F. Zijlstra et al., "A Comparison of Immediate Coronary Angioplasty with Intravenous Streptokinase in Acute Myocardial Infarction," *NEJM* 328 (1993): 680–91.

46. For an account of the history and philosophy of this approach, see Friedman, Furberg, and DeMets, *Fundamentals of Clinical Trials.*

47. J. E. Muller et al., "Let's Not Let the Genie Escape from the Bottle—Again," *NEJM* 304 (1981): 1294–96.

48. "Thrombolytic Agents in Evolving MI," *FDA Drug Bulletin* 14 (1984): 4–5.

49. F. Khaja et al., "Intracoronary Fibrinolytic Therapy in Acute Myocardial Infarction," *NEJM* 308 (1983): 1305–11; J. Anderson et al., "A Randomized Trial of Intracoronary Streptokinase in the Treatment of Acute Myocardial Infarction," *NEJM* 308 (1983): 312–18; and J. W. Kennedy et al., "Western Washington Randomized Trial of Intracoronary Streptokinase in Acute Myocardial Infarction," *NEJM* 309 (1983): 1477–82.

50. 21 USC §355.

51. J. Weinstein, "The International Registry to Support Approval of Intracoronary Streptokinase Thrombolysis in the Treatment of Myocardial Infarction," *Circulation* 68, suppl. I (1983): I-61–I-66.

52. E. Braunwald, "Thrombolytic Therapy in Patients with Acute Myocardial Infarction: Summary and Comments," *Circulation* 68, suppl. I (1983): I-67–I-69.

53. J. W. Kennedy et al., "Streptokinase in Acute Myocardial Infarction: Western Washington Randomized Trial—Protocol and Progress Report," *American Heart Journal* 104 (1982): 899–911.

54. E. R. Passamani, ed., "Limitation of Infarct Size with Thrombolytic Agents," *Circulation* 68, suppl. I (1983): I1–I109.

55. Braunwald, "Thrombolytic Therapy," p. I-69.

56. J. Ross, "Future Directions for Clinical Investigation in Thrombolytic Therapy," *Circulation* 68, suppl. I (1983): I-105–I-109. Quote, p. I-108.

57. B. E. Sobel, "Methodologic Issues in Assessment of Thrombolytic Agents," *Circulation* 68, suppl. I (1983): I-96–I-97. Quote, p. I-97.

58. Department of HHS, Public Health Service, National Institutes of Health, National Heart, Lung, and Blood Advisory Council, "Minutes of Meeting," May 20–21, 1982. Following excerpt is from pp. 5–6.

59. "$12 Million Clinical Trial OKd" by Heart Institute Council, *N.I.H. Week*, May 21, 1982, pp. 3–4, and "Request for Proposal—Thrombolysis in Myocardial Infarction (TIMI)—Clinical Units" (NIH: RFP NHLBI HV82-11, August 20, 1982).

60. T. Astrup and P. M. Permin, "Fibrinolysis in the Animal Organism," *Nature* 159 (May 17, 1947): 681–82.

61. J. R. B. Williams, "The Fibrinolytic Activity of Urine," *British Journal of Experimental Pathology* 32 (1951): 530–37.

62. J. Plough and N. O. Kjeldgaard, "Urokinase: An Activator of Plasminogen from Human Urine," *Biochemica et Biophysica Acta* 24 (1957): 278–82.

63. A. P. Fletcher et al., "The Development of Urokinase as a Thrombolytic Agent," *Journal of Laboratory and Clinical Medicine* 65 (1965): 713–31.

64. Several of the major proponents of the use of tissue plasminogen activator have indicated that it was this feature which made tissue plasminogen activator so attractive to investigators in the

period under question. These claims are advanced in B. E. Sobel, "Coronary Thrombolysis and the New Biology," *JACC* 14 (1989): 850–60, and in J. Loscalzo and E. Braunwald, "Tissue Plasminogen Activator," *NEJM* 319 (1988): 925–31.

65. D. C. Rijken and D. Collen, "Purification and Characterization of the Plasminogen Activator Secreted by Human Melanoma Cells in Culture," *Journal of Biological Chemistry* 256 (1981): 7035–41, and U.S. Patent No. 4,752,603 (June 21, 1988).

66. S. R. Bergmann et al., "Clot-Selective Coronary Thrombolysis with Tissue-Type Plasminogen Activator," *Science* 220 (1983): 1181–83, and F. Van de Werf et al., "Coronary Thrombolysis with Tissue-Type Plasminogen Activator in Patients with Evolving Myocardial Infarctions," *NEJM* 310 (1984): 609–13.

67. Van de Werf et al., "Coronary Thrombolysis," pp. 612–13.

68. Details about the Cohen-Boyer patent and about the controversies it has engendered can be found in Appendix 2 of M. Kenney, *Biotechnology: The University-Industrial Complex* (New Haven: Yale University Press, 1986). Details in the following paragraphs come from the account in R. Teitelman, *Gene Dreams* (New York: Basic Books, 1989).

69. Kenney, *Biotechnology*, pp. 94–96.

70. Details of these early years can be found in Genentech's form 10-K filed annually with the Securities and Exchange Commission. This paragraph relies heavily on details supplied in the 1984 form 10-K (Commission File No. 2-68864).

71. D. Pennica et al., "Cloning and Expression of Human Tissue-Type Plasminogen Activator cDNA in *E. coli*," *Nature* 301 (January 20, 1983): 214–21.

72. M. A. Hlatky et al., "Adoption of Thrombolytic Therapy in the Management of Acute Myocardial Infarction," *American Journal of Cardiology* 61 (1988): 510–14.

73. The minutes are reprinted in *Federal Response to Misconduct in Science* (Washington: GPO, 1989), pp. 229–34. Following excerpt is from p. 234.

74. The details of phase I are gathered from four reports published by the TIMI study group, the references to which are as follows: "The Thrombolysis in Myocardial Infarction (TIMI) Trial: Phase I Findings," *NEJM* 312 (1985): 932–36; "Thrombolysis in Myocardial Infarction (TIMI) Trial, Phase I: A Comparison between Intravenous Tissue Plasminogen Activator and Intravenous Streptokinase," *Circulation* 76 (1987): 142–54; "Thrombolysis in Myocardial Infarction (TIMI) Trial—Phase I: Hemorrhagic Manifestations and Changes in Plasma Fibrinogen and the Fibrinolytic System in Patients Treated with Recombinant Tissue Plasminogen Activator and Streptokinase," *JACC* 11 (1988): 1–11; "The Effect of Intravenous Thrombolytic Therapy on Left Ventricular Function," *Circulation* 75 (1987): 817–29.

75. A good review is N. L. Geller, and S. J. Pocock, "Interim Analyses in Randomized Clinical Trials," *Biometrics* 43 (1987): 213–23, although the TIMI study did not follow their exact approach.

76. F. H. Sheehan et al., "The Effect of Intravenous Thrombolytic Therapy on Left Ventricular Function," *Circulation* 75 (1987): 817–28.

77. Letter of November 26 from Marder to Hood, reprinted in *Federal Response to Misconduct*, p. 213, n. 73.

78. Ibid., p. 215.

79. Ibid., pp. 216–20.

80. D. Stipp, "A Clot-Dissolving Drug Proves Effective in Federal Test of Heart-Attack Patients," *Wall Street Journal*, February 11, 1986.

81. Yusuf, "Fibrinolytic Therapy." Excerpt from p. 556.

82. It is difficult to summarize the views of Yusuf and his colleagues about which trials would be ethical if they involve a placebo control run in light of these data. The reader should review the discussion on pp. 580–82 of the article for their treatment of this complex issue.

83. A good summary is found in D. P. DeBona, "Thrombolysis with Intravenous Human Recombinant Tissue-Type Plasminogen Activator in Acute Myocardial Infarction: The European Experience," *JACC* 10 (1987): 75B–78B.

84. M. Verstraete et al., "Randomised Trial of Intravenous Recombinant Tissue-Type Plasminogen Activator versus Intravenous Streptokinase in Acute Myocardial Infarction," *Lancet*, April

13, 1985, pp. 842–47, and M. Verstraete, "Double-Blind Randomised Trial of Intravenous Tissue-Type Plasminogen Activator versus Placebo in Acute Myocardial Infarction," *Lancet*, November 2, 1985, pp. 965–69.

85. F. Van de Werf and A. E. R. Arnold, "Intravenous Tissue Plasminogen Activator and the Size of Infarct, Left Ventricular Function, and Survival in Acute Myocardial Infarction," *British Medical Journal* 297 (1988): 1374–79.

86. The relevant publications are H. S. Mueller et al., "Thrombolysis in Myocardial Infarction (TIMI): Comparative Studies of Coronary Reperfusion and Systemic Fibrinogenolysis with Two Forms of Recombinant Tissue-Type Plasminogen Activator," *JACC* 10 (1987): 479–90; E. Passamani et al., "The Thrombolysis in Myocardial Infarction (TIMI) Phase II Pilot Study: Tissue Plasminogen Activator Followed by Percutaneous Transluminal Coronary Angioplasty," *JACC* 10 (1987): 51B–64B; TIMI Study Group, "Comparison of Invasive and Conservative Strategies after Treatment with Intravenous Tissue Plasminogen Activator in Acute Myocardial Infarction," *NEJM* 320 (1989): 618–27; TIMI Research Group, "Immediate vs Delayed Catheterization and Angioplasty Following Thrombolytic Therapy for Acute Myocardial Infarction: TIMI-II(A) Results," *JAMA* 260 (1988): 2849–58.

87. The relevant publications are GISSI, "Effectiveness of Intravenous Thrombolytic Therapy in Acute Myocardial Infarction," *Lancet*, February 22, 1986: pp. 397–401; GISSI, "Long-Term Effects of Intravenous Thrombolysis in Acute Myocardial Infarction: Final Report of the GISSI Study," *Lancet*, October 17, 1987, pp. 871–74; and F. Rovelli et al., "GISSI Trial: Early Results and Late Follow-Up," *JACC* 10 (1987): 33B–39B.

88. These principles are contained in such statements as the World Medical Association's Declaration of Helsinki (1964). A comprehensive treatment of these issues is found in R. Faden and T. Beauchamp, *A History and Theory of Informed Consent* (New York: Oxford University Press, 1986), especially Chapters 5 and 6. The quote is from *Lancet*, February 22, 1986, p. 398.

89. Which of these is the better way to state such results is a matter of considerable importance and some controversy. A recent analysis of this issue is J. P. McCormack and M. Levine, "Meaningful Interpretation of Risk Reduction from Clinical Drug Trials," *Annals of Pharmacotherapy* (forthcoming).

90. Its publications include an interim report, "Intravenous Streptokinase Given within 0–4 Hours of Onset of Myocardial Infarction Reduced Mortality in ISIS-2," *Lancet*, February 28, 1987, p. 502, and a final report, "Randomised Trial of Intravenous Streptokinase, Oral Aspirin, Both, or Neither among 17,187 Cases of Suspected Acute Myocardial Infarctions: ISIS-2," *Lancet*, August 13, 1988, pp. 349–60. The details about its consent policy are contained in a letter of August 15, 1990, from Dr. Richard Peto to me.

91. In H. P. Wolff, A. Fleckenstein, and E. Philipp, eds., *Drug Research and Drug Development in the 21st Century* (Berlin: Springer Verlag, 1989), p. 282. Italics added.

92. J. W. Kennedy et al., "The Western Washington Intravenous Streptokinase in Acute Myocardial Infarction Randomized Trial," *Circulation* 77 (1988): 345–52.

93. M. L. Simoons et al., "Improved Survival after Early Thrombolysis in Acute Myocardial Infarction," *Lancet*, September 14, 1985, pp. 578–81.

94. ISAM Study Group, "A Prospective Trial of Intravenous Streptokinase in Acute Myocardial Infarction," *NEJM* 314 (1986): 1465–71.

95. H. D. White et al., "Effect of Intravenous Streptokinase on Left Ventricular Function and Early Survival after Acute Myocardial Infarction," *NEJM* 317 (1987): 850–55.

96. Its major publication is R. G. Wilcox, "Trial of Tissue Plasminogen Activator for Mortality Reduction in Acute Myocardial Infarction," *Lancet*, September 3, 1988, pp 525–30.

97. A. D. Guerci et al., "A Randomized Trial of Intravenous Tissue Plasminogen Activator for Acute Myocardial Infarction with Subsequent Randomization to Elective Coronary Angioplasty," *NEJM* 317 (1987): 1613–18. Quote, p. 1614.

98. M. O'Rourke et al., "Limitation of Myocardial Infarction by Early Infusion of Recombinant Tissue-Type Plasminogen Activator," *Circulation* 77 (1988): 1311–15.

99. National Heart Foundation of Australia Coronary Thrombolysis Group, "Coronary

Thrombolysis and Myocardial Salvage by Tissue Plasminogen Activator Given Up to 4 Hours after Onset of Myocardial Infarction," *Lancet*, January 30, 1988, pp. 203–7. Quote, p. 204.

100. R. G. Wilcox, "Trial of Tissue Plasminogen Activator," p. 526.

101. The original report is R. A. G. Smith et al., "Fibrinolysis with Acyl-Enzymes: A New Approach to Thrombolytic Therapy," *Nature* 290 (April 9, 1981): 505–8. The list of desired properties is found both in that report and in an article by Jeffrey Anderson, a crucial figure in this section; J. L. Anderson, "Development and Evaluation of Anisoylated Plasminogen Streptokinase Activator Complex (APSAC) as a Second Generation Thrombolytic Agent," *JACC* 10 (1987): 22B–27B.

102. J. L. Anderson, "Summary of U.S. Clinical Trials Program for Evaluation of Anistreplase," *Clinical Cardiology* 13 (1990): V33–V38.

103. Its major publications are AIMS Trial Study Group, "Effect of Intravenous APSAC on Mortality after Acute Myocardial Infarction: Preliminary Report of a Placebo-Controlled Clinical Trial," *Lancet*, March 12, 1988, pp. 545–49; AIMS Trial Study Group, "Long-Term Effects of Intravenous Anistreplase in Acute Myocardial Infarction: Final Report of the AIMS Study," *Lancet*, February 24, 1990, pp. 427–31.

104. J. L. Anderson et al., "Multicenter Reperfusion Trial of Intravenous Anisoylated Plasminogen Streptokinase Activator Complex (APSAC) in Acute Myocardial Infarction: Controlled Comparison with Intracoronary Streptokinase," *JACC* 11 (1988): 1153–63. Quote, p. 1161.

105. AIMS Trial Study Group, *Lancet*, March 12, 1988, p. 546.

106. The agenda is reprinted in E. Clarke, ed., *The NDA Pipeline—1987* (Washington: FDC Development Corporation, 1988), pp. V19–V21, while the transcript is available from Caset Associates, 8300 Professional Hill Drive, Fairfax, Virginia. Page numbers following quotations in this section of the text refer to the transcript.

107. "Human Sacrifices," *Wall Street Journal*, June 2, 1987, p. 30.

108. P. R. Kowey et al., "The tPA Controversy and the Drug Approval Process," *JAMA* 260 (1988): 2250–52. Quote, p. 2251.

109. Clarke, *NDA Pipeline*, p. I-123.

110. On this last point, see *Scrips*, no. 1216 (June 24, 1987): 10.

111. H. S. Mueller, et. al. "Thrombolysis in Myocardial Infarction (TIMI): Comparative Studies of Coronary Reperfusion and Systemic Fibrinogenolysis with Two Forms of Recombinant Tissue-Type Plasminogen Activator," *JACC* 10 (1987): 479–90.

112. Figures are drawn from a table printed on November 19, 1987, in the *Wall Street Journal*.

113. They range from Genentech arrogance to FDA in-fighting. A good introduction to these speculations is found in the *Scrips* story cited in note 110.

114. *Wall Street Journal*, June 2, 1987, p. 30.

115. Reuters Business Report, June 1, 1987, BC Cycle.

116. Michael Specter, "Rejection of Heart Drug Was by the Book," *Washington Post*, September 13, 1987.

117. Clarke, *NDA Pipeline*, pp. I-126–I-127.

118. Ibid., p. I-126.

119. Ibid., pp. I-123–I-124.

120. "There May Still Be Hope for tPA," *Chemical Week*, June 17, 1987, p. 17.

121. Clarke, *NDA Pipeline*, pp. I-123–I-124.

122. "Birth of a Blockbuster: How Genentech Delivered the Goods," *Business Week*, November 30, 1987, p. 138.

123. Clarke, *NDA Pipeline*, pp. I-123–I-124.

124. "Genentech: A David that Comes On Like Goliath," *Business Week*, October 30, 1989, p. 165.

125. *NDA Pipeline—1989* (Washington: FDC Development Corp., 1990), p. V-17.

126. The data presented here come from a Health Care Financing Agency document called "Data Sheet: Medicare Payment for Heart Attacks," dated May 25, 1988.

127. Correspondence from Joseph A. Oddis to Henry Waxman, January 13, 1988.

128. Social Security Act §1886 (d)(4)(C), 42 USCA §1395 ww(d)(4)(C).

129. Social Security Act §1886 (e)(2), 42 USCA §1395 ww(e)(2).

130. Summary of Minutes, January 13, 1988, Prospective Payment Assessment Commission.

131. Correspondence of Donald Young to Bill Bradley, February 5, 1988, and Prospective Payment Assessment Commission, *Annual Report*, March 1, 1988.

132. Just such an effect had in fact been observed in two studies whose results had already been announced before the PROPAC meeting, a study by Leigh Hopkins at the Thomas Jefferson University Hospital in Philadelphia (presented at the December 9, 1987, Midyear Clinical Meeting of the ASHP) and a study by Eric Topol at Michigan (an abstract of which was published in *Circulation* 76, suppl. IV [1987]: IV-22).

133. PR Newswire, January 15, 1988.

134. M. Gladwell, "Medicare Stance May Limit Use of Heart Drug," *Washington Post*, March 6, 1988, p. H1.

135. "Bowen Is Weighing tPA Coverage under Medicare," *AHA News* 24 (March 14, 1988): 1.

136. "tPA: Miracle Drug or One of Medicare's Broken Promises?" *AHA News* 24 (March 21, 1988): 4.

137. M. Freudenheim, "Cost Cutters Gain in TPA Debate," *New York Times*, April 5, 1988, p. 26.

138. Ibid., and M. Freudenheim, "Hospitals Fault Limit on Heart Drug Funds," *New York Times*, March 31, 1988.

139. Letter from Kevin Barry to Stephen King, April 21, 1988, and letter from Kathleen Buto to Kevin R. Barry, May 10, 1988.

140. Quoted in *Technology Reimbursement Reports*, March 24, 1989, p. 6.

141. T. Lerner and B. Fradd, *Thrombolytic Therapy: What Users Are Saying* (New York: Shearson Lehman Hutton, September 6, 1988), p. 23.

142. Mark A. Hlatky et al., "Adoption of Thrombolytic Therapy in the Management of Acute Myocardial Infarction," *American Journal of Cardiology* 61 (1988): 510–14.

143. Lerner and Fradd, *Thrombolytic Therapy*.

144. T. H. Grasela and J. A. Green, "A Nationwide Survey of Prescribing Patterns for Thrombolytic Drugs in Acute Myocardial Infarction," *Pharmacotherapy* 10 (1990): 35–41, and B. Brody et al., "The Impact of Economic Considerations on Clinical Decision Making," *Medical Care* 29 (1991): 899–910.

145. The Loran Commission, *A Report to the Community* (Brookline, Mass.: Harvard Community Health Plan, 1989), pp. 8–9.

146. Transcript of Braunwald–Marder debate, 37th American College of Cardiology meeting, Atlanta, March 30, 1988.

147. E. J. Topol and R. M. Califf, "Tissue Plasminogen Activator: Why the Backlash?" *JACC* 13 (1989): 1477–80. Quote, pp. 1478–79.

148. Genentech, Inc.'s, Patent, Court of Appeal (Civil Division), October 31, 1988, p. 105 of Lexis text.

149. E. L. Andrews, "G.A.O. Study Finds Genetic Engineering Faces Patent Delays," *New York Times*, July 19, 1990, p. 1.

150. The basic claims are summarized in *Genentech, Inc. Innov. N.V., and Leuven Research and Development VZW v. The Wellcome Foundation*, United States District Court for the District of Delaware Civ. A. No. 88-330/89-407 JJF (Memorandum opinion, March 8, 1990).

151. The standard enunciated in *Graver Tank & Mfg. Co. v. Linde Air Products Co.*, 339 US 608.

152. United States District Court for the District of Delaware, No. 88-330/89-407 JJF (April 6, 1990).

153. A. Pollack, "Wellcome Dropping Its tPA Heart Drug," *New York Times*, May 11, 1990, p. 3, and Genentech 1991 form 10-K filed with the SEC, p. 7. See also Y. Ko, "An Economic Analysis of Biotechnology Protection," *Yale Law Journal* 102 (1992): 777–804.

154. D. Brahams, "Alteplase (rtPA) Patent Case," *Lancet*, November 26, 1988, p. 1263. A recent analysis of this decision, and of other European and Japanese decisions on tPA and other biotechnology products, is found in L. Maher, "The Patent Environment: Domestic and European Community Frameworks for Biotechnology," *Jurimetrics Journal* 33 (Fall 1992): 67–132.

155. Genetech, Inc.'s, Patent, Court of Appeal, Lexis text, Section 13.17.

156. Ibid., p. 87.

157. Ibid., pp. 132–33.

158. D. Zinman, "Doctors as Stockholders," *Newsday*, September 29, 1987, Discovery Section, p. 1.

159. TIMI Study Group, "Comparison of Invasive and Conservative Strategies after Treatment with Intravenous Tissue Plasminogen Activator in Acute Myocardial Infarction," *NEJM* 320 (1989): 618–27.

160. A. D. Guerci et al., "A Randomized Trial of Intravenous Tissue Plasminogen Activator for Acute Myocardial Infarction with Subsequent Randomization to Elective Coronary Angioplasty," *NEJM* 317 (1987): 1613–18.

161. "Bad Chemistry," *Wall Street Journal*, January 26, 1989, p. 1.

162. *Federal Response to Misconduct.*

163. Ibid., p. 5.

164. The closest they came to considering the issue of meaningful consent is found briefly in the transcript, but having raised it, they let it go (ibid., p. 179). A real opportunity was lost.

165. Ibid., p. 187.

166. "Drug's Testers Had Stock in Its Maker," *Washington Post*, September 30, 1988; M. Mahar, "Taking Stock: Add a Congressional Probe to the Company's Woes," *Barron's*, November 21, 1988, pp. 13, 28–31; "Bad Chemistry."

167. TIMI Study Group, "Comparison of Invasive and Conservative Strategies."

168. B. Healy et al., "Conflict of Interest Guidelines for a Multicenter Clinical Trial of Treatment after Coronary-Artery Bypass-Graft Surgery," *NEJM* 320 (1989): 949–51.

169. Cited in *The Blue Sheet*, January 25, 1989, p. 5.

170. This account is based on D. Zinman, "Far Apart on Ethical Issues," *Newsday*, August 29, 1989, Discovery Section, p. 6, and on J. Palca, "NIH Grapples with Conflict of Interest," *Science*, vol. 240, July 7, 1989, p. 23.

171. T. Weiss, "Research that U.S. Government Is Paying for Should Not Be Tainted by Any Possibility of Bias," *Chronicle of Higher Education*, October 4, 1989, p. A56.

172. D. S. Wheeler, "Health Secretary Kills Guidelines to Bar Abuse among NIH Grantees," *Chronicle of Higher Education*, January 10, 1990, p. A1.

173. D. Baim et al., "The Thrombolysis in Myocardial Infarction (TIMI) Trial Phase II: Additional Information and Perspectives," *JACC* 15 (1990): 1188–92.

174. D. P. DeBona et al., "The SWIFT Study of Intervention versus Conservative Management after Anistreplase Thrombolysis," *Circulation* 80 (1989): II-418 (abstract).

175. E. J. Topol, D. R. Holmes, and W. J. Rogers, "Coronary Angiography after Thrombolytic Therapy for Acute Myocardial Infarction," *Annals of Internal Medicine* 114 (1991): 877–85.

176. See, for example, C. L. Grines et al., "A Comparison of Immediate Angioplasty with Thrombolytic Therapy for Acute Myocardial Infarction," *NEJM* 328 (1993): 673–78.

177. G. Koren et al., "Prevention of Myocardial Damage in Acute Myocardial Ischemia by Early Treatment with Intravenous Streptokinase," *NEJM* 313 (1985): 1384–89.

178. S. W. Sharkey et al., "An Analysis of Time Delays Preceding Thrombolysis for Acute Myocardial Infarction," *JAMA* 262 (1989): 3171–74.

179. An excellent review of all of these studies through the spring of 1992, including a summary of the preliminary reports from the EMIP and MITI trials, is to be found in A. M. Ross, "Prehospital Thrombolysis," *Journal of Myocardial Ischemia* 4 (July/August 1992): 13–20. The final EMIP data have been published as the European Myocardial Infarction Project Group, "Prehospital Thrombolytic Therapy in Patients with Suspected Acute Myocardial Infarction," *NEJM* 329 (1993): 383–89. The final MITI report is W. Douglas Weaver et al., "Pre-Hospital Initiated vs. Hospital-Initiated Thrombolytic Therapy," *JAMA* 270 (1993): 1211–16.

180. In J. W. Marx, "Which Clot-Dissolving Drug Is Best?" *Science* 242 (1988): 1505–6.

181. H. D. White et al., "Effect of Intravenous Streptokinase as Compared with that of Tissue

Plasminogen Activator on Left Ventricular Function after First Myocardial Infarction," *NEJM* 320 (1989): 817–21.

182. E. Rapaport, "Thrombolytic Agents in Acute Myocardial Infarction," *NEJM* 320 (1989): 861–64.

183. M. Waldholz, M. "Genentech Heart Drug Dealt Critical Blow," *Wall Street Journal*, March 30, 1989, p. B4.

184. GISSI, "GISSI-2: A Factorial Randomised Trial of Alteplase versus Streptokinase and Heparin versus No Heparin Among 12,490 Patients with Acute Myocardial Infarction," and The International Study Group, "In-Hospital Mortality and Clinical Course of 20,891 Patients with Suspected Acute Myocardial Infarction Randomised between Alteplase and Streptokinase with or without Heparin," *Lancet*, July 14, 1990, pp. 65–70 and 71–75, respectively.

185. L. K. Altman, "Study Finds a $2,200 Heart Drug No Better than One Costing $76," *New York Times*, March 9, 1990, p. 1.

186. Ibid.

187. *Advances in Cardiology*, published by Gardiner-Caldwell Communications, for Genentech.

188. The preliminary report was presented at the American College of Cardiology meetings in March 1991 and is described in L. K. Altman, "Cheapest Anti-Clot Drug Is Found to Be the Safest," *New York Times*, March 4, 1991, p. B9. The final report is ISIS-3 Collaborative Group, "ISIS-3: A Randomized Comparison of Streptokinase vs. Tissue Plasminogen Activator vs. Anistreplase and of Aspirin Plus Heparin vs. Aspirin Alone among 41299 Cases of Suspected Acute Myocardial Infarction," *Lancet*, March 28, 1992, pp. 753–70.

189. S. Sherry and V. Marder, "Streptokinase and Recombinant Tissue Plasminogen Activator (rtPA) Are Equally Effective in Treating Acute Myocardial Infarction," *Annals of Internal Medicine* 114 (1991): 417–23. Quote, p. 418.

190. L. K. Altman, "Cheapest Drug for Blood Clots Is Called the Safest," *New York Times*, March 27, 1992.

191. M. Waldholz, "Genentech Inc. Pressed by Data on Clot Drugs," *Wall Street Journal*, March 27, 1992, p. B5.

192. Genentech 1991 form 10-K filed with the SEC, p. 5.

193. M. Chase, "As Genentech Awaits New Test of Old Drug, Its Pipeline Fills Up," *Wall Street Journal*, April 30, 1993, p. 1.

194. Two initial sources of detailed information were L. K. Altman, "A Surprise in War between Heart Drugs," *New York Times*, May 1, 1993, p. 6, and "GUSTO Trial Reports 14 percent Mortality Advantage for Genentech's Activase over Streptokinase," *The Blue Sheet*, May 5, 1993, p. 10. The formal report, issued in September, is GUSTO Investigators, "An International Randomized Trial Comparing Four Thrombolytic Strategies for Acute Myocardial Infarction," *NEJM* 329 (1993): 673–82.

195. M. Chase, "Genentech Drug Raises Question of a Life's Value," *Wall Street Journal,* May 4, 1993, p. B6. All the reactions in this paragraph are drawn from her insightful article.

196. The extent of that challenge can be seen in two recent publications. The first is D. Ketley and K. L. Woods, "Impact of Clinical Trials on Clinical Practice," *Lancet*, October 9, 1993, pp. 891–94, which documents a remarkable continued failure to provide thrombolytic therapy to many patients. The other is The Late Study Group, "Late Assessment of Thrombolytic Efficacy Study," *Lancet*, September 25, 1993, pp. 759–66. It provides data needed to challenge those who withhold thrombolytic therapy from those presenting more than 6 hours after the onset of symptoms.

197. Figures are drawn from Genentech's 1985 Annual Report and from its form 10-K filing for 1985 with the Securities and Exchange Commission.

198. Genentech 1987 form 10-K filed with the SEC and 1987 Annual Report.

199. Genentech 1988 form 10-K filed with the SEC and 1988 Annual Report.

200. M. Chase, "Genentech Battered by Great Expectations, Is Tightening Its Belt," *Wall Street Journal*, October 11, 1988, p. 1.

201. A. Pollack, "Taking the Crucial Next Step at Genentech," *New York Times*, January 28, 1990, Business Section, p. 1.

202. T. Lerner, *Genentech* (New York: Shearson Lehman Hutton, August 8, 1989).

203. A. Pollack, "U.S. Biotechnology Leader to Sell Swiss 60 percent Stake," *New York Times*, February 3, 1990, p. 1.

204. Genentech form 10K for 1990 and 1991.

2

Troubling Ethical Issues in the Conduct of Clinical Trials

The case study in Chapter 1 illustrates at least three major ethical issues in clinical trial procedures that troubled investigators conducting the thrombolytic trials and observers of those trials. All three are in fact disturbing issues that warrant further analysis:

1. Under what conditions, if any, is it ethical to withhold from the control group in a placebo-controlled trial of a new therapy an already existing therapeutic intervention which has been proven to be relatively safe and effective?
2. What type of informed consent, if any, should be obtained from research subjects in emergency research?
3. How can clinical trials be structured to avoid problems of conflicts of interest which may arise because of economic factors influencing the investigators?

This chapter will consider all three of these issues. A variety of approaches to each will be examined, and some recommendations will be offered. These recommendations will be used to evaluate what happened in the clinical trials of the thrombolytic agents. But first we will review a series of influential statements of principles and regulations governing research involving human subjects.

This review will have two purposes. First we will see what fundamental values are embodied in these principles and regulations in the hope that they will help us deal with our issues. Then we will examine the extent to which the issues have been adequately dealt with in these principles and regulations.

A Selected Survey of Statements of Principles and Regulations

The early history of reflections about the ethics of human research has been studied by many authors,[1] and we need not redo their work here. The crucial point they have shown is that the Nuremberg Code, presented in 1948 in the trial of Nazi physician-experimenters, was the first major set of principles governing the ethics of research on human subjects.[2] Its ten principles can be stated as follows:

1. Voluntary consent of the human subject (based upon sufficient knowledge) is essential.
2. The experiment should be designed to yield fruitful results unprocurable by other means.
3. The experiment should be based upon supporting animal experimentation and other studies which justify its performance.
4. Unnecessary suffering and injury should be avoided.
5. No experiment should be conducted when there is a reason to believe that death or disabling injury will occur, except when the researcher also serves as research subject.
6. The degree of risk should never exceed the importance of the problem to be solved.
7. Subjects should be adequately protected against even remote possibilities of injury, disability, or death.
8. The experiment should be conducted by highly qualified persons using the highest degree of skill and care.
9. Experimental subjects should be free to withdraw throughout the experiment if they judge continuation to be impossible.
10. If the experimenter judges that continuation of the experiment is likely to result in injury, disability, or death to the subject, the experiment should be terminated.

A review of these ten principles makes it clear that two major values are operative in them. Principles 1 and 9 seem to be rooted in a commitment to individual liberty and autonomy. Patients can be enrolled in trials only if they agree voluntarily to participate and if their agreement does not bind them since they must always remain free to withdraw when they judge withdrawal to be appropriate. Principles 2–8 and 10 seem to be rooted in more consequentialist concerns, concerns that the research not be too harmful to the patient (principles 5 and 10), that it should minimize possible harm (principles 4, 7, and 8), and that it should be justified because the benefit of the research outweighs even the minimized harm that may occur (principles 2, 3, and 6). Moreover, since all of these principles must be satisfied if the research is to be considered licit, the Nuremberg Code does not justify research simply because patients give informed consent; it calls upon researchers to eschew certain research as too risky in and of itself or in relation to the potential benefit even if patients would give their voluntary informed consent to participating. Satisfying the demands of liberty and autonomy for valid informed consent is necessary for research to be licit; it is not, according to the Nuremberg

Code, sufficient. Equally true, satisfying the demands with respect to risks and benefits of consequentialist analysis is necessary but not sufficient for the licitness of the research. Only satisfying both is sufficient.[3]

This approach to the licitness of research on human subjects will be very important in our later discussion, and it is by no means uncontroversial. It might, after all, be challenged in two very different ways. One insists that satisfying the demands of autonomy is all that should be required; on this account, any research, however risky, is licit if the subjects give their informed voluntary consent to participation in the research since that consent ensures that the rights of the subjects have not been violated. The other challenge insists that satisfying the consequentialist demands is all that should be required; on this account, any research, even if done without consent, is licit if the benefits justify the risks since that favorable risk-benefit ratio makes the research worth doing.

It seems to me, however, that both of these challenges make the same mistake and that the Nuremberg Code and all the codes which follow it are right in imposing both sets of requirements. The common mistake made by both challenges is their concentration on only one moral requirement; they thereby fail to recognize the multiplicity of the demands made by morality. While the first challenge is correct in its claim that research to which subjects give voluntary informed consent cannot (because of that consent) violate the rights of the subjects, that correct claim does *not* entail the conclusion that such research is therefore automatically morally licit. Other moral considerations, including the fact that the research is too risky, may make it illicit; some actions which violate the rights of no other individual are still morally illicit actions. While the second challenge is correct in its claim that research satisfying the consequentialist concerns is research worth doing, that correct claim does *not* entail the conclusion that such research is therefore automatically morally licit. Other moral considerations, including the fact that the subject has not consented, may make it illicit; some beneficial actions are still morally illicit actions. Research must therefore satisfy both the demands of autonomy and the demands of consequentialism before it can be morally licit.

The Nuremberg Code is a set of principles and not a code of regulations, so its silence both about the process by which its principles will be enforced and about the detailed implications of these principles is not surprising. It certainly does not say anything that specifically addresses our issues. But it does embody certain values, and both its explicit principles and their underlying values will be of importance to us throughout this chapter.

A second major statement of principles is the Declaration of Helsinki, adopted by the World Medical Association in 1964 and revised in 1975, in 1983, and again in 1989.[4] The same values are operative in this declaration, although there is a crucial difference in its treatment of autonomy and liberty. While principle 9 of part I of the declaration reiterates the requirement that research presupposes for its licitness free and informed consent, an exception is made in some cases of clinical research (research which holds out the promise of direct benefit to the subjects who are also patients). To quote the text of the crucial clause II.5: "If the doctor considers it essential not to obtain informed consent, the specific reasons for this proposal should be stated in the experimental protocol for transmission to the independent committee." Not much is said about why a doctor might consider it essential not to obtain informed consent or about what standards any independent review should adopt in considering such proposals; we shall return to these issues later.

Several other features of the Declaration of Helsinki deserve special attention. First, it does address the question of the process by which its principles should be enforced. One of its principles (I.2) is that all research involving human subjects should be submitted to an independent committee "for consideration, comment and guidance." It says little about the composition of this committee and about its powers. Can it, for example, veto a research protocol? Still, this is an important procedural point that became the foundation for much of what happened throughout the world, as such committees proliferated. Second, it does say something about one of our important issues, the question of the control group. In the very important principle II.3, the Declaration of Helsinki mandates: "In any medical study, every patient—including those of a control group, if any—should be assured of the best proven diagnostic and therapeutic method." Naturally, many questions will arise as to when diagnostic and therapeutic methods are the "best proven" and cannot therefore be denied to a control group, but these ambiguities should not take away from the significance of the initial principle.

These major internationally recognized statements of principles, the Nuremberg Code and the Declaration of Helsinki, were supplemented in 1982 and 1993 by proposed international guidelines developed collaboratively by the World Health Organization (WHO) and the Council for International Organizations of Medical Sciences (CIOMS). Also, regulations and policy statements have been developed in many countries. All of them are based upon the same values as the Nuremburg Code and the Declaration of Helsinki, although they sometimes add values such as justice, and they sometimes recategorize these values, for example, seeing respect for autonomy as part of a broader respect for persons. It is these commonly accepted values that we will be invoking in attempting to resolve our issues.

We turn then to the second task of this preliminary section, the survey of regulations and principles in the United States and elsewhere. Our goal is to determine the extent to which these regulations have adequately resolved our issues.

There are two sets of overlapping, but not identical, American regulations involving experiments on human subjects. One, from the Food and Drug Administration, governs research to be used in support of applications for FDA approval of drugs and devices. The other, from the Department of Health and Human Services, governs research funded by the NIH and other federal agencies, whether in their own facilities or at other institutions. In practice, it governs all research at those institutions.

Both sets of regulations date from 1981 (although the DHHS regulations have been supplemented by 1983 regulations governing research involving children).[5] Both are modifications of earlier regulations by both agencies, drafted in response to the work of the National Commission for the Protection of Human Subjects of Biomedical and Behavioral Research, a body which was created by the National Research Act of 1974 and which did its work between 1974 and 1978.[6] The earlier history of the attitudes of these agencies to issues of human experimentation is of great interest, but we shall ignore that history here and concentrate on the philosophy of the National Commission and the response of the agencies.

One side note of importance. As Robert J. Levine pointed out in 1979,[7] the National Commission opted for a single set of regulations administered by a single agency which would, for all practical purposes, govern research in the United States, and the very existence of these separate rules (even if they overlap considerably) is itself somewhat questionable. Even recent efforts to produce one uniform set of federal regulations have not been fully successful.[8]

One of the congressional charges to the National Commission was to identify the basic ethical principles governing research involving human subjects. The process of identifying those principles began in 1976 at a conference held at the Belmont Conference Center of the Smithsonian Institution and concluded with the publication of the Belmont Report, which summarized those deliberations.[9] That report identified three major principles and offered one application of each. Other applications of the three principles—such as a requirement for compensation to those injured in the research as an application of the principle of justice—are possible, but they were not identified in the report. The report listed the following:

Principles	*Application*
Respect for persons	Informed voluntary consent
Beneficence	Assessment of risks and benefits
Justice	Fair selection of subjects and protection of vulnerable subjects

The first two of these principles and their corresponding applications are familiar from both the Nuremberg Code and the Declaration of Helsinki. The third, which is an important addition, represents the recognition that research can be illicit if its benefits and burdens are unfairly distributed, especially if the burdens fall disproportionately on vulnerable subjects (the institutionalized, the very sick, racial minorities, and the economically disadvantaged).

With these principles in mind, we turn to the 1981 regulations. Both sets of regulations incorporate the idea that research must be approved by an independent committee (called in the regulations an institutional review board, or IRB).[10]

And both sets of regulations incorporate the very same requirements for IRB approval.[11] These requirements are set out in Table 2.1, whose left-hand side represents the requirement and whose right-hand columns are my attempt to relate the requirement to the principles and applications drawn from the Belmont Report. With one very important exception, the protection of privacy and confidentiality, whose absence from the Belmont Report is clearly an error, the FDA-DHHS requirements are a clear outgrowth of the principles of the Belmont Report and represent a very significant amplification of, and advance over, the Declaration of Helsinki and the Nuremburg Code.

The similarity of the two sets of regulations extends to the definition of informed consent, since each provides for the following points:

1. Consent shall be obtained under circumstances which allow sufficient opportunity to consider whether to participate and which minimize coercion or undue influence.
2. Information shall be provided in lay language.
3. There can be no waiver of liability for negligence.
4. Patients shall be told: (a) that they are being asked to participate in research of a specific type for a specific time which involves specific elements which are experimental; (b) the risks of or discomforts from participation; (c) the benefits from participation; (d) the available alternatives; (e) the measures to protect confidentiality; (f) the compensation that will be available if injury occurs; (g) whom to contact about questions or problems; (h) that participation is voluntary and that they may withdraw without penalty at any time; (i) a variety of other things that may be appropriate in specific cases (including additional costs, if any).[12]

Table 2.1 Relation of 1981 Regulations to Belmont Report

Requirement	Principle	Application
Risks to subjects are minimized	Beneficence	Assessment of risks
Risks to subjects are reasonable in relation to anticipated benefits	Beneficence	Assessment of risks
Selection of subjects is equitable	Justice	Fair selection of subjects
Informed consent is obtained	Respect for persons	Informed consent
Informed consent is documented	Respect for persons	Informed consent
Study is monitored to protect subjects	Beneficence	Assessments of risks and benefits
Privacy and confidentiality are protected		
Additional safeguards are provided for vulnerable subjects	Justice	Protection of vulnerable subjects

Our review of the overlapping sets of federal regulations makes it clear that there is in place today in the United States a very substantial set of procedural and substantive regulations governing research on human subjects, regulations which go a long way toward protecting both the well-being and the autonomy of these subjects. It is not clear, however, that these regulations deal effectively with our three issues. Let us look at each of them separately.

What about the issue of withholding from a placebo control group existing therapeutic interventions that have been proven to be effective? The FDA regulations and supporting material have much to say about this issue, while the DHHS regulations are silent about it. To begin with, the official FDA regulations recognize that placebo controlled trials may not be necessary in order to have the required substantial evidence of effectiveness. They recognize (in 21 CFR §314.126) several alternatives, including most crucially comparing the group getting the new drug with a control group getting the therapy whose efficacy is known (active treatment concurrent controls). Moreover, in accompanying FDA Clinical Investigator Information Sheets, the agency goes so far as to say that "placebo-controlled trials, whatever their advantages in interpretability, are obviously not ethically acceptable where existing treatment is life-prolonging."[13] Nevertheless, it is clear that the FDA strongly favors placebo-controlled trials. The very sentence just quoted continues with the claim that "there are relatively few situations where this is the case." Moreover, the whole thrust of the packet sent to clinical investigators on the issue of placebo-controlled versus active-controlled drug study designs is to emphasize the preferability of placebo-controlled trials over active-controlled trials. We will review the arguments offered for this preference in the next section of this chapter. For now, it is sufficient to say that the FDA clearly prefers placebo-controlled trials, although it does recognize the theoretical legitimacy of active-controlled trials and their ethical inevitability when existing treatments are life-prolonging. In all of this, the FDA attitude seems in opposition to the Declaration of Helsinki with its absolute affirmation of the right of all patients, including those in the control group, to receive the best proven diagnostic and therapeutic method. In any case, it is clear that the ambiguities in the FDA attitude and the silence of the DHHS regulations means that the issue of placebo control groups has not been adequately resolved in the current U.S. regulations on research.

The FDA regulations do seem to address the question of emergency research. Its regulation 56.104(c) exempts "emergency use of a test article" from the requirement of IRB review, and informed consent is not required (according to 50.23) if the human subject is confronted by a life-threatening situation, the subject cannot give informed consent, there is not sufficient time to contact the subject's representative, and no approved or recognized therapy provides an equal or greater likelihood of saving the life of the subject. However, the FDA has made it clear that it interprets these regulations to not apply to anticipated emergency research (for example, emergency room research) but to the unanticipated emergency. To quote from their IRB information sheets:

> Use of a test article in an investigation designed to be conducted under emergency considerations (e.g., emergency room research) usually does not qualify for the emergency use exemption. In these circumstances, a protocol is designed well before the study is initiated and the IRBs have ample time to review the study and provide for informed consent.[14]

Part of this is quite understandable. If we are dealing with emergency room research, one can develop in advance a protocol which can be reviewed and approved by an IRB and there is no need to waive the requirement of IRB approval before the research is conducted. But what is difficult to understand—and this is crucial for our purposes—is how the FDA expects the IRB to provide for informed consent when the patients coming in cannot give that consent and there is no time to contact any patient representative. Does the FDA want to confine the research protocol to patients whose representatives are available? What if the experimental treatment is the patient's best hope? These are crucial questions which neither the FDA regulations nor their information sheets answer.

The DHHS regulations are even more silent on these questions. The most relevant provisions I can find are provision 46.116(f) that "nothing . . . is intended to limit the authority of a physician to provide emergency medical care" and provision 46.116(c), which allows research without informed consent when "the research could not practicably be carried out without the waiver or alteration." Whether these provisions allow emergency room research without informed consent is unclear, since there is always the option of treating all but confining the research to patients who arrive competent to give consent or with representatives who can provide consent on their behalf. The Office of Protection from Research Risks has concluded that they do not, and that the emergency patients treated innovatively without consent cannot be considered research subjects. This silence in the formal DHHS regulations about emergency research, combined with the ambiguities in the FDA regulations, means that the issue of consent to emergency research has not been adequately resolved in the current U.S. regulations on research involving human subjects.[15]

Neither agency has adopted regulations about the last of our issues, the issue of regulating trials to avoid conflict-of-interest problems. Although both agencies have had in place regulations limiting conflicts of interest involving their own staff,[16] they have not (at least until very recently) dealt with our third issue. So, in conclusion, it is clear that the current U.S. regulations are seriously incomplete in that they don't adequately deal with any of our issues.

One final observation before leaving these American regulations. Although drafted by American agencies, they have international ramifications. For the FDA, the crucial issue is whether it will accept studies conducted outside the United States in support of applications for approving drugs and devices if those studies did not conform to FDA regulations protecting human subjects or were not conducted under a permit (an investigational new drug [IND] permit) obtained from the FDA. The FDA's basic response is:

> Foreign clinical research is required to have been conducted in accordance with the ethical principles stated in the "Declaration of Helsinki" . . . or the laws and regulations of the country in which the research was conducted, whichever represents the greater protection of the individual.[17]

DHHS policies on this matter are somewhat less categorical. The relevant regulation says:

> It also includes research conducted or funded by the Department of Health and Human Services outside the United States, but in appropriate circumstances, the secretary may, under paragraph (c) of this section, waive the applicability of some or all of the requirements of these regulations for research of this type.[18]

Unfortunately, no criteria are stated for which requirements can be waived under which circumstances. There has been much discussion of this issue,[19] and some critics have categorized these provisions as examples of ethical imperialism. I find myself, however, convinced by the rather persuasive argument presented on behalf of its own policy by the FDA:

> FDA recognized that standards for protection of human subjects vary from country to country and that the United States should not and cannot impose its standards on other countries. However, *minimum* standards to assure human subjects protection are required if the FDA is to accept the data from investigational studies not conducted under an IND or an IDE.[20]

I would add only that the minimum requirements (defined as conformity with the Declaration of Helsinki) are also the internationally accepted standards incorporated and strengthened in the recent WHO-CIOMS Proposed International Guidelines. So this is not a question of the United States imposing its unique standards on the world.

Having reviewed the American regulations, we turn to the principles and regulations found in other countries to see if they have offered a better resolution of our three issues. Because of its large pharmaceutical industry, we shall focus primarily but not exclusively on Great Britain. Although Great Britain has a very large and internationally important drug industry, it had no formal system of legally required premarketing testing and approval of drugs (similar to the FDA system in America) until the Medicines Act was passed in 1968 and went into effect on

September 1, 1971.[21] Even today, as a result of the 1981 Clinical Trials Exemption Scheme, clinical trials can begin without formal approval of the relevant division of the Department of Health so long as it is notified about the proposed trial and does not object in a very limited period of time. Not surprisingly, given such a new and less demanding scheme, there had been no formal regulations issued from the Department of Health governing human research, except for a 1975 circular which, following the advice of the Royal College of Physicians, called for the health authorities to arrange to set up ethical committees (the analogue of American IRBs) to review research projects.[22] In 1989, however, the Department of Health issued a draft of proposed guidelines for review of research by local research ethics committees, and those guidelines were finalized in the summer of 1991.

The proposed governmental guidelines[23] refer to some of the same values and principles we discussed in our examination of the American material, but they do so in a much weaker fashion. The process of protecting patients is the review of research proposals by an independent committee, and the appointment of such committees is now mandated, as it is in America. The topics to be considered by the committee are risks and benefits to patients, obtaining consent, and protecting confidentiality; thus many of the underlying values are the same as they are in America. But there is not even a strict requirement that the risks to the patient be outweighed by the benefits from the research. And, more crucially, implied consent is recognized as an alternative to explicit consent, consent may be documented in the charts rather than by a patient signing a consent form, and it is claimed that in therapeutic research it may be inappropriate to explain all the details of certain treatments for the purpose of gaining consent. In all of these areas, the proposed governmental requirements for the licitness of research, and especially its requirements for informed consent, are quite lax. But it may well correspond to traditional British research practice, if the recent controversy about British breast cancer trials is any indication of practice.[24] Whether this governmental response is adequate to the emerging professional standards in Great Britain (to which its proposed regulations obliquely refer) is questionable, as we shall see in a moment.

We turn to an examination of these professional standards to get a fuller sense of the British views on this topic. While the *Handbook of Medical Ethics* of the British Medical Association devotes four pages to research on human subjects, it offers very little by way of substantive standards except a reference to the Declaration of Helsinki.[25] This is no doubt a reflection of the general philosophy that "codes, regulations, and laws help to keep standards of ethical behavior high, but volunteers and patients are best protected by ethical conduct." Far more explicit, particularly on issues of informed consent, is the Guidelines on Good Clinical Research Practice of the Association of the British Pharmaceutical Industry, which in 1988 identified the many elements of informed consent.[26] But perhaps the most valuable guidance comes from a series of documents recently issued in two reports from the Royal College of Physicians in 1990[27] and three reports from the Medical Research Council in 1991 and 1992.[28] We will examine each set of reports separately, first looking at their general standards and then looking at what they have to say about our issues.

The standards recommended by the Royal College of Physicians in its new guidelines are clearly far more demanding than the proposed governmental guidelines. These standards mandate that research committees must find that there is a favorable balance of benefits from the knowledge to be obtained over risks to patients, that the risks to the patients have been minimized, and that these risks are minimal. In a very careful discussion, the guidelines present the limited circumstances in which patients can be subjected to more than minimal risk.[29] Moreover, its views about informed consent are quite different from those found in the proposed governmental regulations. With five exceptions (nonintrusive observational research, innocuous research into comprehension, examination of anonymous specimens, research based on medical records, and emergency research, which we will return to later), informed consent is required,[30] and written consent is the norm for all but the most minor of research procedures.[31] Simplification of information is permissible only so long as it does not lead to understating any risks or glossing over inconveniences or discomfort.[32] Finally, randomization should (except in special circumstances) be done only after consent is obtained, and that consent should be based upon the patient's being told of the alternatives under study.[33] All these issues are discussed with great sensitivity, and many practical suggestions are made that can only enhance patient autonomy in the process.

The Royal College of Physicians report addressed several of our questions. One of its five exceptions to the requirement of obtaining informed consent is research on the management of unexpected overwhelming emergencies (one example, close to our case study, is sudden cardiac arrest). Their views are nicely put in the following passage:

> Research of this sort seems to represent the only exception to the rule that prior consent is always required in research which may involve minimal or greater risk to the patient. It should be undertaken only if the Research Ethics Committee has given approval to proceeding without prior consent. . . . It will usually be right to inform the patient and relatives of what has taken place. The Research Ethics Committee should again give special attention to what the patient should be told. In the case of research which continues after the unexpected initiating event, consent to continued participation should be sought from the patient or near relative as soon as possible in the usual way.[34]

These views represent a considerable advance over the FDA's vague counsel to IRBs to "provide for informed consent."

There is also an extensive discussion of conflict-of-interest questions.[35] Interestingly enough, the focus is not on investigators having equity positions in the company whose drugs are being studied, the topic that has generated so much interest in the United States. It is, instead, on financial inducements which may play an improper role in any clinical trial, particularly in leading clinician-researchers to apply pressure on patients to be entered into trials, the very question raised by the Galin case discussed in Chapter 1. One of its recommendations is that there should be an absolute ban on payments made by a sponsor to investigators if those payments are on a per capita basis (the more patients enrolled, the higher the fee). Such an arrangement is felt to be unethical because it might lead a doctor to unduly pressure patients into participating. Even if the payment is to the institution rather than to the practitioner, such payments are inappropriate unless they simply cover expenses and provide no element of profit to the institution. Finally, when payments are not on a per capita basis but require that a minimum number of patients be enrolled, the Research Ethics Committee (which must be informed of the payment) must be satisfied "that the number is a reasonable one which is likely to be easily achieved by patients volunteering, bearing in mind the nature of the research and the normal work load of the clinicians." Another requirement is that "the scheme of payment should not consist of a series of steps proportional in some way to the number of patients participating." As far as I know, no treatment of this issue in such a comprehensive manner has been produced by any other regulatory or advisory group.

The Royal College has less to say about the issue of withholding proven treatment from the control group. There is one paragraph (7.100) which addresses this issue, a paragraph which is in contrast to the absolute ban of the Declaration of Helsinki on withholding such therapy and which comes closer to the FDA view:

> Withholding effective treatment for a short time, whether or not it is substituted by a placebo, can sometimes be acceptable in order to validate a technique of measurement or confirm the sensitivity or discrimination of a therapeutic trial design. An investigator who proposes to do this should explicitly justify his intention and the intended research procedure to the Research Ethics Committee. Patient consent is necessary, and the patient may agree that he need not know precisely when this will take place.

Consider two questions left unanswered by this statement: Is it sufficient that the patient consent, or must this withholding be limited to cases in which the possible ill-effects of the treatment being withheld are quite limited? In particular, can treatments of proven efficacy be withheld on life-threatening conditions, even with the consent of the patient? These are, of course, crucial questions to which we shall return, since they are directly relevant to our analysis of the ethical validity of the placebo-controlled trials of the thrombolytic agents.

In short, then, the most recent statements by the Royal College of Physicians are a resounding affirmation and extension of all the fundamental values we have been discussing. In many of the details, and in particular in connection with our three issues, it moves ahead of the United States in carefully analyzing problems and developing standards to resolve them.

The three statements from the Medical Research Council incorporate the same general values and policies. They also require approval of the research by a research ethics committee and mandate obtaining informed consent even in therapeutic research. The Medical Research Council has explicitly rejected its own earlier view—still incorporated in the Department of Health Guidelines—that therapeutic research can sometimes proceed without fully informed consent.[36] But these statements, as useful as they are, have nothing to say about our three issues. So in Great Britain it is only the Royal College of Physicians that has made an important contribution to the discussion and resolution of our issues.

We turn from Great Britain to an examination of some recent developments on the European continent. A 1988 survey of France, Germany, Sweden, and Switzerland (four countries with substantial drug industries) showed a wide variety of patterns of regulation involving legislation, industrial and professional standards of self-government, and the local use of research ethics committees.[37] Standards also varied considerably from one country to another. All of this will presumably be superseded by a newly issued recommendation of the Committee of Ministers of the Council of Europe to member states concerning medical research on human subjects.[38] That document calls upon member states to adopt legislation in conformity with its principles or to otherwise ensure their implementation. The principles in question are very close to those found in the DHHS and FDA regulations in the United States and in the new statements from the Royal College of Physicians in Great Britain. They call for independent review with special attention to risks and benefits assessment, to informed and specific consent, to confidentiality, and to protection of vulnerable subjects. These recommendations, supplemented by earlier guidelines issued by the director-general for internal market and industrial affairs of the European Commission,[39] are already being implemented by new legislation in France and by new national guidelines in Switzerland.[40] I would add only that provisions are made in this European material for emergency research, this being the only one of our three issues explicitly discussed. According to the Committee on Ministers, such research should be carried out without prior consent only if it is planned in advance, approved by an ethics committee, and is intended for the direct health benefit of the patient.

One final observation about both the British and the European material. While there are extensive provisions in this material dealing with disabled subjects, minor subjects, prisoner subjects, and other subjects drawn from vulnerable groups, they have little to say about general equity in the selection of research subjects with special reference to socioeconomically deprived groups or minority groups. This stands in stark contrast with the American regulations, but this neglect may actually say something very positive about the British and European situations. The fear that research may unjustly burden poor patients or minority patients may be a greater concern in the United States and other countries without a national health system or a universal insurance scheme. Poorer "charity" patients may wind up paying for their care by being the subjects of suspect research, and regulations against that may be required. In countries in which there are no "charity" patients because the health-care needs of all legal residents are covered, that concern about equity in the selection of subjects may not be needed.

Let us summarize what we have learned. We have seen the emergence of a consensus that research on human subjects should be governed by the principle of independent assessments of benefits and risks, by the requirement of informed consent, by the protection of confidentiality, and by equity in the selection of research subjects. We have also seen that our three problems are addressed to some degree in various countries, but that there remain major gaps in their treatment even in the most developed policies.

With all of this information in mind, we turn to an examination of our three questions as general issues and specifically in the context of the development of thrombolytic therapy.

The Use of Placebos in Clinical Trials

Framing the Issues

The issues we will be examining in this section are very complex, and it is therefore important that we begin by stating exactly which issues we will be examining and which issues we will not be examining. There has been much discussion in the literature of the use by physicians in their clinical practice of placebos,[41] with the advocates of that use stressing potential physical or psychological benefits and the opponents of that use stressing the deception inevitably present. This is an important issue, but it is not an issue of research ethics and we will not be examining it in this book. Our discussion will be confined to clinical trials of new interventions, where one group (the control group) is receiving just a placebo. No deception need be involved in such cases, since the informed process for the clinical trial should make clear to all participants that at least some of them (those randomized to the placebo control group) will be receiving a placebo rather than the intervention being tested. Nevertheless, this use of placebos raises the ethical question of whether it is legitimate to not provide the intervention to the control group. This is the question we will be considering in this section. It was raised by the many clinical trials of intravenous thrombolytic agents discussed in Chapter 1 which withheld from the placebo control group any thrombolytic agent, and it really involves two separate but related issues.

The first issue is whether it is ethical to withhold from the control group a therapy whose efficacy and safety have already been sufficiently demonstrated to receive approval by the relevant regulatory agencies for use in the clinical setting in question. This issue was raised by all the placebo-controlled trials of the intravenous use of thrombolytic agents except Anderson's multicenter APSAC trial, since they all involved a placebo control group which did not receive intracoronary strepto-kinase (SK) even though it had been approved for use after a myocardial infarction because of its demonstrated efficacy in reducing mortality. All these trials might have followed the lead of multicenter APSAC, which compared the efficacy of APSAC against a control group that received intracoronary SK, but they chose instead to use a placebo control group. Was that decision ethical?

The second issue is whether it is ethical to withhold from the control group a therapy that has not yet been approved by the relevant regulatory agencies for use in the clinical setting in question but which has been shown in one or more trials to be effective and safe in that clinical setting. This issue was raised by all of the placebo-controlled trials of the intravenous use of thrombolytic therapy which began or were continued after the publication in 1985 of the Yusuf analysis[42] of the pooled data about intravenous SK and the publication in 1986 of the data from the GISSI trial,[43] since both these publications reported that the use of intravenous SK after a myocardial infarction produced a significant reduction in mortal-ity. All these trials could have followed the lead of the NIH, which canceled the originally planned TIMI-II trial of tPA against a placebo control group because it felt that the issue of the safety and efficacy of intravenous thrombolytic therapy was settled. Alternatively, they could have run trials of intravenous tPA or APSAC against a control group receiving intravenous SK. The trials in question did nei-ther; they continued or began placebo-controlled trials of some thrombolytic agent administered intravenously. Was that decision ethical?

These issues are not new. They were already raised in Henry Beecher's classi-cal article about the ethics of clinical research, published in 1966.[44] The Beecher article, which stimulated much of the scrutiny of research ethics in the United States, discussed 22 examples of questionable research. The first three involved the withholding of treatments of known efficacy from placebo control groups. In one of those studies, typhoid fever was not treated in the placebo control group. Our case study shows that these issues are far from resolved, despite all of the activity which has resulted from Beecher's article, and that they need further exami-nation.

Beecher's article also reminds us that our issues are far from purely academic. In comparing the death rate in the treatment group to the placebo control group,

Beecher calculated that the decision to run the trial resulted in 23 excess deaths in the control group. In the trials of the thrombolytic agents, as in the trials he was discussing, there were more deaths in the placebo control group. Following his example, we can calculate the number of deaths in question. If none of the placebo-controlled trials should have been run because of the previous approval of intra-coronary SK, then the trials in question involved 497 additional deaths in placebo control groups that should not have existed. If placebo control groups were per-missible until the Yusuf and GISSI data demonstrated the efficacy of intravenous SK but not afterward, then the trials that continued or were begun later involved 261 additional deaths in placebo control groups that should not have existed. The details of these calculations can be found in Appendices B and C to Chapter 1. There is certainly room for differing judgments about some of the details. What is clear, however, is that many lives might have been saved if the placebo controlled trials were not run, so our issues are far from academic.

Couldn't these ethical issues be set to rest if researchers simply employed more active-controlled trials? Why don't researchers use them more often, thereby avoid-ing the need to confront these difficult issues? There are good answers to these questions, and they need to be understood at this point in order to appreciate the full difficulty of these issues.

One of the best accounts of the problems encountered by active-controlled trials is to be found in a series of three documents distributed by the FDA as part of its Clinical Investigator Information Sheets.[45] The series consists of an official FDA statement followed by reprints of two articles by Dr. Robert Temple of the FDA Three arguments are presented as to why active-controlled trials encounter diffi-culties. They all begin with the observation that active-controlled trials are tests of the hypothesis that there is no difference between the efficacy of the approved drug and the new drug being tested, and they run as follows.

1. Active controlled trials are often too small to ensure that a clinically signifi-cant difference, if it exists, will be detected. The more important even a small difference would be (say, if it is a difference in mortality), the larger the sample size needed to ensure with a sufficiently high probability that the difference, if it exists, will be detected. These larger trials may be too expensive and/or cumber-some to run, and smaller trials cannot establish that the new drug is as good as the older approved drug.

2. Sloppy trial design or execution often obscures differences. In placebo-controlled trials, when you want to demonstrate a difference (the drug being tested works better than the placebo), you have an incentive to avoid these errors due to sloppiness. In active-controlled trials, when you want to demonstrate that there is no difference (the drug being tested works as well as the older drug being given to the control group), you have no such incentive.

3. Showing that two drugs in an active-controlled trial are equally efficacious does not establish that the new drugs works, even if the older drug against which it has been tested has been shown to work in the past. To quote Temple:

> Because the positive control is known to be an effective agent, we usually conclude, if equivalence is shown, that both agents were effective. This seems reasonable at first glance, but a closer look reveals a crucial assumption, namely, that the control drug was effective in the particular study in question. The assumption cannot be tested from data in the study; it is based on past performance, an implicit historical control. . . . Recognizing the assumption, we can consider whether it is valid. In fact, it is not necessarily valid, because many effective agents are not demonstrably effective every time they are tested. . . . To summarize the above discussion, the fundamental principle, when considering a positive control design is this: if we cannot be very certain that the positive control in a study would have beaten a placebo group, had one been present, the fundamental assumption of the positive-control study cannot be made and that design must be considered inappropriate. Any condition in which large spontaneous or placebo-responses occur, or in which there is great day-to-day variability (or imprecision of measurement), or in which effective drugs are not easily distinguished from placebo, should be considered a poor candidate for a positive control study. (pp. 49–50)

Several points need to be made about this impressive battery of arguments. First, none of these objections would be objections to clinical trials employing active control groups designed to prove that the new drug is better than the older drug given to the active control group. Such active-controlled trials are like placebo-controlled trials, because in these active-controlled trials we are testing the hypothesis that there is a difference between the drug being tested and the control group, rather than the hypothesis that there is no difference. Therefore, none of the stated objections arise. Second, the first two objections can be met if the active-controlled trial is well-designed and implemented and of adequate size; only the third objection is an objection in principle to such trials. Finally, as Temple points out, the third objection becomes progressively less serious as we have more reason to believe that the drug supplied to the active control group would have beaten a placebo group.

Temple's own conclusion from his arguments is that "any trend toward greater reliance, for fundamental evidence of effectiveness, on positive control trials has a substantial potential for eroding the advances of the last two decades in our ability to assure ourselves of the effectiveness of drugs that are proposed for marketing" (p. 48). This seems too strong. Perhaps it would be better to just conclude that there are costs (because of trial size considerations) and potential problems (because of possible design problems and unwarranted assumptions) that we confront whenever we adopt an active-controlled design. Naturally, these costs and potential problems will have to be weighed against the risks to the control group in a placebo-controlled trial of not receiving effective therapy.

In a series of articles, A. L. Gould has argued for using information from previous placebo-controlled trials about the response to the placebo as a further control in a current active-controlled trial.[46] This approach makes the reliance on a historical control group even more explicit than the implicit reliance found in standard active-controlled trials. Gould's approach offers still another alternative whose costs and potential problems will have to be weighed against the risks to the control group in a new placebo-controlled trial when deciding what type of trial to run.

Withholding Intracoronary Streptokinase

Keeping in mind the need both to save lives by avoiding placebo control groups and to run good trials by using them, we turn to the first of our issues: should placebo-controlled trials of the intravenous administration of thrombolytic agents have been conducted after FDA approval of intracoronary streptokinase in 1982? Some might argue that this is a very straightforward question. The Declaration of Helsinki, which is the foundation of all later codes of research ethics, specifically mandates, as we have seen, that every patient, including those in the control group, should be given the best proven therapeutic methods. With the approval of intracoronary SK by the FDA in 1982, it became one of those best proven therapeutic modalities, which should not have been withheld from the control group. There was, of course, a need for trials of the intravenous administration of SK and other thrombolytic agents, but they should have been conducted as active-controlled trials with intracoronary SK as the active control.

This argument from the standards of the Declaration of Helsinki is straightforward but unconvincing because it rests upon the Declaration's absolute ban, a ban whose absoluteness can be questioned. Suppose that all of the following conditions are met: (1) withholding the proven therapy for the period of the clinical trial is unlikely to produce any significant long-term losses for the patient; (2) the patient is aware that the therapy in question is proven to be efficacious and may be withheld as part of the trial and nevertheless agrees to participate in the trial; (3) conducting the trial as a placebo-controlled trial rather than as an active-controlled trial produces considerable scientific gains and/or substantially lessens the cost of conducting the trial. If all of these conditions (drawn from, but not identical with, the conditions mentioned by the FDA and by the Royal College of Physicians) are met, then both the requirements of respecting patient autonomy and of protecting patients from excessive risks are met, and the research in question would be morally licit. The Declaration of Helsinki's absolute ban cannot be accepted and cannot therefore serve as the basis for a sound argument.

A recent study illustrates these points.[47] The authors examined data from drug trials submitted to the FDA to support the approval of various beta blockers and calcium antagonists for the treatment of chronic angina. Most of these trials involved a placebo control group which received only sublingual nitroglycerin as needed for the period of the trial (2 to 23 weeks) despite the approval of various antianginal agents. The study showed that there was no difference in the risk of undergoing a serious adverse event between the treatment group and the placebo group. In light of that finding, and subject to the condition that the patients give full consent, the authors conclude, in agreement with our previously noted criteria, that further trials of such agents could proceed with use of a placebo control group despite the approval of various antianginal agents.

While adequate as a reply to the argument from the Declaration of Helsinki, these observations are insufficient to justify the placebo-controlled trials of the intravenously administered thrombolytic agents. Myocardial infarctions are after all life-threatening conditions, and intracoronary SK had been approved because it reduced mortality. Condition (1) was *not* satisfied in our case, so the placebo-controlled trials which withheld intracoronary SK cannot be justified by the same criteria that would justify placebo-controlled trials of antianginal agents.

It is worth noting, as was pointed out in the previous section, that the FDA, which disagrees with the Declaration of Helsinki, does agree that placebo-controlled trials are unethical where existing treatment is life-prolonging. The authors of the above cited study agree as well: "It is clear that a placebo group cannot be used when existing treatment is known to favorably affect survival or irreversible morbidity."[48] This raises our question again: In light of the fact that the 1982 FDA approval of intracoronary SK was based on the evidence that it reduced mortality from myocardial infarctions, how could placebo-controlled trials of intravenous thrombolytic agents (which denied to the control group any thrombolytic therapy) have been justified?

I see two possible responses. The first claims that the trials were justified because the patients consented to the possible withholding of thrombolytic therapy. The second claims that despite FDA approval, intracoronary SK had not really been proven to be effective. Let us examine each of these responses separately.

The first response faces several difficulties. To begin with, the earliest large trials (GISSI and ISIS-2) did not obtain the patient's informed consent to withhold intracoronary SK. As will be explained and discussed in the next section of this chapter, GISSI did not obtain any consent and ISIS-2 did not address the alternative of intracoronary SK in its consent process in most countries. Second, as we shall show in the next section, it is far from clear that informed consent is a meaningful process in emergency research such as research on the use of thrombolytic therapy after myocardial infarctions. Given that this is so, it is hard to see how the patient's informed consent, even if it had been obtained, would have been

sufficient to justify withholding all thrombolytic therapy. Third, and most crucial, obtaining informed consent addresses the autonomy requirements for licit
research only; it does not address the consequentialist risk–benefit requirements.
As we saw in the previous section, all analyses of research ethics have properly
insisted that both these requirements must be met. So even if the placebo-controlled
trials had obtained informed consent to not using intracoronary SK as well as to
participating, and even if that was a meaningful consent process, that consent would
not by itself justify those trials exposing the patients in the control group to the
higher risk of death. The research might have been illicit, even if none of the autonomy rights of the patient had been violated.

That leaves the second response. It challenges the claim that intracoronary SK
had been proven to be effective at the time of FDA approval. This issue was already
examined in Chapter 1. We saw there that the May 1982 FDA approval was based
primarily on a company-maintained registry, and that there were serious scientific questions about the data which did not even come from a controlled trial. As
late as 1984, when the FDA published its account of the use of thrombolytic agents
in evolving myocardial infarctions,[49] the best that it could appeal to was the data
from Kennedy's Western Washington trial.[50] Those data are impressive. They came
from a placebo-controlled randomized trial, and they showed a reduction in mortality from the 11.2 percent mortality rate in the placebo control group to the 3.7
percent mortality rate in the streptokinase group. This result is very significant
($p < 0.02$) despite the small number of patients (250) involved. It might nevertheless be argued that the Western Washington trial was too small to justify the
claim that intracoronary SK was so clearly efficacious that a placebo control group
in further trials was unjustified.

This is a possible response, although it is far from convincing. The trouble is
that it requires us to heavily discount not merely the registry, which is easy to do
because of its noncontrolled nature, but also the impressive data from the well-
designed Western Washington trial. It requires us to say that it is sometimes permissible to run a placebo-controlled trial in the context of a life-threatening illness when an approved drug is being withheld from a control group despite the
results of a well-designed trial showing a major reduction in mortality. To return
to Temple's criterion, it requires us to say that had intracoronary SK been used in
these studies, we were not sure it would have better results than a placebo. None
of these claims which discount the results of the Western Washington trial are
very persuasive.

My own conclusion then is that Anderson's group was right in the claim that
no placebo-controlled trials were justified once intracoronary SK was approved.
For the sake of the rest of our discussion, however, we will accept the discounting
of the results from the Western Washington trial and the consequence that placebo-

controlled trials were justified after FDA approval of intracoronary SK. That will enable us to examine our second issue: Were placebo-controlled trials justified even after the first data came in (from GISSI and from the Yusuf analysis of pooled data) about the effectiveness of intravenous thrombolytic therapy?

Withholding Intravenous Streptokinase

Before turning to our specific example, we need to explore the general issue it raises regarding the ethics of withholding from a control group a therapy that has not yet been approved by the relevant regulatory agency for use in the clinical setting in question but which has been shown in one or more trials to be effective and safe in that clinical setting.

Two preliminary points need to be kept in mind. The first is that it is obviously acceptable to withhold an experimental drug at least in those cases in which the subjects in the placebo group are unlikely to suffer significant long-term losses and consent to be randomized in light of that information, since even approved drugs can be withheld in such cases. So our issue is best reformulated as follows: Is it ethical to withhold from a control group a therapy which has not yet been formally approved for use but which has been shown in one or more trials to be effective and safe if the subjects in the control group may suffer significant long-term losses from being in that group?

The second preliminary point is that it is important to distinguish our question from the statistical question as to when preliminary data in a given trial are sufficiently impressive that the trial should be terminated. As noted in Chapter 1, a series of stopping rules has emerged in the statistics literature, and these rules are designed as answers to the statistical question. But that is not our question. Our question is far broader in scope, since it covers data from other trials and not just preliminary data from the trial in question. Our question may arise even before a trial is commenced, when one asks whether it is permissible to begin a trial involving a placebo control group given earlier impressive studies. Our question may arise during the course of a trial, when one asks whether it is permissible to continue a trial involving a placebo control group given newly available impressive data from another trial which has been completed. Our question is therefore not answered by any stopping rule, since our question arises in many cases in which stopping rules are irrelevant. This point has been inadequately stressed in the literature. Moreover, stopping rules are designed only to answer the statistical question as to whether the preliminary data are so good that they must be accepted as significant evidence that the null hypothesis is false rather than as an artifact due to the data being looked at too soon. They are not designed to answer the ethical questions as to whether, in light of the risks to the subjects in the placebo control group from being in that group, it is unethical to continue use of a placebo control group even if there is a real possibility that the data are just artifactual. The answer to the statistical question tells us only about the likelihood of the data being just artifactual; it does not tell us what to do given that likelihood and given the risk of losses to the subjects. So even in those cases in which both our question and the question posed by the statistical stopping rules are relevant, our question examines more issues than those examined by the purely statistical question.

There has been an extensive literature devoted to the ethical issues raised by our question. Unfortunately, most of the standard discussions focus on the setting where researchers are considering stopping a trial earlier than planned because of promising but as yet inconclusive data from their trial. I know of only a few outstanding discussions of how ongoing trials should be affected by data from *other* trials, some from clinical trial groups who faced this issue during the course of their trial and some from theoreticians.[51] However, I think that we will find it helpful in developing a reasoned response to our broader question if we begin by examining various proposals which have been advocated in the standard discussions.

A good point of departure is a classic analysis developed by Dr. Thomas Chalmers in 1967–1968.[52] A striking feature of this analysis is a radical shift of opinion by Chalmers between his initial presentation of his analysis in 1967 and his final published analysis in 1968. The published report contains both analyses. Chalmers originally claimed that it would be unethical to randomize a patient into a trial once there are some data favoring one arm over the other. His argument for that claim was straightforward:

> But what about the rights of the patient who enters a study at a time when one treatment is leading the other, but when the study is being continued because the difference is not significant? One can easily argue that since the difference is not significant, the result can be reversed by further experience. But one can also argue that the welfare of that one patient is more assured if he receives the treatment that is ahead rather than the one that is currently behind in the evaluation. In other words, randomization could be unfair to him because he might be assigned to a treatment that has less than 50 percent chance of being shown to be the correct one. . . . To this problem I can see no solution.[53]

Before publication of his analysis, however, Chalmers rejected this argument and conclusion and put forward the following alternative:

> A second modification in my thinking has developed with regard to how to handle the problem of an impending statistically significant difference between two treatments before the planned conclusion of a study. The dilemma is well outlined above. The only practical solution, not included in the document, is the setting up of a data monitoring committee of clinicians, statisticians, and consumer representatives who

will look at the trends in studies and consider cessation as soon as the results in that study, or other studies reported since the inception of the one in question, indicate that this should be done, and stop the trial whenever it is in the best interests of the participants to do so, recognizing that the patients have agreed in response to the informed-consent document that the study will be continued until a useful answer is obtained.[54]

Chalmers has developed this final analysis in other publications,[55] and the idea of such an independent data monitoring committee is now widely accepted.[56]

It is important to note that there are two separate considerations mentioned in Chalmers's second analysis, the claim that the research is justified by the patient's consent and the claim that the research is justified by the presence of an independent committee which gives its continued approval to the research. The former claim is clearly insufficient. While the patient's continued consent is necessary for the research to be legitimate, it is not, as we have seen, sufficient. Most attention has therefore focused on Chalmers's second claim about the legitimizing role of the independent committee.

As a procedural suggestion, this point is clearly well-taken. Researchers might have a wide variety of interests which would bias their decision in one way or another as to whether certain research should be commenced or continued in light of data becoming available. Putting this decision in the hands of an impartial group of outsiders can help avoid these biases. But however valuable this procedural point may be, it seems to address neither Chalmer's substantive argument nor our substantive issue. Such committees will also need to address the question of when randomized trials are licit in terms of available data and the argument that such trials might be unfair to the patients involved in them. Their existence hardly resolves the issue in question.

Some light is shed on what Chalmers has in mind by consideration of one of his other important articles on this topic.[57] It is clear from this article that a major function of the committee is to enable the patient's treating physician to remain blinded to the data being accumulated in the trial. The legitimacy of continuing the trial, in light of accumulating data, can be regularly examined by the committee, while the patient's clinician, who does not know the accumulating data, is not violating his or her obligation to provide the best therapy by allowing the patient to remain in the trial even if the accumulating data favor one of the approaches being tested. To quote the article:

> If the physician owes it to this next patient to give that patient the therapy most likely to be successful for him, can he include him in the study when he believes that only a few more patients are needed to reach a conclusion that "A" is going to be better than "B"? . . . An apparent solution is to keep the results confidential from the participating physician until a peer review group says that the study is over.

There is much to be said about whether or not this approach resolves the ethical problem of the clinician deciding whether to recommend participation in a trial to his or her patient. It certainly does not solve that problem if the data in question are from other trials whose results are suddenly announced. But whether or not this approach helps with the ethical problem of the clinician, it certainly does not help with our issue, which is not about the ethical obligations of treating physicians to their personal patients. Our problem is an ethical issue faced by the research community organizing and conducting the trial, including any data-monitoring committee, and that entire community, as Chalmers himself recognizes, cannot remain blinded to newly available data.

I turn to two alternative approaches suggested by two philosophers who have addressed these issues, Don Marquis and Benjamin Freedman. Marquis's suggestion comes at the end of an article which is very critical of the ethical licitness of running any randomized clinical trials. His analysis is quite similar to Chalmers's original analysis, and he is very critical (among other things) of Chalmers's later appeal to independent monitoring boards. He ends the article with the following suggestion: "Perhaps what is needed is an ethics that will justify the conscription of subjects for medical research. Nothing less seems to justify present practice."[58]

I have heard this approach advocated by others in discussion, and it is related to Pocock's important claim that we need to emphasize collective as well as individual needs as we deal with this issue,[59] so it needs to be discussed. Applied to our problem, it is the claim that it would be ethical to withhold from a placebo control group a therapy which has been proven safe and effective even if the subjects in the control group may suffer a long-term loss if the gains from running such a placebo controlled trial (as opposed to just an active-controlled trial) are so great from a collective perspective that they would justify conscripting subjects into a trial.

It seems to me that the following observations about this proposal are in order. First, it does go against all the adopted codes and principles of research ethics. Second, it trades heavily upon the analogy to wartime conscription, with the image being that the war against disease is like other wars in which we conscript those who may even die. The analogy is far from appropriate, even if we grant (and this is far from obvious) that conscription into an army is justified. It is a rare disease that threatens our public order in the way in which being attacked by an external enemy does. Moreover, military conscription requires a public determination through the democratic representative process of its necessity, and it is hard to see anything analogous to that in the research setting. Third, we need to remember that active-controlled trials remain an option, even if there are costs and problems associated with them. It is hard to see how the gains from the placebo-controlled trial will be great enough to justify conscription when we have the option of paying the extra costs of the active-controlled trial.

Freedman's suggestion is quite different.[60] He would allow placebo-controlled randomized trials as long as there exists within the expert clinical community no consensus about the comparative merits of the regimens being tested. Only when the accumulated evidence is so strong that no open-minded clinician is in doubt about the comparative merits would the trial in question be unethical.

This sociological approach is very troubling. Unless we simply declare researchers who assess the evidential situation differently from us to be close-minded, we will be forced to accept as licit randomized placebo-controlled trials long after impressive evidence exists for the benefits of receiving the active treatment. Freedman is aware of this objection, and he attempts to meet it as follows:

> Because of the arbitrary character of human judgment and persuasion, some ethical problems regarding the termination of a trial will remain. Clinical equipoise will confine these problems to unusual or extreme cases, however, and will allow us to cast persistent problems in the proper terms.

I find this response unsatisfactory. Our case is not an unusual or an extreme case, and yet feelings about whether the merit of some form of thrombolytic therapy was clear ranged all the way from Anderson's view that it was settled after the Western Washington trial to the view of those who found it unsettled until trials such as ASSET were completed. Such differences exist in many cases. Does that mean, as Freedman's theory seems to entail, that those who stopped trials early or didn't start them on the grounds that further placebo-controlled trials were unethical were wrong, and wrong just because other colleagues disagreed? I think not. I think that we need a more objective approach. I turn therefore to an attempt to develop an objective answer to our question, one that will enable us to decide in an objective fashion when it was and when it was not appropriate to run placebo-controlled trials of the thrombolytic agents.

My point of departure will be an analysis, primarily devoted to the interim data problem, developed by the eminent biostatistician Paul Meier in 1979.[61] Meier began his analysis by restating the constraint that it is illicit to abuse research subjects even if that abuse would lead to significant gains in clinical knowledge. But he suggested that we need to have a better understanding of what constitutes abuse:

> As I hope it is now clear, the key to what I think is wrong with most of the arguments on the ethics of clinical experiments lies in the notion that it is unethical to deny an individual any expected benefit of treatment A over treatment B, regardless of how small that benefit may be or how uncertain. . . . As a matter of normal social behavior, most of us would be quite willing to forego a modest expected gain in the general interest of learning something of value. However, we should want to be assured that what we agree to give up is indeed modest and not a truly large amount.

Applying that approach to our problem, Meier's claim would become the claim that it would be ethical to withhold from a placebo control group a therapy which has been proven safe and effective in at least one trial, even if the subjects in the control group may suffer a long-term loss, if the probability of suffering that loss and/or the significance of that loss is sufficiently low that most of us would judge the gain of getting the treatment a sufficiently modest gain.

This approach seems the most promising of any we have examined, although it depends for its validity on developing an account of what is a sufficiently modest gain and it is not easy to do that. After all, people vary both in their degree of altruism and in their risk-aversiveness, and these variations will affect their sense of how modest is the gain of getting the promising therapy as well as their willingness to undergo the risks of being in a placebo control group. So how are we to set the level of when the gain of getting the promising therapy is sufficiently modest to justify continued trials using placebo control groups?

Two approaches suggest themselves. One, the person-dependent approach, suggests that the acceptable additional risk level from being in the control group is that level of additional risk to which the particular research subject freely and knowingly consents. The other, the person-independent approach, suggests that the acceptable level is that level of additional risk to which a reasonable person of average altruism and risk-aversiveness would freely and knowingly consent. Some combination of these two approaches was adopted by the VA investigators of the early use of AZT who continued their trial after promising results were announced by the AIDS Clinical Trial Group;[62] their sophisticated use of additional informed consent to justify the continuation of their trial is the best exemplar I know of these approaches.

I think that we do need to combine both approaches. After all, the licitness of any particular research project depends upon meeting the demands both of autonomy and of consequentialism. The former will be met if the particular research subject freely and knowingly consents to assuming the additional risk. The latter will be met if the risk-benefit ratio is sufficiently favorable so that the reasonable person of average altruism and risk-aversiveness might find the additional risk acceptable.

We come, after this long discussion, to the following conclusion: it is ethical to withhold from a control group a therapy that has not yet been formally approved but that has been shown in one or more trials to be effective and safe, even if the subjects in the placebo control group are thereby exposed to a greater risk of long-term losses, only if those losses and the probabilities of their occurring are sufficiently small that (1) the subject, informed of all of this, freely consents to being randomized into the trial and (2) reasonable people, of an average degree of altruism and risk-aversiveness, informed of all this, might consent to being randomized into the trial.

This conclusion is related to, but not completely identical with, the position of Robert Levine.[63] Like him, I neither approve nor disapprove of all placebo-controlled trials; some are acceptable and others are not. Like him, I evaluate each proposed placebo-controlled trial in light of all the available data about the risks of being in the placebo control group. My approach differs only because it involves the explicit adoption of conditions (1) and (2).

With this standard in mind, we return to the question of whether further placebo-controlled trials (as opposed to active-controlled trials) of intravenous thrombolytic agents were morally permissible once the data from GISSI and from the analysis of the pooled data demonstrated the safety and efficacy of intravenous thrombolytic therapy. We know, of course, that the NIH-funded investigators conducting the TIMI series of trials concluded that they were not and therefore did not run a placebo-controlled trial of tPA. Were they correct, or were the investigators in other placebo-controlled trials correct in continuing their trials?

In setting the issue this way, I am presupposing that in fact GISSI and the pooled data did demonstrate the safety and efficacy of intravenous thrombolytic therapy. Not all investigators saw it that way. Dr. Alan Guerci, of Johns Hopkins University, who headed one of the placebo-controlled trials which did continue, had the following to say about these issues:

> The Johns Hopkins trial of intravenous tPA began in December 1984. In February of 1986, a group of Italian investigators reported the first convincing evidence that the intravenous administration of any blood clot dissolving medicine (in this case streptokinase) reduced mortality from heart attacks. The reduction in mortality observed in the Italian study was concentrated among patients treated within one hour of the onset of the heart attack and among patients with large heart attacks. The reductions in mortality in these groups were extremely persuasive; the reduction in mortality attributable to intravenous streptokinase for other patients was questionable. Therefore, after deliberation with the Johns Hopkins Institutional Review Board, I and the other Hopkins investigators decided to exclude patients with large heart attacks who presented to the hospital within 90 minutes of the onset of symptoms because we thought that it would be unethical to randomly assign certain of these patients to receive placebo. Genentech, a sponsor of the Johns Hopkins trial, accepted this decision. This decision and its acceptance by Genentech are important because exclusion of these high risk patients exerted a prejudicial effect against Genentech's interests in the outcome of this trial. This is indisputably the case because patients treated with blood clot dissolving medicines early in the course of large heart attacks are likely to gain the most in terms of recovery of the strength of the heart and those treated with placebo would sustain the most damage to the heart. Thus, our decision to exclude these patients from the trial eliminated the type of patients most likely to produce the result which Genentech naturally wanted.
>
> In June of 1986, a group of German, Swiss, and Canadian investigators reported in the *New England Journal of Medicine* that intravenous streptokinase had failed to reduce mortality when compared to placebo in patients with heart attacks. This study did not contain enough high risk patients treated early to refute the earlier

Italian observation, but did serve to support our belief that it was ethically appropriate to continue a placebo controlled trial of tPA.

On February 28, 1987, a letter reporting a highly significant reduction in mortality in nearly 4,000 patients treated with streptokinase or placebo within four hours of the onset of heart attack appeared in the British journal *The Lancet*. As a result of this information, I and the other Johns Hopkins investigators thought that it was no longer acceptable to enroll patients in a placebo controlled trial of thrombolytic therapy within four hours (the time limit used in the Hopkins study) of the onset of a heart attack. This matter was discussed with the Johns Hopkins Institutional Review Board, and the Johns Hopkins trial was terminated in March of 1987. As in the case of the previous protocol modification, this decision was also prejudicial to Genentech's interests because early termination of the study meant a smaller number of patients enrolled and a lesser probability that any difference between patients treated with tPA and those receiving placebo would be statistically significant. Nevertheless, Genentech again accepted our decision.[64]

I must respectfully disagree with Guerci's account. To begin with, his account of the GISSI results is not consonant with the actual data in the GISSI publication. Table 2.2, from that original publication, presents the crucial results. While it certainly shows that the best results were obtained in patients treated within 1 hour of the onset of symptoms, very significant results were also obtained in patients treated less quickly. The reduction in mortality for patients treated within the first 3 hours was significant at the level of 0.0005 and the reduction in mortality for patients treated within 3–6 hours was significant at the level of 0.03. These were, of course, data from an entire trial, not from an interim analysis, so the usual

TABLE 2.2 Mortality by Hours from Onset of Symptoms

Hours	SK % (deaths/n)	Control group % (deaths/n)	p	Relative risk (95% Confidence Internal)	Total % (deaths/n)
<3	9.2 (278/3,016)	12.0 (369/3,078)	0.0005	0.74 (0.63–0.87)	10.6 (647/6,094)
>3–6	11.7 (217/1,849)	14.1 (254/1,800)	0.03	0.80 (0.66–0.98)	12.9 (471/3,649)
>6–9	12.6 (87/693)	14.1 (93/659)	NS	0.87 (0.64–1.19)	13.3 (180/1,352)
>9–12	15.8 (46/292)	13.6 (41/302)	NS	1.19 (0.75–1.87)	14.6 (87/549)
<1	8.2 (52/635)	15.4 (99/642)	0.0001	0.49 (0.340–0.69)	11.8 (151/1,277)

Key: n = no. of patients; NS = not significant ($p > 0.05$).

Source: GISSI, "Effectiveness of Intravenous Thrombolytic Therapy in Acute Myocardial Infarction," *Lancet*, February 22, 1986, p. 399

levels of significance apply, making these results significant. I cannot therefore agree with Guerci's statement about patients presenting more than 1 hour after the onset of symptoms: "The reduction in mortality attributable to intravenous streptokinase for other patients was questionable." Moreover, his account pays absolutely no attention to the data available from Yusuf's 1985 pooled data analysis. That analysis showed, in fact, a continued significant reduction in mortality as long as 24 hours after the onset of symptoms. It certainly would not support any claim that the benefits of thrombolytic therapy were confined to patients presenting in the first hour after the onset of symptoms. A recent reanalysis has reinforced the validity of Yusuf's analysis, arguing that neither GISSI nor ISIS-2 was really necessary because the pooled data from the earlier trials were more than adequate.[65] The actual data available in 1986 support our claim that GISSI and the pooled analysis showed the safety and efficacy of intravenous streptokinase at least for patients presenting within the first 6 hours.

We turn then to the question of the licitness of the trials in light of the data. It will be, I think, useful to examine the attitudes on this question of the investigators in three large placebo-controlled trials, ISIS-2, ASSET, and AIMS. We will see, in that process, how some of the other ideas we have discussed played a role in their thinking. Having done that, we will analyze the issue in light of the standard I have advocated.

The best evidence I can find about the attitude of the ISIS-2 steering committee to our issues appears in a decision they made in January–February 1987 (almost a year after the GISSI results were available) when they were informed by their data monitoring committee that there was evidence beyond reasonable doubt that streptokinase reduced in-hospital mortality among patients presenting within 0–4 hours after the onset of symptoms. The steering committee pointed out that a trial was still needed to answer questions about efficacy in later presenting patients and also to answer some questions about the early presenting patients (would the benefits hold up after discharge and are there some subclasses who should not receive streptokinase). In the end, they decided that "ISIS-II will continue through 1987 and patients (whether within 0–4, 5–12, or 13–24 h. of pain onset) can be randomized if the responsible physician remains, in the light of this and other evidence, uncertain as to whether streptokinase is indicated."[66]

Initially I found it very difficult to understand the basis of their decision. After all, both their preliminary data and the final data from the GISSI trial showed a significant reduction in mortality in the treatment group. Their own data monitoring board found the evidence of efficacy in the group presenting early beyond reasonable doubt. How could a placebo control group involving early presenting patients be justified? The best explanation I can come up with is that they were implicitly presupposing something like Freedman's approach. As long as there were responsible clinicians who remained uncertain as to whether SK was indicated, there was no consensus within the clinical community, and as long as there was no consensus, it was permissible for them (despite the fact that their own monitoring committee said that the evidence was beyond reasonable doubt) to continue to run the trial and randomize early presenting patients of those clinicians. For the reasons indicated in my discussion of Freedman's approach, I find this approach inappropriate. The episode is an excellent example of the risk that this sociological approach gives too much ethical force to residual dissenting opinions.

It is also important to learn what we can from this example about the value of Chalmers's suggestion that an independent data-monitoring board can help deal with these problems. The ISIS-2 trial had such a board, and it was the board's members who identified the early very significant data. As noted in Chapter 1, Sir Richard Doll, the chair of that monitoring board, felt that the decision to continue the trial was in the hands of the steering committee running the trial, not in the hands of the data-monitoring board. My own conclusion from this is that Chalmers's suggestion can help only if the independent reviewers have the power to stop the trial, not just advise on that point.

Other problems can arise when one relies too heavily on Chalmers's procedural proposal of independent review. One of them, the delay problem, is illustrated by the workings of the ASSET trial. The ASSET trial began after the GISSI data were available and continued for a year after the publication of the interim data from the ISIS-2 trial. It involved patients presenting less than 6 hours after the onset of symptoms. ASSET employed a three-person independent monitoring committee. How did that committee help deal with the problem of the legitimacy of continuing to use a placebo control group? I quote from the report:

> The ethical committee did advise, on the basis of the published results of other studies of thrombolysis, that it was no longer reasonable to include patients in a placebo-controlled study, but this advice coincided with the inclusion of the intended total of 5,000 patients.[67]

That advice came then in February 1988, when recruitment was completed, and it came 2 years after the publication of the GISSI data and the pooled data and 1 year after the preliminary ISIS-2 data were published. The conclusion is clear: unless independent review committees move with dispatch—and have the power to stop trials—they will be of little help.

I turn finally to the attitudes of the AIMS investigators to our issues. Their attitudes are of particular interest, because they were running a placebo-controlled trial of APSAC in early presenting patients which began after GISSI and continued for a while after ISIS-2 published its preliminary report, and this was in sharp contrast to the other major trial of APSAC (Anderson's trial), which never used a placebo control group, relying instead on an active control group which received intracoronary thrombolytic therapy.

They describe the decisions of their independent monitoring board as follows:

> The initial proposal was to undertake one interim analysis half-way through the trial. . . . However, in the light of other trials showing highly significant mortality reductions after thrombolytic therapy [references provided to GISSI, the pooled data, and ISIS-2], the data monitoring committee redefined the plans for interim analysis.[68]

In fact, that revised plan led to the trial being stopped after only 1,000 patients were enrolled, instead of the 2,000 originally planned.

Two observations seem to be in place. The first is that the independent committee seems to have functioned in this case. It seems to have responded quickly to ISIS-2 and it seems to have had the power to modify the trial design. The second is that it unfortunately relied upon the wrong tool, namely, interim analyses and stopping rules. As noted previously, such rules only address the question of when the data from a trial are good enough so that we can conclude that the results demonstrate a significant finding, a question which is relevant to deciding to stop a trial because of its own data. They do not even begin to address the question of whether a trial should be initiated or continued in light of data *from other trials*; their use in the AIMS trial in response to that question is just inappropriate. Because of this misunderstanding, the AIMS investigators and independent monitoring committee managed to avoid confronting our issue.

We have argued thus far, contrary to Guerci, that the GISSI data and the Yusuf pooled data analysis demonstrated the efficacy and the safety of thrombolytic therapy at least in patients presenting up to 6 hours after the onset of symptoms. We have also argued that the investigators in three major placebo-controlled trials (ISIS-2, ASSET, and AIMS) failed to adequately address the ethical issues at stake in their continued use of placebo-controlled trials, in large measure because they relied on approaches (the Freedman approach, the Chalmers approach, and the reliance on interim stopping rules) whose validity as a response to our issue is questionable. We turn then to the question of whether these placebo-controlled trials could have been justified in light of our modification of the Meier approach.

Would reasonable patients of average altruism and risk-aversiveness have voluntarily agreed to be in these placebo-controlled trials if they had been informed about the results of GISSI and of the pooled data analysis? I ask the reader to consider the following thought experiment (applied to the ISIS-2 case; a slightly different question would have to be asked about AIMS and ASSET): suppose you were asked in 1986 or 1987 whether you would agree to be in a trial of a new drug to treat your heart attack with a 50 percent chance of getting that drug and a 50 percent chance of not, when an earlier trial plus some other data had shown around a 20–25 percent reduction in death produced by taking that new drug. Would you agree? If not—and I think that most people would decline—is it because you are unreasonable or excessively selfish or too risk-aversive, or is it because you think that it's too much of a risk for you to undergo solely to advance knowledge? If the latter, if because you believe that what you are being asked to give up is more than a modest sacrifice, then you should conclude that the ISIS-2 trial (and analogously the ASSET and AIMS trials) were wrong to enroll patients in a placebo control group after the data from GISSI came out. And if this is true with only the data from GISSI, it is even more true (at least for patients presenting within 4 hours) after the preliminary results from ISIS-2 were available.

But didn't the patients in these trials give voluntary informed consent to being randomized? And if they did, how can it be claimed that reasonable people would not? For ISIS-2, there is a quick response to these questions. For reasons to be discussed in the next section, ISIS-2 had two suggested consent forms, an abbreviated form and a longer form. The information mentioned about GISSI is *not* found in either of those forms. This is not necessarily a criticism of the ISIS-2 forms, since the whole question of informed consent in emergency situations needs extensive discussion, which it will receive in the next section. In relation to ASSET and AIMS, where I do not know whether the information about the GISSI data was included in consent forms, that discussion in the next section will question whether the informed consent relied upon in this defense could be adequate even if the information about GISSI was provided. All of this means that the objectors are wrong in saying that actual enrollment in these trials shows that reasonable, *informed* patients would agree to participate.

One final response needs to be considered. Until nearly the very end of these trials, intravenous SK was not formally approved. Consequently, if the patients in the placebo control group had not been in the trial, they would not have received any thrombolytic therapy, so what harm could the trial do? Leaving aside the possibility of their receiving intracoronary SK, which had been approved, this objection misses the point that, given the availability of SK, many doctors were doing what they had a right to do—providing their patients with intravenous SK outside of trials such as ISIS-2.[69] Thus the placebo patients were being harmed by being randomized.

We have, in this section, addressed two issues. The first was whether there should have ever been any placebo-controlled trials of intravenous thrombolytic therapy or whether all such trials should have employed active control groups receiving intracoronary thrombolytic agents. Our conclusion was that there probably should not have been such trials once the FDA approval of intracoronary SK was supported by the results from the Western Washington trial. The second was whether placebo-controlled trials of intravenous thrombolytic therapy were justified after

GISSI and the publication of the pooled data analysis, even if they had been justified earlier despite FDA approval and the results of the Western Washington trial. Our conclusion was that at least for patients presenting in the first 6 hours after the onset of symptoms, there should not have been active-controlled trials. This conclusion was based upon an adaptation of Meier's approach to these issues, an adaptation which demands that the requirements of both autonomy and beneficence be met before the research in question is licit.

One final observation. My goal in this section has not been to say that there were good researchers who refused to run placebo-controlled trials and bad researchers who were willing to run them. I have proceeded throughout on the assumption that all of the investigators in all of the trials were good people who were operating with the best of intentions. My goal rather was to argue that even good researchers with the best of intentions can make mistaken decisions in this complex area of placebo-controlled versus active-controlled trials, and that this reinforces the need for better guidelines in this area. My hope is that this discussion and the guidelines I have provided may help future investigators make better decisions in this area.

Consent in the Emergency Room

The investigators in several of the major trials of the thrombolytic agents adopted innovative approaches to the requirement of obtaining informed consent. The most notable example was the GISSI trial, where the investigators made a decision not to require informed consent because "the patient's predicament was judged too acute for acceptable application of the procedure."[70] Of equal interest was the approach of the ISIS-2 investigators, who adopted in their protocol the following policy:

> The degree and timing of consent is entirely a matter for individual doctors to decide for individual patients in the light of local requirements and advice from any relevant ethical committees. This will result in a wide range of practices, ranging from formal written consent . . . at one extreme, through various degrees of verbal consent, to, at the opposite extreme, some vague mention of the trial intended merely to offer patients an easy opportunity to *initiate* any discussion they may want.[71]

Their sample consent form provided only some very basic information about the trial supplemented by technical details, but there was also a far more formal and complete consent form intended for use in the United States to conform with FDA and NIH requirements. Only that U.S. form discussed intracoronary streptokinase as an alternative, and even it did not state how effective that alternative was in limiting mortality.

What motivated the adoption of these approaches? Two suggestions come to mind. The first (explicitly stated by the GISSI investigators) was doubts about whether informed consent is meaningful and appropriate in the emergency setting. A similar viewpoint was expressed by Dr. Richard Peto of the ISIS-2 trial: "The American documents were three pages of legalistic junk. That's not the sort of thing you want to push under someone's nose as he's having a heart attack, terrified, with chest pain, on morphine. You want to tell him about the trial, but you want to be humane."[72] The second suggestion, implicit in the ISIS-2 protocol, was the concern that it would be possible to enroll the many thousands of subjects required for the trial only if the burden of all aspects of the trial, including obtaining informed consent, was minimized for the busy professionals at the participating hospitals. Both these issues deserve serious attention, but we will focus our attention on the first issue, which raises many subtle problems.

Our strategy for examining this issue will be as follows. We will first look at the ideal conditions for obtaining voluntary informed consent and the ideal patients from whom to obtain such consent. We will then see why these ideals are unlikely to be met when doing emergency room research involving acutely ill patients with life-threatening illnesses such as myocardial infarctions. After evaluating various suggestions that have been made in the literature and in formal policies for dealing with less than ideal consent in these circumstances, we will develop a new approach based upon an analysis of the reasons for obtaining informed consent. Finally, we will apply this analysis to the clinical trials we have been examining.

I turn first to the issue of the ideal conditions for obtaining voluntary informed consent. A good introduction to these conditions is found in the following requirement present in both the NIH and FDA requirements: "An investigator shall seek such consent only under circumstances that provide the prospective subject or the representative sufficient opportunity to consider whether or not to participate and that minimize the possibility of coercion or undue influence."[73] This statement emphasizes the need for time to consider whether or not to participate, as well as the need for conditions which minimize undue influences, but it provides few guidelines about the time or conditions in question. A fuller analysis of the time issue, with some informal guidelines, is found in the following statement from the Royal College of Physicians:

> It is unreasonable to ask a patient to agree on the spot to take part in research which either involves more than minimal risk or involves extended inconvenience or discomfort. Time should be allowed for the patient to consider the position, to read the Information Sheet in unhurried circumstances and to discuss it with a friend or relative. . . . For research which is low risk or undemanding, it might, for example, be quite acceptable for a patient attending a hospital clinic or a general practitioner to have a cup of tea and to reach a decision within a few minutes. In other circumstances it might seem appropriate for the decision to be declared at a different visit on a different day.[74]

In short, then, a major circumstance required for an ideal consent is that the subject have adequate time, in light of the seriousness of the decision, to consider the information provided and to reach a decision.

We need to be concerned not merely with the ideal conditions for obtaining consent but also with the ideal patients from whom to obtain consent. A quick sketch of an ideal patient pictures a fully competent, rather than an impaired, decision maker. It is of some interest to note that the United States still lacks formal policies for research involving less that fully competent patients analogous to the formal policies we have governing research on children,[75] although the NIH has adopted a policy for intramural research on such subjects.[76] Nor does the United States have a clear and precise account of what a fully competent patient is like, although a great deal—often conflicting—has been written on that question.[77] I have elsewhere defended the view, which I shall just adopt here, that the fully competent patient with respect to a given decision is the patient who, in connection with that decision, is capable of receiving and remembering information, appropriately assessing that information, using that information in making a decision, and making a decision and giving a reason for it.[78]

Putting these points together, I conclude that an ideal consent which fully plays the role of consent in making research licit is a voluntary informed consent given by a fully competent subject who has the time to consider the information before deciding whether to participate in the research. But what if these conditions are not fully met? Is the consent then irrelevant? I think not. It seems to me that all four of the relevant conditions on the consent (that it be voluntary, that it be informed, that it be made by a competent subject, and that the subject have adequate time) can be met to a greater or lesser degree, and that the appropriate thing to say is that the consent has greater force in legitimizing the research to the extent that these conditions are present to a greater degree. Our problem will then be how to analyze the licitness of research where the consent in question involves one or more of these factors present only to a modest degree.

In the mid-1970s Harmon Smith called attention to the fact that the conditions for obtaining ideal informed consent were far from fully met in patients presenting in an emergency room shortly after a myocardial infarction.[79] To begin with, as he pointed out, their physiological condition by itself challenged their competency to give consent:

> Patients with a suspected or confirmed diagnosis of acute myocardial infarction (MI) dramatically illustrate the futility, or at least the highly problematic value, of applying conventional criteria as the unexceptionable surety of valid consent. The signs of MI vary among patients, but ordinarily include all or a combination of the following: hypertension (especially high blood pressure), tachycardia (excessive rapidity of heart action), pallor, hypothermia (abnormally low temperature), and fast breathing or shortness of breath together with pain on breathing. Patients may also be

hypoxic (low oxygen content) and cyanotic (blueishness of skin from cardiac malfunction). They are frequently anxious and afraid; their emotional/psychological condition, together with diminished volumes of oxygen and blood to the brain, contributes commonly to a general disorientation through deteriorated mental function. Sedatives (e.g., morphine or Demerol) may also have affected mental function.

Moreover, as others have pointed out, the emergency nature of thrombolytic research just doesn't allow for the time required as part of the conditions for ideal consent. As the authors of one recent important study said:

> Clearly, the quality of consent given by a patient who has discussed the research protocol at length with his physician and has taken the consent form overnight to study will be entirely different from that obtained from a patient in the midst of an acute medical emergency like myocardial infarction. The patient with an AMI must consent to a research protocol immediately in order to be enrolled and to receive maximal potential benefit from the therapy. There is simply not time to reflect, question, and consult.[80]

These observations are reinforced by some data from interviews of patients who participated in TIMI-I.[81] Of 28 patients interviewed before discharge about their consent, 21 had been given sedatives before consenting, only 13 thought that they were calm at the time, only 7 consented after family participation, and 20 of the 28 signed without reading the consent form. Despite their expressed satisfaction with the process, the meaningfulness of that type of consent is obviously questionable.

For all of these reasons, we may safely conclude, I would submit, that emergency room research involving patients with an acute myocardial infarction cannot be justified on the grounds that voluntary and informed consent has been obtained from a competent patient under ideal conditions. Our question of the licitness of research when one or more of these factors is present only to a modest degree is then extremely relevant to the licitness of emergency room research on patients with an acute myocardial infarction.

A number of possible views might be proposed to deal with this problem. Among them are the following:

1. Research is licit only when all these conditions are fully met and consent is obtained from the subject. All other research, however promising it may be, should be eschewed because respect for the rights of research subjects must be given the highest priority.
2. When the patient's consent does not meet all these conditions, investigators should seek to obtain consent from those family members of the subject who can give consent in a fashion that fully meets all these conditions, and it is

the consent of those family members which validates the research, even if a less than fully valid consent is also obtained from the research subject. Absent a fully valid consent, however, the research in question should not be conducted.

3. At least in those cases in which the research holds out a reasonable chance of providing significant benefits to the patient, research should be considered licit even if neither the patient nor the family member can give fully valid consent so long as either the patient or at least one family member can give consent in a way that partially meets these conditions. The more favorable the risk-to-benefit ratio of the research *to the patient*, the less these conditions can be met and the research still be licit.

4. If the risk-benefit ratio *to the patient* is sufficiently good, research may licitly be conducted without any consent from either the patient or a family member providing that the patient and/or the family is informed afterward and given the opportunity to consent to or to refuse further participation. This approach, for reasons to be discussed shortly, is often referred to as the deferred-consent approach.

It is important to keep in mind that approaches 3 and 4 are not mutually exclusive, since one may combine them so as to claim that, with appropriate risk-to-benefit ratios, the research may be justified either by less than fully valid consent or by deferred consent.

There is something to be said both for and against each of these approaches. The first approach draws its strength from its insistence that the principle of not using people as subjects without their consent be maintained. This insistence is desirable, in part because that principle is a fundamental constraint on licit behavior and in part because it is hard to know when to stop once you start making exceptions to it. Its weaknesses are that it may seriously impede important research on medical problems that typically involve conditions in which ideal consent cannot be obtained and that it may deny to the patients in question the benefits of the new therapies being tested. The second approach draws its strength from its commitment both to the principle of consent (in that the fully valid consent of family members is required) and to the needs of patients and society for research on incompetent subjects (in that patient consent, which cannot be obtained, is not required). Its weakness is that fully valid family consent may also be difficult if not impossible to obtain since the family may have no more time in an emergency to give the issue of participation adequate thought. The third approach draws its strength from its recognition that the benefits to the patient from participating are by themselves important justifications for the research and from its insistence that the principle of consent should nevertheless not be entirely neglected. Its weakness is that it allows strangers to decide on behalf of the patient whether the benefits of the research are sufficient to justify participation, a matter on which reasonable people might disagree. The final approach also draws its strength from its recognition that research may be justified because of its benefits to the patient and from its insistence that the principles of honesty and of obtaining consent when relevant and possible should be maintained. But to an even greater extent than the third approach, it allows research under certain conditions on the basis of others judging that the benefits are sufficient, and this questionable feature is its major weakness.

The emphasis of positions 3 and 4 on the benefits to the patient justifying the research is based upon the suggestion of the European Community noted earlier, while the emphasis of position 4 on deferred consent is based upon the views of the Royal College of Physicians, also noted earlier. But neither of these positions is fully developed, so we turn to the views of two groups involved in conducting emergency research who have developed detailed protocols that merit our consideration because they have utilized these positions.

The first is the approach developed by the Brain Resuscitation Clinical Trial group.[82] The research they were conducting involved a randomized trial of a calcium entry blocker in comatose survivors of cardiac arrest. Three doses of the drug or the placebo were given within 24 hours, with the first given within 30 minutes of restoration of spontaneous circulation. The patient's condition together with the time constraints always precluded obtaining prospective consent from the patient and almost always precluded obtaining prospective consent from the family. The first dose was therefore given before anyone's consent was obtained, but the family (when available) was asked for prospective consent before the next dose was administered (8 hours later). This is, of course, a version of approach 4. The second protocol was developed by a group studying the administration of thrombolytic therapy in ambulances to patients who had suffered a myocardial infarction and were being rushed to the hospital.[83] Their protocol involved a two-stage consent process, an initial consent by the patient in an ambulance to a loading dose of tPA (which was obtained by a paramedic on the basis of a brief read statement) and a full regular consent obtained at the hospital before the rest of the tPA was administered. This is close to approach 3, since a less than ideal consent was still obtained before the research was initiated. Notice, of course, that the patients in the second study had some capacity to give consent, unlike the patients in the first study, and that may help explain the difference in the two approaches. As already noted, 3 and 4 can be treated as supplementary rather than as in conflict with each other. Let us now examine both these protocols with care.

One preliminary observation. Both groups questioned the legality of their protocols in light of FDA and NIH regulations. Unfortunately, their discussions of legality were not helpful. The Brain Resuscitation group argued that their protocol fell under the emergency exception in the FDA regulations, while the thrombolytic therapy group was less sure, in part because tPA was already approved for use in myocardial infarctions. In fact, as we already pointed out early in this chapter, the FDA specifically excludes emergency room planned research from that exception. Similar problems arose in their discussions of the NIH regulations, in large measure because the meaning of the relevant exception is unclear. If such sophisticated groups have trouble ascertaining what the current federal regulations mean, these regulations obviously need to be clarified.[84]

In their most recent publication, the Brain Resuscitation group reported widespread family approval of their use of deferred consent. In 368 families, nearly all gave deferred consent and expressed approval of that mechanism for obtaining consent. Only 13 refused consent for further participation, with the primary reason being a fear that the end result would be the patient's surviving in a highly impaired manner. These data are obviously relevant to assessing the validity of their approach. If, in fact, we can reasonably assume that families will give informed consent afterward, then that assumption might well justify proceeding before one gets the consent. Despite the claims of the Brain Resuscitation group, however, I am far from satisfied that there really was deferred consent of any value. The authors themselves had the following to say:

> Although concerns were often expressed about the safety of the experimental drug, few families requested detailed information regarding this or the study methodology. Even fewer understood the concepts of or need for randomization, blinding, or placebo controls. Many felt relieved that something was already being done and that their relative might get "special" treatment. Families often expressed a desire that the active drug, not the placebo, be given.[85]

In light of all this misunderstanding, due no doubt to the time pressure for consenting to the second dose and to the anxiety naturally felt by the family, it is hard to see what moral force this consent had in justifying the continuation of the research, much less in retrospectively justifying its initiation. Moreover, the last sentence suggests that what the families were actually consenting to was the administration of the drug, not enrollment in a randomized trial, and if that is so, the value of the deferred consent is even more questionable. In short, this important experiment with the use of deferred consent does not support its use as a way of resolving our dilemma. The brain resuscitation experiment may have been morally licit, but if it was so, its licitness was probably not due to the deferred consent.

None of this proves that deferred consent could not in other settings play an important role in justifying certain research protocols. Perhaps when the continuation of the research does not involve any further interventions for a longer period of time, so that the family (or the recovering patient) has the time to understand and consider, deferred consent may have greater value. But the foregoing data give us little reason to be optimistic about the role of deferred consent in validating research in the emergency room setting.

We turn then to the protocol adopted by the group studying the initiation of thrombolytic therapy in ambulances. A good deal of insight into their thinking can be obtained by examining their account of why they did not adopt the deferred-consent approach:

> Deferred consent, however, ultimately proves unsatisfactory for conscious, emergently ill patients such as those with AMI because it treats them initially as though they were incompetent. Although this method of consent may be ethically defensible for a comatose patient, it seems less defensible for AMI patients who are conscious and alert. While it is reasonable to suppose that an acutely ill patient is not thinking as clearly as usual, there is no reason to presume that such a patient is incompetent. Thus, for the problem of prehospital thrombolytic therapy, deferred consent also affords insufficient respect for the rights of persons to consent to or refuse a research protocol.[86]

Their argument comes to the following: (1) the AMI patients in the ambulances are either incompetent (in which case deferred consent may be legitimate) or competent (in which case deferred consent is not legitimate); (2) their problems are not sufficient to justify declaring them incompetent; (3) therefore, we must treat them as competent and get their consent before initiating the experiment.

Given this argument, the trial group felt compelled to get consent in advance. But they also recognized the time constraints on getting consent for the first dosage in the ambulance. That is why they got the more modest consent initially, and a fuller consent later:

> The two-step process also introduces an additional element of sophistication: quality of consent is commensurate with assumed risk. Brief informed consent is obtained when the risks involved are only those of receiving a 20-mg. loading dose. Only after giving a second consent under conventional conditions will the patient receive the remaining dose of tPA and be exposed to the total risk of drug therapy.[87]

With this two-step process, they felt that they had met the demands of autonomy while still being realistic about the possibilities for consent.

This is a well-designed and thoughtful protocol, the most serious attempt in the literature to deal with the issue of consent in emergency research. I am nevertheless troubled by several aspects of it. First, the researchers argue that the patients in question were not incompetent because they were conscious and alert. Those facts are not sufficient to justify the claims of competency, since surely more is required for competency. Smith's previously cited description of the condition of these patients should make us suspicious about a blanket claim of competency. Perhaps it is more reasonable to say that some were competent and some were not and that the solution was deficient in treating all subjects as competent and taking the consent of any as sufficient to legitimize the research. Second, even if we accept the competency claim for all of the subjects, the authors admit in a crucial paragraph (on p. 255) that there was inadequate time for reflection in light of the sense of crisis and stress either for the initial consent or for the later consent. The third and most crucial troubling aspect is the assumption that these patients were either competent or incompetent, which was the basis for development of their protocol. It would have been far better if the trial group had recognized that the subjects had varying degrees of competency and that their consent under the conditions in question had varying moral force and if they had developed a protocol that reflected that recognition.

This is precisely what we shall try to do in the remainder of this section. We will return to our earlier observations that all the conditions for ideal consent (that it be voluntary, that it be informed, that it be made by a competent subject, and that the subject have adequate time to reflect) are at best partially met in research in an emergency setting, and that different consents from different subjects meet these conditions to differing degrees. We shall attempt to develop a theory of legitimate research that reflects these realities. To do that, however, I think we need to first focus on the question of the reasons for obtaining informed consent.

There are, it seems to me, three different reasons for obtaining informed consent from a subject before that subject is enrolled in a research protocol. Two of these reasons, the respect for autonomy and the risk–benefit determination, are also reasons for obtaining informed consent before any medical intervention. The third reason, concern for conflict of interest, is found only in the context of research protocols. Let us review all three of these reasons.

The respect for autonomy reason for obtaining informed consent is based upon the view that each person has a unique authority over his or her body and that as a result of this authority no one else may do anything to that body without the person's consent. Even physicians who are treating that person's illnesses in a standard fashion whose efficacy and safety are well-known may not do so without consent, and a failure to obtain consent is an instance of that moral fault which the law calls a battery. The risk–benefit determination reason for obtaining informed consent is based upon the recognition that medical interventions carry risks as well as benefits, that different people may assess their relative significance differently because they have different values, and that the best (perhaps even the only) way to be sure that the benefits of the intervention outweigh its risks in light of the values of the patient is to obtain the patient's informed consent before performing the intervention. If all this is true even when an intervention is a standard intervention whose risks and benefits are well understood, it is even more true in the case of experimental interventions whose risks and benefits are not well understood. The conflict of interest reason for obtaining informed consent, a reason unique to the research context, is based upon the realistic understanding that physician-researchers may find that their interest as researchers in enrolling subjects in studies brings them into conflict with their obligation as physicians to do what is in the best interest of their patients and that patient-subjects are best served by having the chance to consent or refuse to participate in the light of adequate information.[88]

These reasons provide a powerful foundation for the requirement that research is licit only when fully valid consent is obtained in advance, for it seems that only fully valid consent can fulfill these reasons. This is, of course, what approaches 1 and 2 demand. They differ only on the question of whether fully valid family consent can take the place of fully valid patient consent when the latter is impossible to obtain. Approach 1 claims, of course, that family consent cannot satisfy the protection of autonomy reason and may not be able to satisfy the risk–benefit determination reason. Approach 2 argues, with some justification, that the consent of family members can fulfill all of the functions of the consent of the patients, in part because it seems reasonable that the patient would want his or her family member to make decisions when he or she cannot and in part because it seems reasonable to suppose that the family member's decision reflects what the patient would have decided if he or she could have made the decision. Leaving aside this difference between 1 and 2, it seems at first glance that their approach of demanding fully valid consent before the research is performed is justified.

Further reflection suggests, however, that this conclusion is probably incorrect. One way to see this is to remind ourselves that there exists in the ordinary therapeutic setting an emergency exception to the requirement of obtaining informed consent in advance, and that this exception makes a lot of sense. A good statement of the conditions for that exception and its rationale is to be found in the classic informed-consent case, *Canterbury v. Spence*:

> Two exceptions to the general rule of disclosure have been noted by the courts. Each is in the nature of a physician's privilege not to disclose, and the reasoning underlying them is appealing. Each, indeed, is but a recognition that, as important as is the patient's right to know, it is greatly outweighed by the magnitudinous circumstances giving rise to the privilege. The first comes into play when the patient is unconscious or otherwise incapable of consenting, and harm from a failure to treat is imminent and outweighs any harm threatened by the proposed treatment. When a genuine emergency of that sort arises, it is settled that the impracticality of conferring with the patient dispenses with need for it. Even in situations of that character the physician should, as current law requires, attempt to secure a relative's consent if possible. But if time is too short to accommodate discussion, obviously the physician should proceed with the treatment.[89]

Perhaps that very same exception can be applied in at least some experimental settings as well.

The *Canterbury* court reminded us that when the benefits of the intervention to the patient clearly outweigh the risks (so that it would require truly unusual values, not often found, for an informed patient to refuse the intervention), it is licit to proceed without consent. The risk–benefit determination reason is satisfied since we can assume, with a high degree of probability, that the patient would judge that the benefits are greater than the risks and the respect for autonomy reason is satisfied since we can assume, with a high degree of probability, that the patient would therefore have consented. If, in some experimental setting, the benefit to the patient from participating clearly outweighs the risk of participating, the same justification can be offered. I take this to be the truth which approaches 3 and 4 were trying to capture.

Several observations are possible. First, the crucial point in this justification of proceeding without fully valid consent is that participation in the research must very clearly be in the interest of the emergency patient. The fact that the research is of great social value will not by itself justify proceeding without consent. Perhaps, borrowing a point from our discussion in the preceding section, that will justify the research without consent if, in addition, the risks of participating are so slight that all reasonable people of average altruism and risk-aversiveness would be willing to participate. But this justification generally will apply only to cases where participation is clearly in the interest of the patient. Second, the justification applies only when there is no family member present who can give fully valid consent. Third, a procedure should be available when someone (the patient or a family member) can at a later time give fully valid consent to continue. In this case the fully valid consent should be obtained before the research is continued because, once the possibility of obtaining that consent exists, it is better to rely upon it than upon even reasonable assumptions. It is probably best, however, that we not refer to this consent as deferred consent, with the suggestion that this later consent justifies the earlier participation. That earlier participation was already justified by the very favorable risk-benefit ratio of participating; the later consent is really relevant to justifying the continuation of the protocol. Fourth, the patient or the family member can give or refuse to give in advance partially valid consent. This legitimizes more emergency research, particularly research that does not have a clearly favorable risk-benefit ratio. Such research can be legitimized by a combination of a somewhat favorable risk-benefit ratio and a somewhat valid consent. The more valid the consent, the less we need the risk-benefit ratio to be so clearly favorable. However, a partially valid refusal will challenge the validity of emergency research with a clearly favorable risk-benefit ratio when the patient refuses consent in a somewhat valid manner. Even research with an increasingly favorable risk-benefit ratio will be invalidated as the refusal of consent becomes increasingly valid.

Summarizing this lengthy discussion, we can conclude that research in an emergency setting is justified under a number of conditions. It is justified if fully valid consent can be obtained from the patient or from a family member. It is justified without any consent if the benefits to the patient from participating are so great that they clearly outweigh the risks of participating. It is justified when the risks to the patient from participating are sufficiently small and the social value of the research sufficiently great that all reasonable persons of average altruism and risk-aversiveness would be willing to participate. Finally, it may be justified even when these risk-benefit ratios are not so obviously favorable, providing that one can obtain from the patient or from a family member a sufficiently valid consent, and it may stop being justified despite a very favorable risk-to-benefit ratio as one gets an increasingly valid refusal of consent from the patient or the family member. With this in mind, let us return to the issue of what consent should have been obtained from the patients participating in the trials of the thrombolytic agents.

We will begin our discussion by examining the views of the GISSI investigators who felt that the conditions were not appropriate for obtaining informed consent and therefore proceeded without that consent. In light of our discussion until now, I think that several observations are in order. First, while the investigators were certainly right in claiming that the ideal conditions for obtaining informed consent were not present, that does not entail the conclusion that informed consent had no place in this study. The conditions of obtaining consent from the patient (or from a family member, an option they did not discuss in their paper) may have been less than ideal, but it may still have been possible to have obtained at least a partially valid consent (or refusal) to participate in at least some cases, and that would have helped determine, as we have seen, whether or not the research was licit. Second, even if we grant the assumption about the impossibility of obtaining meaningful and appropriate consent, that does not lead to the conclusion that the research is licit. To make it licit, the investigators would have had to show either that the benefits to the patient of participating very clearly outweighed the risks to the patient of participating, so that they could treat participating as a form of emergency therapy, or that the risks to the patient of participating were so low that they could proceed without consent because all reasonable people would be willing to undertake that risk to help society get the needed information. Third, in evaluating the risks and benefits of participating, they would need to consider the alternatives to participating, which include getting intracoronary and perhaps even intravenous streptokinase without being randomized into a study that might result in getting no thrombolytic therapy at all. That risk of participation, in light of the information available when GISSI began, was sufficiently great that neither of these risk–benefit claims about participation seem plausible. It might well have been very different if this had been an active-controlled rather than a placebo-controlled trial, but it was not. Fourth, in light of all these considerations, it seems that the GISSI investigators made an incorrect judgment in concluding from the emergency nature of their research that they were entitled to proceed without any consent at all.

The ISIS-2 investigators developed a framework for obtaining partially valid consent (only partially valid, because, in addition to all of our regular issues about consent in an emergency setting, their consent form left out crucial information), even though they left the decisions about obtaining that consent to each of the clinical centers. That consent, when obtained, could have helped legitimize their research. One major problem with their approach is that all of the research conducted in centers that did not obtain any consent could not be justified by that consent. Another problem is that given the limited nature of the validity of the consent, even when obtained, it could not have helped legitimize the research unless the risk-benefit ratio to the patient of participating was highly favorable. Given the previously noted risk of being randomized to receive only a placebo, that assessment of the ratio is not very plausible. It becomes even less plausible for the second part of ISIS-2, when both the GISSI data and its own preliminary data were available and emphasized the risk involved in getting a placebo rather than some thrombolytic therapy.

It would be tempting to conclude from these observations that the only correct approach was to get fully valid informed consent before proceeding. I think, however, that this approach, which seems to have been adopted by the ASSET and AIMS investigators, is equally unacceptable precisely because it is unrealistic. For all the reasons pointed out earlier in this section, especially the constraints of time and of the patient's physiological and psychological condition, the likelihood of enrolling for these very large trials enough patients who could give (or whose family could give) fully valid informed consent is not high. So AIMS and ASSET were not justified in their attempt to get fully valid consent.

In the preceding section we raised serious ethical doubts about the legitimacy of having run the trials in question as placebo-controlled trials. Those doubts are reinforced by the considerations raised in this section. As placebo-controlled trials, the trials in question had sufficient risks due to the chance of getting no thrombolytic therapy that they could have been legitimized only by obtaining fully valid consent. But given the factors we have identified, obtaining such a consent was not realistically possible. Therefore, the consent problem was unsolvable for these placebo-controlled trials. We have then a second reason why these trials should have been run as active-controlled trials. For at least some of these trials, partially valid consent could have been obtained, and that might have been sufficient to justify those trials if they had been run as active-controlled trials.

I wish to reiterate that my goal in this section, as in the last section, has not been to judge the people who made these decisions about how to handle the consent issue. My concern has been only with the decisions they reached. I believe that those decisions were in error, and that this error may at least in part have been due to the lack of good theoretical treatments of the issue of consent in the emergency setting. I hope that the theory we have developed in this section, even if complicated, will be of help to future investigators as they consider this very difficult issue.

Conflicts of Interests and the Validity of Clinical Trials

The last of the issues we will be examining in this chapter is the structuring of clinical trials to avoid potential conflicts of interests between the economic interests of investigators and the interest of society at large in obtaining scientifically valid results from clinical trials. This problem has received extensive discussion in the last few years, a discussion which was greatly stimulated by the revelations in 1987–1988 of the stockholding in Genentech by clinical investigators in the tPA trials. Some have been concerned with looking into the behavior of those investigators in the tPA trials, but that will *not* be our focus of attention. As before, our concern is not with particular individuals but with the broader policy issue. We are using the example of the trials of the thrombolytic agents to discuss a far broader issue. This observation is particularly important, for as we shall shortly see, many have been led by excessive attention to the details of stockholding in Genentech to miss the broader issues and to propose solutions that are incomplete.

Our strategy for examining the issues surrounding conflicts of interests begins with an examination of the reasons for being concerned with conflicts of interests; I argue that this concern is very different from the concerns about scientific fraud and misconduct that have also attracted much interest recently. The real reasons for concern will be fully illustrated by examples drawn from the trials of thrombolytic agents. We will then argue that the conflict-of-interest issue is far broader than the stockholding question and that the various proposals that have surfaced (which focus on stockholding and other relations with drug companies) are therefore inadequate. We will end by offering new proposals for dealing with this set of problems.

The original *Newsday* article which called attention to the stockholding by clinical investigators in Genentech discussed the possibility that this type of conflict of interest might lead to actual fraud in research, to the publication of incorrect data.[90] The report of Congressman Weiss's subcommittee at the end of its hearings, which combined investigations into fraudulent misconduct with investigations into conflicts of interest, entitled "Are Scientific Misconduct and Conflicts of Interest Hazardous to Our Health?" also may have encouraged the view that conflicts of interest are troubling because they will lead to fraudulent data.[91] But I want to argue, following up on certain suggestions already made in Chapter 1, that this concern with fraudulent data is not central, precisely because the design of clinical trials makes it difficult to perpetrate frauds. Instead, the concern should be with how conflicts of interests may lead investigators, perhaps unconsciously, to make inappropriate decisions about the design and conduct of clinical trials.

Many of the standard features of modern clinical trials are designed at least in part as protection against fraud. The fact that patients are randomly assigned to the various treatment arms in a clinical trial means that the investigators cannot assign more favorable cases to their favorite treatment. The fact that the trial is "double-blinded"—that neither the subjects nor the investigators know which treatment the patient is getting—makes it difficult for the investigators to improve the data on patients getting their favorite treatment, although not always impossible, since you can sometimes know from other clinical data which treatment a subject is getting. The fact that the clinical data are often gathered and analyzed by an independent group (a central lab and/or data analysis group) prevents investigators from fraudulently manipulating the data. I do not want to suggest that these measures are foolproof. What I do want to say is that if fraud were the real concern raised by conflicts of interests, we would do best to focus on improving these features of modern clinical trials to make fraud highly unlikely.

What then is the concern with conflicts of interests? It seems to me that the concern grows out of the recognition that there are many decisions that have to be made about both the design and implementation of a clinical trial, and that these decisions provide ample opportunity for those with a conflict of interest to make decisions that aid the case for their favored treatment. This may be a conscious process, in which case we are dealing with personal guilt, or it may be an unconscious process, in which case we may not be dealing with personal guilt. Whatever may be the case about the personal guilt, the social problem of how to minimize these inappropriate decisions remains.

Some of these decisions have to do with the design of the clinical trials. The following questions must be answered:

1. Which treatments will be tested in the proposed trial and which treatments will not be tested?
2. Will there be a placebo control group as well, or will the treatments be tested against each other or against some active control group?
3. What will be taken as the favorable end points (the results which constitute the evidence of efficacy of the treatment) and what will be taken as the adverse end points (the results which constitute the evidence of the dangerousness of the treatment)?
4. What will be the conditions for inclusion or exclusion of subjects from the trial?
5. What provisions will be made for informed consent, and what information will be provided as part of the informed consent process?

Other decisions concern the actual conduct of the clinical trial. They include the following:

6. Under what conditions will the trial be stopped or modified because there have been too many adverse end points in one or more arm of the trial or because the preliminary data have shown that one of the treatments is clearly the most favorable treatment?
7. Under what conditions will the trial be stopped or modified because of newly available results of other trials?
8. Which patients who meet the entry criteria will actually be enrolled and which will not?

These are only some of the many questions which inevitably will arise in the design and implementation of clinical trials. The answers to them will profoundly affect the results of the trial, with some answers being more favorable to one treatment rather than another. In some cases the answers to these questions will be straightforward, so the opportunity for flawed decision making will be modest. In other cases the answers will be far from obvious, and there will be tremendous potential for conflicts of interests leading, consciously or unconsciously, to flawed decision making. That, to my mind, is why we need to be concerned with conflicts of interests.

These are not merely theoretical concerns. In fact, many of these decisions, made in the design and the conduct of the clinical trials of the thrombolytic agents, were quite controversial, so the potential for flawed decisions resulting (consciously or unconsciously) from conflicts of interests was very real. I will now illustrate the existence of that potential by listing a series of highly controversial decisions involving all of the trials of thrombolytic agents, not just TIMI. Please note that I am not claiming here that any of these decisions were flawed, although I have argued that about some of them earlier in this chapter. I am certainly not claiming, here or elsewhere, that any of them were produced by conflicts of interests. All I am claiming is that the existence of these types of decisions opens the possibility of conflicts of interests leading to flawed decision making, and that these examples illustrate why we need to be concerned about conflicts of interest.

Let us review the eight types of questions listed above. Questions of type 1 involve deciding which treatments to test and which treatments not to test. The TIMI trials provide good examples of these types of controversial decisions. The initial decision to take tPA as a serious candidate for study so soon after its synthesis, the decision to drop intracoronary administration from further study, the decision to run a preliminary TIMI-I trial and to then run all the rest of the studies involving only the winner of TIMI-I, and the decision to not study APSAC are all good examples of controversial decisions of type 1.

Questions of type 2 involve deciding whether to use placebo control groups. Nearly all of the trials, as seen earlier in this chapter, are good examples of these types of controversial decisions, ranging all the way from Anderson's unwillingness to run any placebo-controlled trials and TIMI's decision not to run any after the results of GISSI, to those (including the Johns Hopkins group) who were unwilling to run them after the preliminary results from ISIS-2 became available, to those (including ISIS-2 itself, AIMS, and ASSET) that continued such trials even afterward.

Questions of type 3 involve deciding what to take as favorable and adverse end points. In the thrombolytic trials, the choice of the favorable end point was quite controversial, with some trials taking survival as the end point while other trials employed surrogate end points. Of particular significance was the controversial decision of TIMI-I to use reperfusion as the favorable end point rather than other surrogate end points such as ejection fraction. The tremendous importance of this type of decision making will become even clearer in Chapter 3 when we examine the criteria for drug approval. Questions of type 4, involving decisions about inclusion and exclusion criteria, are closely related to questions of type 3. If you want large trials, like the European trials (GISSI, ISIS-2, AIMS, and ASSET), you must include nearly everyone; if you are running smaller trials with surrogate end points (like TIMI-I), you can employ stricter inclusion and exclusion criteria, and these can be quite controversial.

Questions of type 5 involve decisions about the informed-consent process. Nearly all of the trials, as seen earlier in this chapter, involved controversial decisions of this type. GISSI and ISIS-2 obviously made a controversial decision to modify the standard informed-consent process, but the decision of the other trials to proceed in the emergency setting with a normal consent process is, as we have argued above, equally controversial.

Questions of type 6 involve decisions about the early stopping of trials in light of their own data. The decision to stop TIMI-I because of its reperfusion data and the decision not to stop ISIS-2 in spite of its own very impressive survival data are good examples of controversial decisions of this type. Questions of type 7 involve decisions about trial abandonment or modification in light of new data from other trials. The decisions to continue ISIS-2, AIMS, and ASSET, even after the preliminary ISIS-2 data, and the conflicting decisions to stop the Johns Hopkins trial and some of the Australian trials in light of those data, are good examples of controversial decisions of this type, as is, of course, the decision not to run the originally planned placebo-controlled TIMI-II trial in light of the GISSI data.

Questions of type 8 are raised in the day-to-day decisions by clinicians as to which of their patients are eligible to participate in the clinical trials. A good example of decisions of this type is the controversial decision discussed in Chapter 1 to admit Mrs. Galin to the TIMI trial.

This very lengthy review clearly demonstrates that the thrombolytic trials illustrated just how many controversial decisions have to be made in the design and conduct of clinical trials. There is clearly a tremendous potential for conflicts of interests to lead, consciously or unconsciously, to flawed decision making. The conflict-of-interest issue is then the problem of how to develop policies that will minimize that potential.

As noted in Chapter 1, two approaches have emerged in the literature. The first is the disclosure approach, as found, for example, in the following policy of the *New England Journal of Medicine*:

> The Journal expects authors to disclose any commercial associations that might pose a conflict of interest in connection with the submitted article. All funding sources supporting the work should be routinely acknowledged on the title page, as should all institutional or corporate affiliations of the authors. Other kinds of associations, such as consultancies, stock ownership or other equity interests, or patent-licensing arrangements, should be disclosed to the Editor in a covering letter at the time of submission. Such information will be held in confidence while the paper is under review and will not influence the editorial decision. If the manuscript is accepted, the Editor will discuss with the authors how best to disclose the relevant information.[92]

This policy covers, of course, a wide variety of potential conflicts of interests, and it attempts to deal with them by requiring disclosure, in the expectation that those who read the resulting publications will be alerted to the potential conflict of interest and will adopt an appropriately cautious attitude to the resulting publication.

A second, very different approach was described in an influential article published at the same time as the disclosure policies were being promulgated. The authors of the article (headed by Dr. Bernadine Healy) were the leading investigators in a multicenter trial funded by the NIH. Their approach, the elimination approach, claimed that the best way to deal with conflicts of interests is to ban the commercial relations which generate the conflicts. The policy is formulated as follows:

> Investigators involved in the post-CABG [coronary artery bypass graft] study will not buy, sell, or hold stock or stock options in any of the companies providing or distributing medication under study . . . for the following periods: from the time the recruitment of patients for the trial begins until funding for the study in the investigator's unit ends and the results are made public; or . . . until the investigator's active and personal involvement in the study or the involvement of the institution conducting the study (or both) ends. Each investigator will agree not to serve as a paid consultant to the companies during these same periods. . . . Certain other activities are not viewed as constituting conflicts of interest but must be reported annually to the coordinating center: the participation of investigators in educational activities supported by the companies; the participation of investigators in other research projects supported by the companies; occasional scientific consulting to the companies on issues not related to the products in the trial and for which there

is no financial payment or other compensation; and financial interests in the companies over which the investigator has no control, such as mutual funds and blind trusts.[93]

This approach has attracted much attention since then, in part because Healy had been one of the investigators in the Johns Hopkins tPA trials who owned shares in Genentech, so this policy represented a major shift in her views, and in part because she subsequently served as director of the NIH while it was attempting to develop policies on this matter.

In September 1989, the NIH proposed a policy on this issue which was an expansion of the elimination approach. In addition to banning equity holdings and paid consultancies, it required that companies sharing the costs of research with the NIH not be in a position to influence the research plan or get advanced access to the information. After much controversy, those policies were put on hold, and, as of September 1993, new policies are still being developed.[94]

There is much that needs to be said about the details of these approaches, about their respective merits and demerits, and about ways of combining aspects of both of them. But that will not be our concern in the remainder of this section, although I heartily endorse some combination of these approaches. What I want to do instead is to identify a fundamental presupposition of both approaches and suggest some broader policies that will need to be adopted in light of the fact that the presupposition in question is almost certainly incorrect.

The presupposition in question is that the conflict-of-interest problem arises primarily out of the commercial relation between clinical investigators and drug companies whose products they are investigating. The disclosure policy of the *New England Journal of Medicine*, for example, is concerned with the "commercial associations" of the investigators and emphasizes disclosures of equity interests, consulting fees, and so on. The NIH proposal and Healy's earlier policies are concerned primarily with prohibiting stockholding, consultancy fees, and so on. This is quite understandable when one remembers that the attention to this issue grew out of particular allegations about the relation between certain investigators and Genentech. But as understandable as it may be, I would like to suggest that the conflict-of-interest problem extends beyond these commercial relations.

I have argued that the conflict-of-interest problem arises when (1) controversial decisions must be made in the design and conduct of clinical trials and (2) flawed decisions may result from biases due to the investigators' financial interests. It is obvious that condition (1) will be satisfied in the case of many clinical trials whether or not the investigators have any commercial relations with any drug companies. But it seems to me that condition (2) may also be satisfied even when these commercial relations are not present, because of problems growing out of grant funding. If this is correct, both approaches are at best incomplete solutions because their fundamental common presupposition is false.

To explain why condition (2) may be satisfied even if the investigators have no equity interests, consultancies, or other commercial relations with any drug company, let us begin by reflecting on the grants funding the trial in question. The clinical centers involved in the trial receive substantial support from the funding source, which pays the salaries of staff and of investigators, helps cover the expenses of the administrative structure of the center, and even offers the possibility of a profit (especially if one considers the marginal cost of running the trial). If that support is cut off, there can be substantial financial losses to the center as well as career losses to the investigators. This certainly has a potential impact upon decisions involving questions of type 6 or 7, questions of stopping trials. Similarly, investigators may be affected in their decisions about patient eligibility, decisions involving questions of type 8, since a failure to enroll enough patients may lead to a lessening of support or even to the center being eliminated from the trial. Thus it is easy to see how there is the potential for flawed decisions due to conflicts of interests in the conduct of a trial because of the benefits of grant funding, even if the investigators have no commercial relations with the relevant drug companies. The same point is true, in a different and slightly more subtle fashion, when it comes to decisions involving the design of trials. Different trial designs, involving different decisions concerning questions of types 1–5, are likely to have greater or lesser appeal to the crucial decision makers in the drug company or the public agency, and those who seek grants may be influenced in their decisions in the desire to maximize the chances of funding. I see no reason to believe, then, that condition 2 is only, or even primarily, satisfied when the investigators have close commercial connections to the companies whose products are being tested.

I would like to suggest, as an alternative to the common presupposition, the following view about conflicts of interests. Conflicts of interests are a matter of concern whenever conditions 1 and 2 are satisfied. Both of these conditions can be satisfied when the investigators have stocks in, or receive consulting fees from, some drug company whose product is being tested, but they can also be satisfied when the trial in question is being funded by a grant either from a drug company or from some public agency. We need to develop policies that are sensitive to all these possibilities. The current proposals, disclosure and/or elimination of commercial relations, are therefore incomplete even if meritorious.

One discussion which has focused on these broader concerns is found in the policies of the Royal College of Physicians which were briefly outlined early in this chapter. Let us turn then to a careful examination of these policies.

The main thrust of those policies is to avoid situations in which researchers are induced by financial considerations to pressure patients to participate in clinical trials. That is why the Royal College would totally ban per capita payments to physicians (payments in proportion to the number of subjects recruited). That is also why the Royal College would allow research grants conditional upon recruiting a minimum number of patients only if the independent committee reviewing the research protocol determines that it is reasonable to assume that the clinic in question can get that number of volunteers in light of the nature of its patient load and the nature of the research.

All of these are quite reasonable policies, and their adoption would go some way toward minimizing the potential for conflicts of interests in questions of type 8, questions about subject eligibility and subject enrollment. Moreover, these policies have the virtue of focusing on what I have identified as a neglected topic, the shaping of decisions to maximize financial gain from grants. Nevertheless, they are far from complete solutions to our problem, since they focus just upon question 8. This is understandable in the context of the report from the Royal College, since this report is devoted to protecting the interests of patients who are also research subjects. But can we learn from these recommendations about steps which can be used more generally? I think that we can.

At a crucial point in the discussion concerning payments to institutions as opposed to physicians, the Royal College has the following to say: "Payment for recruitment should not exceed a reasonable estimate of the cost of studying the patient together with any legitimate expenses. There should be no element of profit to the institution or department related to the number of patients recruited."[95] This is the crucial point. As noted, grants often cover more than the marginal costs of research, so they constitute a source of additional revenue to institutions. This is part of the way in which grants (as well as equity holdings and consultancies) are the source of potential conflicts of interests.

We need better information about income from grants if we really want to minimize the potential for conflicts of interests. In an important recent study, Shimm and Spece estimated that at their institution, an investigator can harvest a profit of $75,000–$225,000 from a drug-company study involving 50 patients.[96] Their estimation is not entirely convincing, since they derived it by simply subtracting the salary of a data coordinator ($25,000) from the income derived from the drug company (50 patients at $2,000–$5,000 per patient), not considering other marginal expenses. They themselves point out that the calculation will be different if these other marginal expenses are counted. Moreover, I am not convinced that they are right in their claim (unsupported by data) that there is not a similar potential in federally funded research. This skepticism is related to the recent controversies about indirect costs. Nevertheless, they have done a great service by beginning the attempt to identify the true institutional gains from grant income.

The development of the details of guidelines for avoiding conflicts of interests resulting from grant income lies beyond the scope of this book, since one can develop them only in response to a detailed examination of a wide variety of fundamental accounting issues about institutional profits from grants. The crucial policy point is, however, clear. Profits to individuals or institutions from grants can be just as much a source of conflicts of interests as equity holdings or consultancy fees, and we need to control the former as much as the latter.

One needs to be realistic about how much such guidelines could accomplish. Even if they resulted in grants producing no direct financial profit to institutions or individuals, securing grants and implementing research under them would still be in the professional and/or financial interest of both individual researchers and their institutions, which is inevitable and probably desirable. But guidelines of the sort I am advocating would at least minimize the extent to which controversial decisions about the design and implementation of research are influenced, consciously or unconsciously, by the prospect of direct financial gain.

Let me add one other observation. In reviewing questions 1–8, it is clear that many of these questions are the very questions that we discussed earlier in this chapter. To the extent that society adopts some of the results of our analysis about when placebo-controlled trials and emergency research are justified, and incorporates them into appropriate regulations and/or guidelines, it will limit the extent of discretion about these matters, thereby also limiting the occasions for the operation of conflicts of interests. In this final way, the topics of this chapter relate to each other.

In summary, we have argued in this section that conflicts of interests are to be avoided not because they lead to fraud but because they can be the source of flawed decisions when there are controversial questions about the design and implementation of research protocols. We have also argued that grant support can be just as much a source of conflicts of interests as equity holdings, so that the current emphasis on equity holdings and paid consultancies is misleading. Finally, we have suggested that what is required is a ban on individual and institutional direct profits from grants, whether from industry or from the government, as well as the more familiar bans on equity holding and paid consultancies and the requirement of full disclosure.

Conclusions

There is something very paradoxical about what we have seen in this chapter. On the one hand, the whole area of experimentation on human subjects has been studied extensively for many years, and there exist in many countries extensive regulations and/or policy statements covering the protection of such subjects. On the other hand, none of our three issues has been extensively discussed in these regulations and/or policy statements, although some of their ideas have been helpful at certain crucial points in our analysis. This gap in their treatment of these issues may help explain the very diverse attitudes that existed to these issues in the clinical trials of the thrombolytic agents.

On the question of placebo-controlled trials, we argued that they are justified in fewer cases than normally allowed and we concluded that most of the placebo-controlled trials of the thrombolytic agents were inappropriate. On the question of emergency research, we argued that a more balanced and realistic approach needs to be adopted toward obtaining consent for such research and we concluded that none of the trials of the thrombolytic agents dealt with this issue adequately. Finally, on the conflict-of-interest question, we argued for a broader understanding of the possibilities of such conflicts and for more demanding regulations to minimize those possibilities and we concluded that the emphasis on the example of the trials of the thrombolytic agents has led to an excessive concern with the conflicts engendered by equity holdings. Perhaps our arguments were not always successful, but they certainly demonstrate, I believe, that all of these questions are hard questions and that we need to advance beyond what is currently said about them.

Notes

1. See, for example, the extensive literature cited in Ruth R. Faden and T. L. Beauchamp, *A History and Theory of Informed Consent* (New York: Oxford University Press, 1986), Chapter 5 notes 1–8. The classical text is R. J. Levine, *Ethics and Regulation of Clinical Research,* 2nd ed. (New Haven: Yale University Press, 1988).

2. The full text is reprinted in Levine, *Ethics and Regulation,* pp. 425–26.

3. This way of combining the two avoids, I believe, many of the problems raised by E. Marshall in "Does the Moral Philosophy of the Belmont Report Rest on a Mistake?" *IRB* 8 (1986): 5–6.

4. The revised declaration is found in Levine, *Ethics and Regulation,* pp. 427–29.

5. The FDA regulations appear in the *Code of Federal Regulations*, primarily in 21 CFR §50, "Protection of Human Subjects," and 21 CFR §56, "Institutional Review Boards." The NIH regulations are found in 45 CFR §46, "Protection of Human Research Subjects." Those regarding children are found in 45 CFR §46, pt. D, "Additional Protections for Children Involved as Subjects in Research." *Federal Register* 48 (March 8, 1983): 9818–20.

6. P.L. 93-348.

7. R. J. Levine, "The Commission's Recommendations and the FDA's Proposals," *IRB* 1 (1979): 1–2, 12.

8. The most recent effort is found in the uniform rules published in the *Federal Register* 56 (June 18, 1991): 28003–32.

9. National Commission for the Protection of Human Subjects of Biomedical and Behavioral Research, "The Belmont Report," *Federal Register* 44 (April 18, 1979).

10. The FDA requirement is founded in 21 CFR §56.103; the NIH requirement is found in 45 CFR §46.103.

11. The FDA requirements are found in 21 CFR §56.111; the NIH requirements are found in 45 CFR §46.111.

12. The FDA requirements are found in 21 CFR §§50.20 and 50.25; the NIH requirements are found in 45 CFR §46.116.

13. *FDA Clinical Investigator Information Sheets* (Washington: FDA, May 1989), p. 38.

14. *FDA IRB Information Sheets* (Washington: FDA, February 1989), pp. 44–45.

15. The Office of Protection from Research Risks (OPRR) opinion is found in *OPRR Reports* 91-01 (May 15, 1991). A different but complementary analysis of the U.S. regulations on emergency research is found in R. J. Levine, "Deferred Consent," *Controlled Clinical Trials* 12 (1991): 546–50. My only disagreement is that Levine does not consider the implications of the above-quoted *FDA Information Sheet* about emergency research.

16. A very useful summary of what they did before the most recent discussions is found in T. L. Kurt, "FDA Issues Concerning Conflicts of Interest," *IRB* 12 (1990): 6–9.

17. 21 CFR §312.120.

18. 45 CFR §46.101(A2).

19. Compare, for example L. H. Newton, "Ethical Imperialism and Informed Consent," *IRB* 12 (1990): 10–11, with M. Angell, "Ethical Imperialism?" *NEJM* 319 (1988): 1081–83.

20. *FDA IRB Information Sheet* (Washington: FDA, February 1989), p. 18.

21. J. P. Griffin, "Medicines Control within the United Kingdom" in J. P. Griffin, ed., *Medicines Regulation Research and Risk* (Belfast: Queens University Press, 1989), pp. 1–25.

22. L. Bergkamp, *Regulation of Medical Experimentation with Human Beings in Western Europe* (Amsterdam: Institute for Social Medicine, 1988), pp. 5–7, and Royal College of Physicians, *Guidelines on the Practice of Ethics Committees in Medical Research Involving Human Subjects* (London: Royal College of Physicians, 1990), p. 1.

23. Printed in the *Bulletin of Medical Ethics* 53 (October 1989): 13–17. Details about the final regulations are found in the *Bulletin of Medical Ethics* 71 (September 1991): 3–5.

24. On these issues, see Anonymous (later revealed to be Evelyn Thomas), "Research without Consent Continues in the U.K.," *Institute for Medical Ethics Bulletin* 40 (July 1988): 13–15, and M. Baum, et al., "Ethics of Clinical Research," *British Medical Journal* 299 (1989): 251–53.

25. British Medical Association, *Handbook of Medical Ethics* (London: B.M.A., 1986), pp. 30–33. Quote, p. 30.

26. Association of the British Pharmaceutical Industry (ABPI), "Guidelines on Good Clinical Research Practice," *Institute for Medical Ethics Bulletin* 40 (July 1988): 8–9.

27. *Guidelines on the Practice of Ethics Committees in Medical Research Involving Human Subjects* and *Research Involving Patients,* both published by the College in London in January 1990.

28. They are "The Ethical Conduct of Research on Children," reprinted in the *Bulletin of Medical Ethics* (March 1992): 8–9, "The Ethical Conduct of Research on the Mentally Incapacitated," reprinted in the *Bulletin of Medical Ethics* (March 1992): 9–10, and "Responsibility in Investigations on Human Participants and Material and on Personal Information," reprinted in the *Bulletin of Medical Ethics* (December 1992): 18–23.

29. The discussion of these topics in *Research Involving Patients*, Sections 5.8–5.26, is outstanding.

30. Ibid., Section 7.6.

31. Ibid., Section 7.17.

32. Ibid., Section 7.13.

33. Ibid., Sections 7.102–7.106.

34. Ibid., Sections 7.73–7.74.

35. Ibid., Sections 7.85–7.87.

36. "Responsibility in Investigations," p. 19

37. Bergkamp, *Regulation of Medical Experimentation.*

38. This document, R(90)3, has been published in the *Bulletin of Medical Ethics* 56 (March 1990): 8–10.

39. EC Document III 3976 88-EN.

40. For details, see the *Bulletin of Medical Ethics* (October 1989): 4–6.

41. See, for example, H. Brody, *Placebos and the Philosophy of Medicine* (Chicago: University of Chicago Press, 1977), and S. Bok, *Lying* (New York: Vintage Books, 1979), Chapters 14–15.

42. S. Yusuf et al., "Intravenous and Intracoronary Fibrinolytic Therapy in Acute Myocardial Infarction," *European Heart Journal* 6 (1985): 556–85.

43. GISSI, "Effectiveness of Intravenous Thrombolytic Therapy in Acute Myocardial Infarction," *Lancet,* February 22, 1986, pp. 397–401.

44. H. K. Beecher, "Ethics and Clinical Research," *NEJM* 274 (1966): 1354–60.

45. "Placebo-Controlled and Active Controlled Drug Study Designs," pp. 36–54 of a May 1989 document entitled *FDA Clinical Investigator Information Sheets,* obtainable from the FDA. The two articles by Robert Temple incorporated into this document are "Government Viewpoint of Clinical Trials," *Drug Information Journal,* January–June 1982, pp. 10–17, and "Difficulties in Evaluating Positive Control Trials," *Proceedings of the American Statistical Association, Biopharmaceutical Section,* 1983. All citations in the text refer to the FDA reprint.

46. A. L. Gould, "Another View of Active-Controlled Trials," *Controlled Clinical Trials* 12 (1991): 474–85, is the most accessible account. A more technical account can be found in A. L. Gould, "Placebo Comparisons in Active-Controlled Trials," *Proceedings of the American Statistical Association, Biopharmaceuticals Section,* 1986, pp. 1–10.

47. Glasser, S. P. et al., "Exposing Patients with Chronic Stable Exertional Angina to Placebo Periods in Drug Trials," *JAMA* 265 (1991): 1550–54.

48. Ibid., p. 1550.

49. "Thrombolytic Agents in Evolving MI," *FDA Drug Bulletin* 14 (April 1984): 4–5.

50. J. W. Kennedy, "Western Washington Randomized Trial of Intracoronary Streptokinase in Acute Myocardial Infarction," *NEJM* 309 (1983): 1477–82.

51. Among the clinical groups, I would mention A. Laupacis et. al., "How Should Results from Completed Studies Influence Ongoing Clinical Trials?" *Annals of Internal Medicine* 115 (1991): 818–22, A. Fletcher et. al., "Implications for Trials in Progress of Publication of Positive Results," *Lancet,* September 11, 1993, pp. 653–57, and M. S. Simberkoff et. al., "Ethical Dilemmas in Continuing a Zidovudine Trial after Early Termination of Similar Trials," *Controlled Clinical Trials* 14 (1993): 6–18. Among the theoreticians, the most important recent discussion is S. J. Pocock, "When to Stop a Clinical Trial," *British Medical Journal* 305 (1992): 235–40.

52. T. C. Chalmers, "The Ethics of Randomization as a Decision-Making Technique and the Problem of Informed Consent," reprinted in N. Abrams and M. Buckner, *Medical Ethics* (Cambridge: MIT Press, 1983), pp. 514–18

53. Ibid., p. 517.

54. Ibid., p. 518.

55. L. W. Shaw and T. C. Chalmers, "Ethics in Cooperative Clinical Trials," *Annals of the New York Academy of Sciences* 169 (1970): 487–95.

56. L. M. Friedman, C. D. Furberg, and D. L. Demets, *Fundamentals of Clinical Trials,* 2nd ed. (Littleton, Mass.: PGS Publishing, 1985), pp. 213–14.

57. Shaw and Chalmers, "Ethics in Clinical Trials." Following excerpt is from p. 493.

58. D. Marquis, "Leaving Therapy to Chance," *Hastings Center Report* 13 (August 1983): 40–47. Quote, p. 47.

59. Pocock, "When to Stop a Clinical Trial."

60. B. Freedman, "Equipoise and the Ethics of Clinical Research" *NEJM* 317 (1987): 141–45. Following excerpt is from p. 144.

61. P. Meier, "Terminating a Trial—The Ethical Problem," *Clinical Pharmacology and Therapeutics* 25 (1979): 633–40. Following excerpt is from p. 637.

62. Simberkoff, "Ethical Dilemmas."

63. R. J. Levine, *The Ethics and Regulation of Clinical Research,* 2nd ed. (New Haven: Yale University Press, 1988), Chapter 8.

64. Letter of Alan Guerci, written in October 1990 to an unknown addressee, distributed on December 17, 1990, by Senior Associate Dean David Blake to all participants in a PRIMR Conference at which I spoke.

65. J. Lau et al., "Cumulative Meta-Analysis of Therapeutic Trials for Myocardial Infarction" *NEJM* 327 (1992): 248–54.

66. ISIS Steering Committee, "Intravenous Streptokinase Given within 0–4 Hours of Onset of Myocardial Infarction Reduced Mortality in ISIS-2" *Lancet,* February 28, 1987, p. 502.

67. R. G. Wilcox et al., "Trial of Tissue Plasminogen Activator for Mortality Reduction in Acute Myocardial Infarction," *Lancet*, September 3, 1988, pp. 525–30. Quote, p. 526.

68. AIMS Trial Study Group, "Effect of Intravenous APSAC on Mortality after Acute Myocardial Infarction," *Lancet*, March 12, 1988, p. 546.

69. M. A. Hlatky et al., "Adoption of Thrombolytic Therapy in the Management of Acute Myocardial Infarction," *American Journal of Cardiology* 61 (1988): 510–14.

70. GISSI, "Effectiveness of Intravenous Thrombolytic Therapy," p. 398.

71. ISIS Protocol, May 1985, p. 7.

72. Quoted in *Pediatrics* 88 (1991): 489.

73. 45 CFR §46.116 and 21 CFR §50.20.

74. *Guidelines on Research Involving Human Subjects*, Section 7.16.

75. 45 CFR §46, pt. D.

76. J. C. Fletcher et al., "Consent to Research with Impaired Human Subjects," *IRB* 7 (1985): pp. 1–6.

77. An excellent summary and analysis is to be found in A. Meisel, *The Right to Die* (New York: John Wiley and Sons, 1989), Chapter 7.

78. B. A. Brody, *Life and Death Decision Making* (New York: Oxford University Press, 1988), pp. 100–104.

79. H. L. Smith, "Myocardial Infarction—Case Studies of Ethics in the Consent Situation," *Social Science in Medicine* 8 (1974): 399–404. Following excerpt is from pp. 399–400.

80. P. S. Grim et al., "Informed Consent in Emergency Research," *JAMA* 262 (1989): 252–55. Quote, p. 253.

81. I. S. Ockene et al., "The Consent Process in the Thrombolysis in Myocardial Infarction (TIMI-Phase I) Trial," *Clinical Research* 39 (1991): 13–17.

82. N. S. Abramson et al. "Deferred Consent," *JAMA* 255 (1986): 2466–71, and N. S. Abramson et al., "Deferred Consent: Use in Clinical Resuscitation Research," *Annals of Emergency Medicine* 19 (1990): 781–84.

83. Grim et al., "Informed Consent."

84. In August 1993 the Office of Protection from Research Risks of the NIH issued a report (93-3) denying the validity of deferred consent under the NIH regulations.

85. Abramson et al., "Deferred Consent: Use in Research," p. 783.

86. Grim et al., "Informed Consent," p. 254.

87. Ibid.

88. This reason may not always be unique to the research setting. In some contexts of reimbursement, physicians may for economic reasons be tempted to do more than what is in the interest of their patients (the fee-for-service context) or less than what is in the interest of their patients (the HMO context). In other contexts of reimbursement, however, these conflicts of interest are minimized in the nonexperimental encounter of patient and physician.

89. *Canterbury v. Spence* 464 F.2d 772.

90. "Doctors as Stockholders," *Newsday*, September 29, 1987, Discovery Section, p. 1.

91. Committee on Government Operations, *Are Scientific Misconduct and Conflicts of Interest Hazardous to Our Health?* (Washington: GPO, September 10, 1990).

92. "Information for Authors," *NEJM* 320 (1989): 952.

93. B. Healy et al., "Conflict of Interest Guidelines for a Multicenter Trial of Treatment after Coronary-Artery Bypass-Graft Surgery," *NEJM* 320 (1989): 949–51; quote, p. 951. An even stricter version of this approach was adopted by the GUSTO investigators. A description is found in E. J. Topol et al., "Confronting the Issues of Patient Safety and Investigator Conflict of Interest in an International Clinical Trial of Myocardial Reperfusion," *JACC* 19 (1992): 1123–28.

94. "Requests for Comments," *N.I.H. Guide for Grants and Contracts,* vol. 18 (September 15, 1989). The 1993 NIH reauthorization act calls for identifying circumstances that may lead to bias and for "responding to, reducing, managing, or eliminating" them. This goes beyond the disclosure approach that the NIH was planning as an alternative to the originally proposed policy. This

difference is likely to lead to further delays. In the meantime, the FDA is considering adopting a policy on these issues. All of this is explored in *The Blue Sheet*, June 23, 1993, pp. 5–6, and July 7, 1993, pp. 2–3.

95. *Research Involving Patients*, Section 7.87.

96. D. S. Shimm and R. G. Spece, "Industry Reimbursement for Entering Patients into Clinical Trials," *Annals of Internal Medicine* 115 (1991): 148–51.

3

Troubling Ethical Issues in the Approval of New Drugs

Our case study in Chapter 1 illustrated that the drug approval process can be highly controversial, in part because so much hinges on it economically as well as medically. Much of the controversy we documented in the case study centered around specific problems encountered in the approval of streptokinase and tPA, including the advisory committee's lack of access to certain NIH data and the poor timing of its meeting. These specific problems will not be the focus of our attention in this chapter. Instead, our attention will center on two more fundamental issues that came up in the earlier discussion:

1. How should the goals of effectiveness and safety be balanced in the drug approval process?
2. How should the demands of adequate evidence and the demands of speedy approval be balanced in the drug approval process?

Two preliminary observations about these questions are in order.

The first is that these two questions, while obviously related, are different. Question 1 relates to the content of what must be established before a drug is approved for marketing. We want drugs that are effective. We want drugs that are safe. But effective drugs often carry with them risks, and these risks must be balanced against the benefits derived from the effectiveness of the drugs. Question 1 asks what is an appropriate balance between these two goals, an appropriate risk-benefit ratio, in order for a drug to be approved. Question 2 relates to the evidence for that content which must be present before a drug is approved. We want firm evidence that there is a favorable risk-benefit ratio. We want good drugs to be approved as quickly as possible. But getting firm evidence often requires waiting for more evidence and produces delays in the approval process, and the benefits of further evidence must be balanced against the losses of the drug not being available for those who might benefit from it. Question 2 asks what is an appropriate balance between these two demands on the evidence in the drug approval process. Throughout this chapter we refer to question 1 as the *content question* and question 2 as the *epistemic question.*

The second preliminary observation is that these questions are value questions requiring a moral analysis, and not technical administrative questions to be settled on purely administrative grounds. To begin with, the very existence of a drug approval process, which ensures that drugs are not available on the open market until they have received approval, is a governmental limitation on the freedom of patients and clinicians who might want to use the drug even if it is not approved. All such limitations on freedom require a moral justification. It is unlikely that such a justification will be forthcoming if the system involves inappropriate answers to our two questions. It is best, I believe, to see answering these two questions as part of the process of designing a liberty-limiting system which can in the end be morally justified. Moreover, part of the role of any good moral analysis is that it helps us balance important individual and social values. Our two questions are precisely about how important individual and social values should be balanced, so we have every reason to expect that a good moral analysis will be of help to us in answering them.

This chapter begins with a selective history of the drug approval process in the United States, a history that emphasizes the evolving responses to our questions and that evaluates these responses in light of their success in dealing with our questions. It then turns to some international comparisons designed to examine alternative answers to our questions. The final section of this chapter presents a new approach. At the end of the analysis we return to our case study to draw important conclusions about the FDA's approval of tPA and streptokinase.

The Development of the FDA Regulatory Scheme in the United States

The history of the development of drug regulation in the United States has been extensively studied.[1] Here we need to say very little about the pre-1962 history since we will focus on the answers to our two questions provided by the regulatory scheme that came into existence as a result of fundamental legislation passed in 1962 which restructured the drug approval process and which remains in existence today. We will examine the legislation and the regulations implementing it, criticisms of it which emerged in the 1970s, the FDA's responses to those criticisms in the early 1980s, further developments in the late 1980s in response to the AIDS crisis, and recent initiatives to further modify the system.

The 1962 Legislation and the Regulations Interpreting It

The first significant federal legislation regulating the sale of drugs was passed in 1906. At that time, physicians' prescriptions were not required to purchase drugs, and many patent medicines were being sold on the basis of exaggerated claims about their efficacy. In response to muckraking articles published in popular magazines documenting these fraudulent claims, Congress passed a law prohibiting the adulteration or mislabeling of drugs (as well as foods) which were sold in interstate commerce. Further scandals led to major additional legislation in 1938. One of the first classes of drugs developed at the very beginning of the pharmaceutical revolution that transformed the practice of medicine was the sulfa drugs. The Massengill Company marketed a liquid form of sulfanilamide, using diethylene glycol as the solvent to make it easier to administer to children. Unfortunately, it turned out to be poisonous, and more than 100 children died. In response to this scandal, Congress passed a law requiring that no drugs could be sold in interstate commerce until the seller had submitted a new drug application (NDA) which demonstrated that the drug was safe for its intended use. It also allowed certain exemptions to the earlier labeling requirements, exemptions which the FDA interpreted to apply to drugs that could be sold only with a doctor's prescription, thereby creating the current system whereby most drugs cannot be purchased over the counter.

The crucial 1962 legislation was also spurred by scandals. Senator Estes Kefauver had been holding hearings in the 1950s about the prices of drugs and the profits of drug companies, hearings that in the end led to no legislation in those areas. The legislation he introduced, however, did require that drugs be shown to be effective, and not merely safe, before they were approved for sale in interstate commerce. This part of the proposed legislation passed in 1962. The 1962 legislation imposed the additional requirement that drugs could not be tested on human beings for safety and effectiveness without the drug company's submitting an application to the FDA (an investigational new drug [IND] application) and getting it approved. There is no doubt but that these elements passed because of the thalidomide scandal. Thalidomide had never been approved for use in the United States, primarily because of the concern of Dr. Frances Kelsey, an examiner for the FDA, but it had been distributed for testing, and that did result in a small but very well-publicized outbreak of phocomelia (children born with hands or feet attached to the body by short stumps rather than proportionately sized arms or legs) in the United States. The problem was far greater in Germany, where the drug had been widely used. Although the new requirement of proving effectiveness would not necessarily have made a difference in the thalidomide tragedy, the requirement of pretesting submission might have made a difference, and both requirements were seen as strengthening the drug regulatory scheme in response to this scandal.

What system of drug regulation and what answers to our questions emerged in the United States as a result of this 1962 legislation? The system is easier to describe[2] than the answers, so let us look at each separately.

The first step in the system is that the sponsor of a drug must submit an IND notice to the FDA. This notice, which is required before testing in humans can begin, must contain information about the composition of the drug, about pre-clinical testing of its safety (including animal studies), about the protocol of the planned testing, about the qualifications of the investigators, and about the provisions for obtaining informed consent. Unless the FDA objects within 30 days (or a longer period if further information is requested), clinical tests on human subjects can commence. These tests are normally divided into three phases. Phase I tests for safe dosage ranges, for toxicities, and for pharmacological information in a limited number of subjects. Phase II tests for initial data on effectiveness for a specific clinical condition, and it also involves a limited (but larger) number of patients. Phase III tests for both safety and effectiveness in a much larger number of subjects using the dosages for which approval will ultimately be sought. Phase III tests are run only if the results of Phases I and II tests are encouraging. Finally, if the results of all the tests are satisfactory, those who have sponsored the study file a new drug application (NDA) with the FDA. This application must contain information about the investigations, about the composition of the drug and the procedures used to produce it, and about the proposed labeling to be used for the drug. In theory, the FDA has 180 days to respond to the filing, but that period is open to extension. The drug can be marketed only after all of the components of the application are found acceptable by the FDA. In making that determination, the FDA draws upon the expertise of advisory committees, but the final decision belongs to the staff. The very description of the process suggests that it can be lengthy; data will be presented below to show just how lengthy it can be.

What standards are employed in the final determination? In other words, what answers have been adopted to both our content question and our epistemic question? There is very little material in the 1962 statute concerning the content question. The most that you get is the initial requirement that the data must show "whether or not such drug is safe for use and whether such drug is effective in use."[3] The actual language of the statute on the epistemic question as applied to effectiveness is as follows:

> As used in this subsection . . . the term "substantial evidence" means evidence consisting of adequate and well-controlled investigations, including clinical investigations, by experts qualified by scientific training and experience to evaluate the

effectiveness of the drug involved, on the basis of which it could fairly and responsibly be concluded by such experts that the drug will have the effect it purports or is represented to have. . . .[4]

Applied to the safety question, the statute talks of "adequate tests by all methods reasonably applicable."

There are two observations that immediately come to mind as one looks at the statutory answers. The first is that they are quite vague. How much evidence is mandated, for example, by the fairly-and-responsibly-be-concluded test? What is an adequate and well-controlled test? What is a reasonably applicable method? The second observation is that the answers do not really address the balancing aspects of our questions. The answers to the epistemic question are framed in standards which, however vague they are, do not even mention the possible losses resulting from demanding further evidence. The answer to the content question does not even recognize the possibility of trade-offs between safety and effectiveness, as the two are just treated as separate requirements.

To what extent are these shortcomings remedied in the regulations interpreting these statutory answers? Leaving aside for a moment certain very recent regulations (the post-1987 regulations, which will be discussed below), we turn to the traditional FDA regulations[5] for answers to our questions.

Unfortunately, the regulations are not all that helpful on the content question. There is, to be sure, at least some recognition (especially in 21 CFR §314.50) that there is a risk-benefit ratio relating to the trade-off between safety and effectiveness which is central to the standard for approval, but there is no discussion of how that ratio should be established and assessed. This is not because there has been a lack of awareness of this issue. As early as 1966, in an internal report identifying issues that the FDA confronted,[6] of the three major policy issues identified, one asked: "Where should the balance be struck between benefits and hazards in the approval of the new drugs?" It is rather that the FDA has resisted specifying a general approach to assessing risk-benefit ratios. To quote Commissioner Schmidt testifying in 1974: "Risk-benefit assessment in the last analysis is a refined and discriminative judgment, the most critical of our mixed scientific and regulatory responsibilities. It is not readily describable in general terms."[7]

The regulations are more helpful on the epistemic question. In a crucial section (314.126), a section which dates back to regulations issued after much controversy in 1970,[8] the FDA downplayed the fairly-and-responsibly-concluded-by-the-experts definition and provided a substantial definition of adequate and well-controlled trials as the definition of the evidence required:

> The Food and Drug Administration considers these characteristics in determining whether an investigation is adequate and well-controlled. . . . Reports of adequate and well-controlled investigations *provide the primary basis* for determining whether

there is "substantial evidence" to support the claims of effectiveness for new drugs and antibiotics. (italics added)

Among the requirements on the trial are the requirements that it be controlled, that there be well-defined selection criteria, that patients be randomized, that biases be minimized by such measures as blinding the assessors of the outcomes, and that the data be analyzed according to standard statistical techniques. Nowhere is it suggested that these criteria might be relaxed because of the possible benefits of earlier approval of the drug. So while the epistemic question is given a much fuller answer in the regulations than in the 1962 statute, the important trade-off issue is really neglected.

The Criticisms of the 1970s

The results of the 1962 legislation cannot be fully understood simply by examining the language of the statute and of its interpreting regulations. One must also look at its actual operation. Fortunately, few systems have been more carefully studied and investigated than the FDA drug approval scheme.[9] We turn therefore to those studies in the hope of learning more about how our questions have been answered in practice.

It is fascinating to note how these studies have gone in very different directions. Until recently, the congressional investigations have for the most part focused on claims that the FDA has been too lax in the drug approval process. Congressman L. H. Fountain (1964–1982), Senator Gaylord Nelson (1967–1980), and Senator Edward M. Kennedy (1973–the present) held hearings to consider allegations that unsafe and/or ineffective drugs were being approved by the FDA, which was not adequately protecting the public's health. Former FDA commissioner Schmidt expressed his sense of the thrust and impact of those hearings as follows:

> For example, in all of FDA's history, I am unable to find a single instance where a Congressional committee investigated the failure of FDA to approve a new drug. But, the times when hearings have been held to criticize our approval of new drugs have been so frequent that we aren't able to count them. . . . The message to FDA staff could not be clearer. . . . The Congressional pressure for our negative action on new drug applications is, therefore, intense.[10]

On the other hand, much of the scholarship has suggested that the FDA has been far too restrictive and that the United States has paid a high economic and health cost due to the delays in the approval of useful drugs. We will focus on those academic critics, and the responses to them both by the FDA and its defenders, in part because that literature contains more data as opposed to anecdotal charges, in part because it addresses our trade-off issues, and in part because it led to many of the changes made by the FDA in the 1980s.

Two scholars, from very different backgrounds, started this scholarly critique of the FDA as being too restrictive. The first was Sam Peltzman, an economist who did his research under a grant from the Center for Policy Study at the University of Chicago.[11] Peltzman was part of the Chicago school of political economists who were highly critical of government regulation. The second was William Wardell, a British-trained physician who did his research as a Merck International Fellow in Clinical Pharmacology at the University of Rochester School of Medicine.[12]

Peltzman's main conclusions were that the adoption of the 1962 law was followed by a more than 50 percent reduction in the introduction of new drugs and that there was economic evidence that this reduction was due to a decline in the flow of useful new drugs. Moreover, his studies showed that there had been a disproportionate increase in the cost of bringing new drugs to the market. Peltzman concluded that market forces present in the pre-1962 marketplace had done a good job in keeping ineffective drugs off the market and that consumers had paid a high price for the new 1962 laws. Unfortunately, his analysis was purely economic, offering little information of a clinical nature, so its impact on those outside the field of economics was limited.

Wardell's work was far more influential precisely because it was clinically relevant. Wardell contrasted drug introduction in the United States and Great Britain during the period 1962–1971, the first 10 years after the new legislation governing FDA approval of new drugs. In looking at the 82 new drugs that were mutually available at the end of that period, he was interested in the lag time between availability in the two countries, and he concluded that Great Britain had a balance of 61 drug-years of prior availability. In looking at the 98 new drugs that were exclusively available in one of the countries, 77 were available in Great Britain while only 21 were available in the United States. In short, Wardell's first conclusion was that new drugs became available for use far more quickly in Great Britain than in the United States under the new FDA law of 1962.

That conclusion, by itself, was not sufficient to establish that there was a problem in the United States. Defenders of the FDA, mindful of the thalidomide tragedy, might well conclude that Wardell's data only showed that the FDA was doing its job of protecting U.S. patients from drugs that might be dangerous or ineffective and which needed further testing. To meet this potential challenge, Wardell reviewed the drugs in question to determine the costs and benefits to U.S. patients from delays in their being available.

Wardell focused attention on a number of drugs that were unavailable in the United States but were available in Great Britain, drugs such as propranolol for the management of angina and hypertension (he was later to emphasize its use after myocardial infarctions), cromolyn sodium for the prophylactic management of allergic asthma, bactrim as an antibacterial agent, and some of the newer benzodiazepines. His own conclusion, shared by many, was that this type of analysis showed that U.S. patients paid a high price for the drug lag. He went further and claimed that the root of the problem was the demand of the 1962 statute that effectiveness be established before a drug can be marketed:

> The important difference between Britain and the United States is that, while efficacy was not ignored in the British regulatory process, the policy has so far been that matters of efficacy—especially relative efficacy—and the control of drug use in the context of specific patients are not the prerogative of a regulatory agency, but are far better left to the medical profession aided by the free processes of scientific publication, debate, and education.[13]

It goes without saying that not everyone accepted Wardell's conclusions. Newly appointed FDA commissioner Dr. Donald Kennedy published in 1978 a blistering attack on the concept of a drug lag, arguing that the true cause in the decline in the introduction of new drugs was a depletion of the stock of scientific breakthroughs (the knowledge-depletion hypothesis), while the true cause of any lag between the United States and elsewhere, if one existed, was a better understanding in the United States of what was needed to adequately test drugs.[14] But the tide had clearly turned against such a viewpoint, and pressure was on to reform the workings of the FDA to speed up the drug approval process. After legislative proposals failed in the 1979–1980 period, the FDA turned to regulatory reforms.

The Reforms of the 1980s

Some of the changing attitude on reform reflected the drive toward deregulation that was sweeping Washington in the 1980s. Some of it was due, however, to the impetus provided by two major reports, one produced by the GAO[15] and one (called the McMahon report) produced at the request of Congressmen James H. Scheuer and Albert Gore, Jr., for the House Committee on Science and Technology.[16] Both of these reports were influenced by the work of Peltzman and Wardell. Let us briefly review their findings, their recommendations, and the FDA's response to them.

The main findings of the GAO report were: (1) the average approval time for an NDA (over and above the time for testing after the issuance of an IND) was 20 months, much more than the statutory period of 6 months; (2) new, important drugs were available elsewhere before they were available in the United States; and (3) factors contributing to these long approval times included imprecise FDA guidelines, poor working relations between the FDA and the industry, and intense scrutiny by Congress and the public, reinforcing FDA conservatism. The report noted that the FDA had committed itself to improving the approval time, especially for drugs that were judged to offer important new advances. It recommended that these goals should be monitored to ensure that they occurred, that the FDA should formally clarify its policy to accept foreign data, that it should provide more timely feedback to manufacturers about the deficiencies in their applications, and that it should improve its postmarketing surveillance. The FDA accepted (in Appendix V of the report) all of these recommendations and expressed its intent to implement them as it rewrote its regulations.

This discussion was helpful, but it did not address our fundamental questions 1 and 2, the questions about whether or not the FDA's conservative stance on drug approvals represented the best trade-offs. The closest the report came to addressing these questions was in its discussion of the proposals in unpassed legislation from 1979 and 1980 to have different standards for drugs that represented major therapeutic advances in life-threatening or severe illnesses, a provision that both it and the FDA approved. To quote the report:

> The need for complete testing to ensure that drugs meet the established standards of safety and efficacy has sometimes caused lengthy delays in the availability of drugs that represent major advances in treating serious illnesses. . . . FDA believes this proposed authority [to approve such drugs with only significant rather than substantial evidence] would not compromise the safety of the drug since the Secretary of HEW will have to make a risk–benefit assessment similar to that made for all drugs before FDA approval. The Secretary will have less evidence of effectiveness, but the evidence will have to be sufficient to justify that the drug is safe (the benefits outweigh the risks) and offers major therapeutic advantages for patients with life-threatening or severely debilitating illness or injury.[17]

This remarkably valuable passage makes it clear that the FDA had come to fully accept the view that the requirement of safety is really the requirement that there be a proper risk-benefit ratio. This means that the FDA had come to see that our content question is the right question to ask. Equally important, this passage makes it clear that the FDA had also come to see that there were losses in delaying approval of new drugs, especially when they involved significant advances in the treatment of life-threatening or serious illnesses, and that those possible losses could justify lessening the evidential requirements for approval. This means that the FDA had come to see that our epistemic question is the right question to ask.

Two cautionary remarks are in order here. There is no evidence in the report or in the FDA response to it that the recognition of the need for trade-offs implicit in our two questions would have a broader impact upon the FDA than in its approval of this special class of drugs. The report itself indicated that these special provisions might apply to only 2 percent of drugs. Second, it is important to remember that the legislation in question did not pass; we shall see how long it took before provisions were made for expedited approval of even this special class of drugs. In short, although very valuable, the discussion in the 1980 GAO report hardly constituted either a breakthrough in the understanding of a proper philosophy for drug approval or the beginnings of new policies for even the special case of therapeutic breakthroughs for life-saving or severe illnesses.

A similar appraisal is appropriate, I believe, for the 1982 McMahon report. Its emphasis was on the entire drug-development process, and not just on the final approval process, in part because it was concerned that it was taking an average of 13 years from the time a new chemical entity was synthesized until an NDA for it was approved. This broader look at the entire process was justified. Moreover, the recommendations of that report on the IND and testing process (the requirements for issuing an IND should be simplified, nongovernmental bodies should be used for issuing INDs, the FDA should actively help sponsors plan their clinical trials, and provisions should be made for the therapeutic use of investigational drugs as needed), on the NDA process (NDAs should be streamlined, outside experts should be used more effectively, postmarketing surveillance should be strengthened, foreign data should be employed, and the standards for approval should be clarified), and on FDA management (FDA needs adequate resources, it should improve its interaction with industry, and it should track time for approval) were all quite useful. Nevertheless, the report was in my judgment unsatisfactory primarily because it didn't address the fundamental content and epistemic trade-off issues. It did have some useful things to say (on pp. 56–62) by way of criticizing the FDA's insistence that rather than examining the total evidence, approvals must be based on two clinical trials, each meeting all standards for adequate trials. But even that section didn't address the trade-off issues raised by our epistemic question.

In short, the major reports of the early 1980s laid the foundations in an already receptive environment for reform of the FDA's regulations, but neither that environment nor the reports in question prepared the FDA for a fundamental reexamination of its standards for approval. It is not surprising, therefore, that the FDA reforms of the mid-1980s involved no such fundamental reexamination of those standards.

Already in the 1970s, the FDA had begun to modify its own procedures to speed up the process of drug approval. It ranked drugs according to their potential therapeutic significance (from 1A, the most significant, to 3A, the least significant), and it gave priority to the approval of drugs with greater significance. Moreover, it began meeting with drug companies after Phase II of clinical trials to plan the Phase III trials so that appropriate data would be produced. These were, however, less formal and very partial reforms. The process of producing more formal and complete reforms began in 1979, when the FDA published in the *Federal Register* a series of concept papers and held a public meeting to discuss them.[18] It ended in 1985 (with the publication of a rewrite of the regulations governing new drug applications, the "NDA Rewrite") and in 1987 (with the publication of a rewrite of the regulations governing FDA review of investigational new drug applications, the "IND Rewrite").[19] I believe that these rewrites, while useful in minimizing some administrative problems and expediting some drug approvals, totally failed to address the fundamental issues raised by the content and epistemic questions, thereby making no fundamental changes.

There are several major themes in these rewrites. One is their emphasis on continuing dialogue between FDA staff and drug sponsors. Conferences are targeted for key steps in the approval process and provisions are made for other communications as needed. Standardized formats are provided for both IND and NDA submissions to facilitate handling and approval. There are new regulations clarifying the use of foreign data and the expectations for the various stages of clinical trials. Finally, dispute resolution, timing of responses, and postmarketing surveillance issues are clarified. In short, the rewrites dealt with most of the procedural issues raised in the GAO report and in the McMahon report. But fundamental issues about the standards for approval were not addressed. The closest you get to any discussion of these issues is a notice by the FDA that the industry had wanted a codification of the substantive standards for approval but that the FDA preferred to rely upon conferences in each case together with guidelines for various types of drugs.[20]

Have these changes made a difference? Recent data from a study that compares NDA review times in the period 1978–1989, looking at trends in each of three 4-year periods (1978–1981, 1982–1985, 1986–1989),[21] raise questions about the impact of the NDA rewrite, the first of the rewrites. If the NDA rewrite had a favorable impact upon expediting drug approval, we should see a decrease in the NDA review time, the time from submission of the NDA until the time of actual approval, in the period after 1985 (when the NDA rewrite was issued). In fact, with the exception of the therapeutically least important drugs, NDA review time increased significantly in the period 1986–1989, as shown in Table 3.1, derived from the study in question. The authors of the study, who were attempting to present a positive picture of recent FDA developments, noted this problem; their proffered explanation was that the type of drugs approved in the later period were drugs that typically take longer to approve, such as neuropharmacological drugs. The

Table 3.1 NDA Review Time

	1A Drugs	1B Drugs	1C Drugs
Total mean approval time (months)	22.5	28.7	38.4
1986–1989 mean approval time (months)	27.1	34.0	36.0

best they could say, using that explanation, was that "it is not possible to conclude, based on the current data, that the FDA's review of important new drugs in recent years has slowed."[22] Two comments are in order here. The first is that there is certainly no evidence in their data of improvement after the NDA rewrite. The second is that there is no reason to take the historical record of long approval time for neuropharmacological drugs as justified. Perhaps the best conclusion is that there is no evidence of any improvement since the NDA rewrite and good reason for being concerned that mere procedural reforms will not do the job. The earliest data on post-rewrite FDA behavior in the period 1986–1989 suggests then that more fundamental reforms were required.

This failure in the early and mid-1980s to address fundamental issues was not due to a failure on the part of scholars writing at that time to identify these issues and to propose alternative solutions to them. For example, Henry Grabowski and John Vernon, two economists from Duke University, published an important study in 1983. It identified the trade-offs involved in both the content and epistemic issues, clarified the pressures that led the FDA to adopt a conservative stance to approval, and proposed either turning the FDA from an approver of drugs into a certifier of information about drugs (a proposal we shall discuss more fully later) or changing the standards for approval to allow for earlier approval while further studies were being conducted.[23] Similarly, Peter Temin, professor of economics at MIT, advocated much greater reliance on physician and patient choice in determining drug therapy (another proposal which we will discuss more fully).[24] Rather, the debate in Congress and the FDA after the failure of the 1979–1980 legislation stayed away from these fundamental issues and focused merely on procedural reforms. This emphasis resulted in the rewrites and in the failure to make sufficient improvements. But then came AIDS, which transformed the whole discussion.

Responses to the AIDS Crisis

Our concern here is not with all the issues raised by the AIDS epidemic but just with its impact upon the drug approval process. We shall try to assess the effect of the AIDS epidemic on the understanding of the need for changes in the drug approval process and the extent to which it has focused attention on the need to address our two fundamental questions. Others have already pointed out that AIDS has made a tremendous difference in this area. Writing in *Medical World News* in 1989, Susan Jenks said, "AIDS activists, ready to 'talk or be handcuffed,' have provided the pivotal push for action on simplifying a regulatory maze and speeding access to new drugs. The effects are being felt, and experts say drugs for all life-threatening diseases will benefit."[25] In a fuller and more scholarly treatment of the impact of AIDS on the drug regulatory process, Harold Edgar and David Rothman concluded as follows:

> What, then, should we expect of drug regulation in the future? . . . The history that
> we have been tracing suggests that the tilt is, and will be, to a consumer-rights ori-
> entation. Perhaps the events of the past two years represent a strategic retreat on the
> part of the FDA that will ward off a more total defeat, but it is highly unlikely that
> the FDA will soon again enjoy the authority that it possessed in the 1960s and
> 1970s.[26]

Our analysis will attempt to relate that "consumer-rights" orientation suggested by Edgar and Rothman to new answers to our two fundamental questions.

Three sorts of drugs would be very helpful in dealing with the AIDS epidemic. Two (a vaccine to prevent the spread of HIV and a cure that would kill all the viruses in infected individuals) seem to be a long way off. Most attention has focused on drugs that preserve the functioning of the compromised immune system for as long as possible and/or treat the infections that are the actual causes of the death of patients with AIDS. Sadly, so many of the drugs initially studied (access to which, even without FDA approval, was demanded by some activists) turned out to be worthless. Such drugs as cyclosporin A, HPA-23, and ribavirin have each had their day of favorable publicity followed by an aftermath of disappointment.[27] AZT changed that, paving the way for the changes at the FDA which we need to examine.

The history of AZT can be briefly summarized as follows.[28] Azidothymidine, or AZT, had been developed in 1964 under a grant from the National Cancer Institute as a potential cancer treatment, but it proved to be inefficacious for that purpose. Studies in late 1984 and early 1985 suggested that it inhibited duplication of the AIDS virus, and Burroughs Wellcome filed an IND application in May 1985 so that clinical testing could begin. Phase I trials proved to be promising, so Phase II trials began in February 1986. The trials involved 282 patients, half of whom got AZT while the other half got a placebo. At the end of 6 months, one patient in the AZT group was dead, while 19 were dead in the placebo control group. The trial was stopped on the grounds that it was unethical to continue to deny treatment to half the patients. Whether or not AZT really makes a difference in the long run, it was life-preserving in the short run. An NDA was filed in December 1986 and approved in March 1987, subject to the proviso that there be extensive postapproval surveillance. From the time the trial was stopped until the application was finally approved, the drug was made available to more than 4,000 patients even though it was still under an IND.[29]

Two concepts emerged from this history. First, in desperate situations very promising drugs might be distributed while final testing and review were continuing; second, such drugs might be approved after Phase II testing with extensive postapproval surveillance. The former idea was codified in 1987 as the Treatment IND program while the latter idea was codified in 1988 as the Subpart E program.[30]

It is these two programs that constitute the initial FDA responses to the AIDS crisis, and we need to look at them carefully.

Both programs are confined to drugs designed to treat specific diseases. The Treatment IND regulations apply to immediately life-threatening ("a stage of a disease in which there is a reasonable likelihood that death will occur within a matter of months or in which premature death is likely without early treatment") or serious (not defined in the regulations) diseases. The Subpart E regulations apply to life-threatening ("likelihood of death is high unless the course of the disease is interrupted" or "potentially fatal outcomes, where the end point of clinical trial analysis is survival") or severely debilitating ("cause major irreversible morbidity") diseases.

The Treatment IND program allows drugs to be used outside clinical trials in treating such illnesses providing that there is no comparable or satisfactory alternative drug or treatment available and providing that the drug is being investigated in controlled trials or all trials have been completed and the sponsor is actively pursuing marketing approval. In the case of serious illnesses, the FDA may deny a request for a Treatment IND "if there is insufficient evidence of safety and effectiveness to support such use." In the case of an immediately life-threatening illness, the FDA may deny a request for a Treatment IND only if "the available scientific evidence, taken as a whole, fails to provide a reasonable basis for concluding that the drug (A) may be effective for its intended use in its intended population or (B) would not expose the patients to whom the drug is to be administered to an unreasonable and significant additional risk of illness or injury." The latter requirement is far less demanding than the former. In a very important passage, the FDA had the following to say in support of this new standard against some of its critics:[31]

> Because of the different risk–benefit considerations involved in treating such diseases, FDA continues to believe there needs to be a separate standard for drugs intended to treat immediately life-threatening diseases . . . the level of evidence needed is well short of that needed for new drug approval—and may be less than what would be needed to support treatment use in diseases that are serious but not immediately life-threatening.[32]

The Subpart E Program allows for drugs designed to treat life-threatening or severely debilitating illnesses to receive final approval more quickly by employing new procedures (a post-Phase I conference designed to produce combined Phase II–III trials sufficient to secure approval) and new standards for approval. Some of the changes in the standards, while quite important, refer to specific technical issues. The commentary accompanying the actual regulations makes it clear, for example, that the FDA will accept active-controlled trials and will not necessarily demand more than one trial. But the crucial change in the standards is the more general point found in the following regulation:

> FDA's application of the statutory standards for marketing approval shall recognize the need for a medical risk–benefit judgment in making the final decision on approvability. . . . FDA will consider whether the benefits of the drug outweigh the known and potential risks of the drug and the need to answer remaining questions about risks and benefits of the drug, taking into consideration the severity of the disease and the absence of satisfactory alternative therapy.[33]

In this standard, we find the FDA building into its regulations something that it had never previously formally implemented—the recognition that the standards for final drug approval must be sensitive to the trade-offs found in both the content and the epistemic questions. It is because these trade-offs are recognized as inevitable and appropriate that the FDA could also say in the opening section of the new regulation that "these procedures reflect the recognition that physicians and patients are generally willing to accept greater risks or side effects from products that treat life-threatening and severely debilitating illnesses, than they would accept from products that treat less serious illnesses."[34] It is this passage that best reflects the consumer-rights orientation referred to by Edgar and Rothman. This orientation became possible only because of the explicit FDA acceptance of the legitimacy of the trade-offs involved in our two questions.

To summarize our account until now, I think that we can say the following: the 1962 statute and its interpreting regulations were insensitive to the trade-offs involved in the content and the epistemic questions. The deficiencies critics pointed out in the post-1962 regulatory scheme reflected the lengthy approval process and the drug lag, while attention focused primarily on procedural reforms of the sort recommended in the GAO and McMahon reports and adopted in the rewrites. The AIDS epidemic focused attention on more substantive changes in the standards for availability and approval and led to the explicit acceptance of our trade-offs as both legitimate and inevitable.

The Most Recent Developments

How have these new changes worked out in practice? Have they led to further innovations? Most important, have they led to any further discussion of how the trade-offs should be made? To answer these questions, we need to review some of the important developments between 1988 and 1993.

Three major developments deserve attention. The first is the actual implementation of the Treatment IND program and the Subpart E program. The second is the development of still another program, the Parallel Track program. The third is the appearance of two additional reports, the Lasagna Report of August 15, 1990, and the November 13, 1991, Report of the Council on Competitiveness, and the implementation of some of their recommendations in one additional program, the Subpart H program.

The FDA issued a report on the Treatment IND program's actual implementation in the period from June 22, 1987, to June 10, 1993.[35] It showed two Treatment INDs issued at the end of 1987, six in 1988, nine in 1989, two in 1990, five in 1991, three in 1992, and one in the first half of 1993. Of the 28, only 9 were for drugs to treat AIDS (trimetrexate for PCP [*Pneumocystis carinii* pneumonia], ganciclovir for CMV [cytomegalovirus] retinitis, aerosolized pentamidine for PCP prevention, erythropoietin for AZT-related anemia, ddI [dideoxyinosine] and ddC [dideoxycytidine] for patients intolerant to AZT, AZT for children, Atovaquone for certain patients with PCP, and Mycobutin for prophylaxis against MAC [*Mycobacterium avium* complex] bacteremia). The others were for the treatment of various cancers (9 drugs) and for a variety of other illnesses (infections in renal transplants, severe obsessive compulsive disorder, severe Parkinson's, respiratory distress syndrome in newborns [2 drugs], Gaucher's disease, spasticity, constitutional delay of growth, Alzheimer's dementia, and multiple sclerosis). So the first thing to note is that the Treatment IND program, while developed as a response to the AIDS crisis, has been implemented in a way that reflects a broader realization that a consideration of trade-offs needs to be made in the case of other diseases as well. The second thing to note is that most of the drugs given a Treatment IND before 1992 were finally approved by the end of 1992, although in some cases that final approval process took more than 2 years after the initial issuance of the Treatment IND.[36] There are, of course, two ways to look at this point. The positive way suggests that this shows the value of the Treatment IND program, which is making drugs available several years earlier than they would have otherwise been available. The negative way suggests that the Treatment IND program, by taking some of the pressure off the FDA for quicker final approval, has allowed the traditional delays in final approval to continue. Much more study is needed on this point. The third thing to note is that any full evaluation of the Treatment IND program would require a careful study of the applications for a Treatment IND that were not approved, but that information is not available. Of relevance here is the fact that of the 12 drugs approved in 1990 or 1991 which received an FDA 1A designation, indicating that they are a significant therapeutic gain, the majority had not previously been available on a Treatment IND. Similarly, of the 11 drugs approved in 1992 which received an FDA priority review designation (its new designation for drugs that represent a significant gain), 7 had not previously been available on a treatment IND.[37] This is an issue that clearly needs further study. The final point to note is the smaller number of Treatment INDs issued in the period 1990–1993. In short, then, there are some signs that the Treatment IND program is serving to respond to some of the real concerns raised by the general trade-off issues, but there are also many concerns about its operation, especially between 1990 and 1993.

The evaluation of the Subpart E program is an even more complicated question. In part this is due to the fact that there is often no clear statement of when an approval is a Subpart E approval. This problem was already noted by Kahan and Read, in their landmark study of these issues in 1990:

> Unlike treatment INDs, which the FDA publicizes quite effectively, products that have been approved on the basis of phase 2 trials [Subpart E approvals] have not been announced. Informal discussions with FDA staff indicate there are [in early 1990] none. The FDA's recent approval of ganciclovir is arguably a phase 2 approval, maybe even phase 1.[38]

This is unfortunate because the Subpart E program is, of course, far more revolutionary than the Treatment IND program, for approval under it makes a drug available on the market to be used as physicians and patients agree. It is, however, possible to begin such an evaluation, and that is what we will now do.

We are fortunate to have some baseline data for such an evaluation. Around the time of the approval of the Subpart E program, the FDA did an important study of 30 drug approvals in the period January 1, 1980–June 30, 1988, that it felt might have been eligible for Subpart E approval if such a program had existed.[39] Interestingly enough, both tPA and streptokinase are included in the list. The data tell us about approvals of such drugs after the FDA prioritization program and after the rewrites but before the Subpart E program. All future studies of the Subpart E program can use these data as baseline data. For our purposes, the crucial point to note is the speedup in the approval process in the 1986–1988 period as compared to the 1980–1985 period for these drugs (as opposed to the broader class of 1A drugs, for which, as we saw, there was no evidence of any speedup). The average NDA review time had decreased from 2.3 to 1.8 years, and the total development time decreased even more rapidly, primarily because NDAs were being submitted even before the pivotal trials were completed. Consequently, any future evaluations of the Subpart E program will need to compare the results under that program to the results of the earlier FDA efforts that had already produced significant improvements.

The second thing we can do in evaluating the Subpart E program is to consider two applications for approval that were submitted in 1991. One of them, the application for the approval of ddI for the treatment of AIDS, was successful, and probably represents the first *clear-cut* case of Subpart E approval. The other, the application for the approval of tacrine for the treatment of Alzheimer's disease was initially denied, but tacrine was approved for a Treatment IND and was eventually approved. This contrast will be useful for a preliminary evaluation of the Subpart E program, in part because some have argued that the contrast shows that the FDA is not serious about drug approval reform outside of the context of AIDS.

Thus the *Wall Street Journal* had the following to say in an editorial shortly after the FDA advisory committee turned down the tacrine application:

> An FDA advisory committee's decision last Friday not to approve the Alzheimer's drug tacrine (or THA) is overwhelming evidence of what we have long suspected: The FDA's efforts to reform its drug-approval process is a bureaucratic hoax. The agency's AIDS effort, such as the "fast-track" approval of AZT, was primarily a shrewd bureaucracy's response to great political pressure, including a presidential AIDS commission. Persons suffering from cancer, Alzheimer's and other tragic diseases can forget it.[40]

I think that this account is a mistake and that there are better reasons for the difference in the treatment of the two. An examination of the development of these drugs and of these differences will teach us a lot about the initial use of the Subpart E program.

DDI is a drug that inhibits the AIDS virus from duplicating itself. In that way, it resembles AZT in being a response to the AIDS virus and not just to the infections to which patients with AIDS are subject. Phase I studies involving ddI had shown some clinical improvement, so Phase II and III clinical trials were begun by the NIH's AIDS Clinical Trial Group after careful consultation with the FDA about their design. These trials compared ddI to AZT in patients who had received AZT for either a short or a long period of time or compared ddI to a placebo in patients intolerant to AZT. At the same time, under two additional programs (to be discussed later as examples of the parallel-track program), over 20,000 patients who had been intolerant to AZT or who had deteriorated on AZT were given ddI and their status was also followed. On July 18–19, 1991, the FDA's Antiviral Drugs Advisory Committee met to consider an application by Bristol-Myers Squibb for the approval of ddI. Final data from the NIH trials involving survival time and progression to AIDS would not be available for at least another year, and the results from the Treatment IND patients involved no data from nonhistorical controls. But there were significant data from the NIH trials showing that the immune systems of the patients taking ddI were doing better than the immune systems of the patients taking AZT because the ddI patients had higher CD4 lymphocyte counts. On the basis of that finding, and despite the fact that crucial trials were still continuing, the committee, with some dissents, recommended the approval of ddI for patients who were intolerant to AZT or who were deteriorating despite the use of AZT. On October 9, 1991, the FDA approved ddI, despite lingering concerns about side effects (pancreatitis) and continuing uncertainties about the long-term significance of the data about improvements in the status of the immune system.[41] It also recommended that the trials continue.

This approval certainly makes sense in the context of the Subpart E program. There was extensive consultation after Phase I about the design of the trials and of the drug distribution program. The approval was for a situation which is life-threatening and for which there are no alternatives (since the patients are intolerant of AZT or are deteriorating despite its use). While there were no data about prolongation of life, there were significant data about the surrogate end point of improvement of the immune system. Further studies about length of survival continued, as called for in the Subpart E program. So while there were real questions about ddI, it seems as reasonable a case as is likely for a Subpart E approval, and the process for getting that approval was followed very carefully.

The postapproval history of ddI is worth noting. Subsequent data from AZT-ddI trials published in 1992 suggested that ddI produced a significant delay in the onset of new AIDS-defining events, especially in patients who already had used AZT.[42] This was seen as support for the Subpart E program. At the same time, the use of surrogate end points such as CD4 counts remained controversial. This controversy was heightened by the recent publication of preliminary data from the Concorde trial of the use of AZT by asymptomatic AIDS patients; despite improved CD4 counts, there were no long-term differences in outcomes. Some, particularly European researchers, have expressed increasing doubts about the use of such end points. Others, such as Dr. David Kessler of the FDA, continue to support their use in accelerated approval programs. Kessler expressed his viewpoint as follows: "There's no question that one day we are going to be wrong. Everyone needs to keep their eyes wide open."[43]

Tacrine was quite different. The initial report of its usefulness in alleviating some of the symptoms of Alzheimer's disease[44] had been severely criticized by the FDA[45] on significant methodological grounds. More recent trials failed to show significant improvement or showed hepatocellular injury.[46] Moreover there had been no close consultation with the FDA in planning trials. Finally, the trial data presented to the advisory committee in March 1991 and again in July 1991 about improved functioning was far from unambiguous. Therefore, despite the fact that Kessler, the head of the FDA, urged the advisory panel at its July meeting to use the same criteria it used in the case of AIDS drugs,[47] it is not surprising that the advisory committee voted against approval. What emerged as the alternative to approval was a close collaboration between the company and the FDA on a carefully controlled trial and a significant Treatment IND program. This seems to me like a very reasonable compromise in light of our trade-offs given the history of tacrine, and it did lead to the approval of tacrine in 1993.[48]

What can we say then about the Subpart E program's early history? We know that we have baseline data for studying its effectiveness. We know from the case of ddI that it will speed up some approvals. We know from the case of tacrine that not every request for approval will be granted. And we know from the controversy surrounding these cases that the criteria for the appropriate trade-offs on both the content question and the epistemic question are far from settled at this point.

We have so far looked at the first of three 1988–1993 developments that deserve our attention, the actual implementation of the Treatment IND and Subpart E programs. We turn now to the second of those developments, the parallel-track program. A good way to understand that program is to return briefly to one aspect of the testing of ddI.

As noted previously, while a variety of Phase II and III trials comparing ddI to AZT were being conducted, over 20,000 additional patients who could not take, or would not benefit from, AZT were also receiving ddI. Officially, this was being done under the Treatment IND program in conjunction with older compassionate-use programs, with the data supporting this use being the limited data on safety and efficacy from the Phase I studies. In May 1990, the FDA proposed a set of regulations, the "parallel-track regulations,"[49] that would formalize this approach, allowing patients who could not be enrolled in trials access to drugs while Phase II and III trials of those drugs were continuing. These proposed regulations were finalized in April 1992.[50] The following are important points to note. (1) The new program, unlike the Treatment IND program and the Subpart E program, is confined to drugs for the treatment of AIDS. The main arguments given for this were that it is best to try this new approach in one disease as a pilot program, and AIDS made sense in light of the need of the patients and the willingness of the AIDS community to participate in both tracks (the trials and the treatment). (2) The FDA said that the main difference from earlier programs was that "the evidence for effectiveness is less than that generally required for a Treatment IND" and that "all drugs distributed under the parallel track mechanism will be under a study protocol. . . . However, most of the data essential for market approval will come from the controlled clinical trials." (3) These regulations represent a further commitment to expediting availability of drugs in light of the obvious trade-offs we have been discussing, but they contain no more information about how the trade-offs are to be made. The evidence required is simply described as "sufficient information," and this is hardly a satisfactory resolution of the trade-off issues involved in the epistemic question. Safety and efficacy are treated separately, so there is certainly no answer in the proposed regulations to the trade-off issues involved in the content question. This is, of course, not surprising, as the far more advanced Treatment IND and Subpart E programs did no better, but it remains disappointing. (4) Patients are allowed to participate in the parallel track, as opposed to the clinical trial, only if they cannot participate in the controlled clinical trial (because they do not meet the entry criteria, they are too sick, participation would cause undue hardship, or the trial is fully enrolled) or they cannot take standard treatment (because it is contraindicated, cannot be tolerated, or is no longer effective). During the comment period on the proposed regulations, one comment suggested that these requirements could be dropped if a patient wanted to choose the experimental treatment and was fully informed of its risks. This suggestion was explicitly rejected in the comments accompanying the final regulations on the grounds that "PHS [Public Health Service] does not agree that informed consent can completely substitute for the eligibility criteria set forth in the policy statement, which provide additional protection for individuals against uncertainties from drugs still in the early stages of development." The significance of this last point will emerge shortly.

We turn finally to the third of the 1988–1993 developments that deserve our attention, the appearance of two additional reports about the FDA, the Lasagna report and the Report of the Council on Competitiveness, and of the Subpart H regulations to implement at least part of these reports. Let us analyze each of them separately.

The National Committee to Review Current Procedures for Approval of New Drugs for Cancer and AIDS, chaired by Dr. Louis Lasagna, was appointed in 1988 at the request of then Vice President George Bush to study how to expand access to new drugs for AIDS and cancer. Much of its 1990 report was devoted to procedural issues.[51] It recommended, for example, that institutional review boards could play a useful role in the earlier approval of drugs. Other portions of its report endorsed the then-emerging Treatment IND and parallel-track proposals. But there are two sections of its report that are particularly important for our story, because they represent an attempt to better articulate the acceptable trade-offs in this area. The first is the committee's concrete recommendation that effectiveness could be established by showing improvement in surrogate end points, such as tumor regression in cancer or improved immune system status in AIDS, rather than waiting for sufficient data about survival rates. The second is the broader recommendation that substantial evidence of effectiveness, even if it is not definitive, be sufficient for approval. The committee's view was that this was all that Congress had intended in 1962. The interaction between this view on the trade-off questions and the consumer-orientation approach discussed earlier is nicely illustrated in the following statement in the final report:

> The committee recognizes that, by making new drugs available for marketing at this early stage, when there is substantial evidence but not yet definitive evidence of effectiveness, there is an attendant greater risk of serious adverse reactions that have not yet been discovered. Cancer and AIDS patients have made it clear to the committee, however, that in light of the seriousness of the diseases involved, they are willing to accept this greater risk. Earlier approval of new drugs will mean that the patient will bear greater responsibility, along with the physician, for understanding and accepting the risks involved.[52]

The significance of this observation about accepting responsibility, and its relation to various scholarly proposals for further changes in the drug approval process, will be discussed later in this chapter.

The other report came from the Council on Competitiveness.[53] The council was chaired by the vice president, and its mission, as its name indicates, was to modify federal regulations so as to make American industry more competitive in the international marketplace. Its sponsorship of the report lent support to the concern expressed by George Annas, among others, that the whole set of regulatory changes we have been analyzing is designed to help the drug industry rather than patients.[54] While understanding his grounds for suspicion, I want to emphasize that the sponsorship of the report is different from its merits, and the merits and deficiencies of the proposals in the report need to be addressed independently of the question of the sponsorship of the report.

I think that it can fairly be said that a number of features of this report are quite far-reaching. The report addressed the entire drug approval process, both accelerated Subpart E–type approval and regular approval, and not just an accelerated approval process for AIDS and cancer drugs. It set specific performance goals for both types of approvals, reducing average development time of drugs approved under accelerated approval from 9.75 years to 5.5 years and average development time of drugs approved under regular approval from 9.75 years to 7 years. Some of this was to be accomplished by procedural reforms, including using external reviewers for reducing the backlog in standard areas, using both advisory boards and institutional IRBs to fulfill some of the tasks currently performed by FDA staff, and computerizing FDA work with the help of industry grants. These procedural changes were overshadowed by fundamental philosophical changes reflected in the report. The most important of these was the complete acceptance of the trade-offs involved in our epistemic question as legitimate. To quote the report:

> FDA will make a deliberative effort to interpret the statutory requirement of efficacy in a manner that maximizes rather than limits a drug's potential for approval and *takes into account the risks to human life and health that may result from delay of new treatments.*[55]

The first part of the statement is troubling, because it talks about maximizing a potential which might not deserve to be realized because of safety concerns. The second part is exactly right, however, because those risks from delay may be of greater significance than the risks from allowing earlier approval and they certainly must be taken into account. In light of this changed philosophy, the report made a number of additional substantive recommendations about the criteria for approval. One of them was an endorsement of the Lasagna report's support of the use of surrogate end points. Another was the recommendation that the FDA rely upon foreign approvals once common standards are developed. The third was the recommendation that Subpart E accelerated approval be extended to any condition, whether or not it is life-threatening or severely debilitating, if there is no satisfactory alternative therapy.

This report immediately attracted considerable concern. Three influential Democrats, Senator Edward Kennedy and Representatives John Dingell and Henry Waxman, sent a letter on November 13, 1991, to Commissioner David Kessler of the FDA describing the new proposals, especially those about the use of outside experts and of foreign data, as "thinly veiled efforts to weaken the agency, and [to] undermine the very purpose for which it was created." They called for a delay in implementation until Congress could assess the proposals. Hearings were held by Congressman Ted Weiss on March 19, 1992, and a critical report was issued by his subcommittee on October 9, 1992, after the congressman's death.[56] These proposals were also opposed by more than 80 percent of the leading medical officers at the FDA who responded to a poll conducted by the Public Citizen Health Research Group,[57] although it should be noted that the response rate to the poll was less than 40 percent and the group which conducted the survey is a long-standing opponent of attempts to ease the FDA regulatory process. The responding medical officers saw these proposals as lowering standards and making the process too vulnerable to industry influence.

While this controversy continued, the FDA issued on April 15, 1992, a proposed set of regulations (the Subpart H or accelerated approval regulations) that expanded the Subpart E regulations by incorporating some of the suggestions from these two commissions. These regulations were finalized on December 11, 1992.[58] The Subpart H program, which applies to all life-threatening or serious illnesses, is broader than the Subpart E program, which applies only to life-threatening or severely debilitating illnesses, but it is not quite as broad as the recommendations of the Council on Competitiveness, which would apply to all drugs. The Subpart H program applies to new treatments that "provide meaningful therapeutic benefit to patients over existing treatment." This is broader than the Subpart E program, which applies only to cases where no satisfactory alternative exists. Finally, following the recommendations of both commissions, the Subpart H program explicitly authorizes approval based on surrogate end points, postmarketing studies to be required where needed, and restrictions to be placed upon distribution in certain cases. While these were only proposed regulations in April 1992, they were used, at the request of Commissioner Kessler, as the basis for the approval of the use in certain circumstances of a third anti-AIDS drug, ddC.[59]

We have seen that the AIDS epidemic transformed the discussion of reforming the drug approval process by emphasizing the substantive issues of how to make the appropriate trade-offs between safety and efficacy and between getting more data or earlier approval rather than the procedural issues emphasized in earlier discussions. Our review of the post-1987 developments revealed that this shift of emphasis has continued, although there has also been a continuing interest in procedural reforms. Thirty years after the 1962 legislation transformed the drug approval process in the United States, we are as a matter of official policy now recognizing that such approvals of drugs involve trade-offs and that we need as a society to think through the question of what trade-offs we want to make.

How should these trade-offs be made? Are the new programs in place (Treatment IND, Subparts E and H, and parallel track) improvements in the drug approval process, leading to the right trade-offs, or dangerous weakenings of that process, leading to the wrong trade-offs? Are even more fundamental changes needed? And what does all of this tell us about the approval in 1987 of streptokinase and tPA? We shall return to these questions in the final section of this chapter. Before doing so, however, we need to look carefully at foreign alternatives.

Alternative Regulatory Schemes in Other Countries

The United States is not the only country which has struggled with the difficult trade-offs that are the focus of this chapter. In this section we look at the experience of other countries to see what we can learn from their approaches.

In the literature on drug approval, there has been considerable attention devoted to the European experience, particularly the British experience. Much of this attention has focused on the outcomes of the regulatory process, on when various drugs are approved in different countries. This type of discussion grows out of the drug lag literature briefly discussed in the last section. There has been much less attention devoted to the differences in the processes themselves and in the standards for approval embodied in them. I shall try to show in this section that much less is understood about these differences and that this means that international comparisons will at best suggest alternatives rather than present clear-cut alternatives.

Let us begin our international comparisons by returning to the drug lag literature, which first focused attention on drug approval procedures in Europe. As we saw in the last section, that literature was stimulated by the appearance of Wardell's studies of the approval of drugs in the United States and in the United Kingdom between 1962 and 1971, studies that he later extended through 1976. Wardell's conclusions were that drugs became available far more quickly in the United Kingdom than in the United States, that some of these delays were very costly to American patients, and that British patients were not suffering as a result of quick approvals of drugs that turned out to be dangerous. As important as those studies were, they are of less guidance for us today since so many changes have occurred in the drug approval process both in the United States (the many procedural pre-AIDS changes) and in the United Kingdom (the adoption in 1971 of the current formal regulatory scheme). Fortunately for us, a much more recent analysis is available, so we will begin with a critical discussion of that analysis.

Kaitin and his colleagues studied drug introductions in the United States and in the United Kingdom from 1977 (the first year after Wardell's studies, and well after the current formal U.K. scheme was introduced) through 1987 (by which time all the pre-AIDS changes at the FDA had occurred).[60] Using several different measures, they concluded that the drug lag was still a real phenomenon. More new drugs were first introduced in the United Kingdom. Some 76 percent (114) of the U.S. new drugs that were mutually available were first introduced in the United Kingdom, while only 35 percent (41) of the British new drugs that were mutually available were first introduced in the United States. The United Kingdom had a much higher mean lead time for mutually available drugs. The mean lead time for mutually available drugs was 60.7 months for drugs first introduced in the United Kingdom as opposed to 28.9 months for drugs first introduced in the United States. Finally, there were more of these drugs exclusively available in the United Kingdom (70) at the end of 1987 than in the United States (54). These problems were particularly pronounced in the areas of respiratory, cardiovascular, central nervous system, and anticancer drugs. Of particular concern is the finding that there was no significant overall change in the mean lag time between 1977–1982 and 1983–1987. Even more ominous is their finding that the drug lag was a serious problem even for drugs rated by the FDA as important therapeutic gains (1A drugs). Some 75 percent of these drugs that were mutually available were first introduced in the United Kingdom (as opposed to 72 percent of the mutually available 1B drugs and 79 percent of the mutually available 1C drugs), and the mean lead time for the mutually available 1A drugs first introduced in the United Kingdom exceeded the mean lead time for the mutually available 1A drugs first introduced in the United States by 40.4 months (as opposed to 39.8 months for 1B drugs and 29.7 months for 1C drugs).

How serious is this continued drug lag problem? Are American patients at least benefiting from the stricter regulatory scheme by not being exposed to more dangerous drugs that are being made available in the United Kingdom? Kaitin and his colleagues addressed both of these questions. They pointed out that the delay in the approval of 1A drugs (which, by the FDA's own account, represent important advances) is particularly indicative that American patients are paying a serious price for delays in the drug approval process. As far as safety is concerned, they found little difference between the two countries as measured by postapproval discontinuations of approval (a less than perfect measure). During 1977–1987, there were eight discontinuations in the United Kingdom and five in the United States, nearly all involving nonsteroidal anti-inflammatory drugs. This pattern is quite similar to what was found for the discontinuations in the period 1964–1983 by other scholars.[61] This marginal increase in safety hardly seems to compensate for the extensive delay in the availability of important therapeutic advances. So the Kaitin analysis at least suggested that the United States might do well to see what it can learn from the drug approval experience of the United Kingdom.

The Kaitin analysis has not gone unchallenged. Several FDA officials collaborated in a response (hereafter called the FDA response) that raised both methodological and substantive critiques of the Kaitin study, a response that provoked a counterresponse by Kaitin.[62] There are many issues raised in that debate, but I want to focus on one, the question of whether the latest data show that the drug lag is disappearing.

The FDA response puts the issue as follows:

> The trend shifts in favor of the United States, however, in the most recent 1984 through 1987 period. Here, despite a temporary U.K. lag time advantage of 1 year for the 15 NCEs [new chemical entities] of this era that are at present mutually available, the U.S. has registered a 1.8 to 1 advantage (37 versus 20) in the larger pool of 57 exclusively available NCEs. This, as we have seen in the previous periods, is the factor that drives and defines eventual drug lags. For these drugs, the passage of time now counts against the United Kingdom, just as it counted against the United States in earlier periods. If we follow the trend of the 1984 through 1987 period to the end of 1988, it conforms with these predictions. We find a virtual tie in the drug lag. . . . These data are consistent with the notion that 1984 may have been a pivotal year in the history of drug-introduction patterns between the United States and the United Kingdom.

The importance of this claim requires that it be analyzed more carefully.

Kaitin, in his response, is skeptical. He sees this trend as a statistical artifact due to the FDA response's looking at the shorter period 1984–1987 rather than the longer period 1983–1987 that he looked at. What is special, according to Kaitin, is that 1983 was a year in which the United States had introduced far fewer drugs than the United Kingdom. As he puts it, "moving the 1983 data to the first period has the effect of making the earlier interval look worse while making the more recent interval look better." There is certainly truth to this claim. If you look at the number of exclusively available drugs at the end of 1987—a crucial figure because it may well be the factor that drives the later lag—and go back to looking at the entire period 1983–1987, the U.S. advantage in exclusively available NCEs becomes much smaller (38 to 31). At the same time, it also remains true that the FDA response has noted a new trend, for this remains the first period in which the United States shows any advantage. Does this mean that the gradual reforms of the 1980s, the pre-AIDS reforms, really made a difference?

Several observations are in order here. First, very few of the drugs which were first introduced in the United States were major therapeutic breakthroughs: 14 were 1C drugs, 18 were 1B drugs, 2 were unranked biologicals, and only 3 were 1A drugs, the drugs that are the major therapeutic advances. Second, the FDA response's claim that 1984 was a pivotal year in the history of American drug regulation is implausible in light of the data presented at the beginning of this chapter that showed no lessening of drug approval time in the United States through 1989. Finally, there is a simpler explanation of the 1984–1987 data showing more initial approvals in the United States. It is that drug introductions rapidly declined in the United Kingdom in 1984–1987, thereby making the American situation look better even though there was no actual improvement in the process of U.S. drug approval in that period. This hypothesis seems very plausible in light of Table 3.2. This decline in the number of approvals in the United Kingdom was accompanied by a tremendous increase in the time required to secure approval. And both phenomena were due to increasing staff shortages at a time when tremendous new burdens, related to a mandated review of older drugs and a new system of review for parallel imported products, were being placed on the process.[63] In short, then, if future analyses eventually show a decline in the comparative U.S. drug lag in the post-1987 period in light of the earlier U.S. approvals in the 1984–1987 period, it will probably be due to problems in the United Kingdom rather than improvements in the United States. In fact, however, data still to be discussed suggest that those problems in the United Kingdom have been resolved, and that the drug lag will remain.

I believe that we can learn even more if we go beyond the drug lag literature's discussion of the outputs of the U.K. process and examine its actual workings. As I indicated at the beginning of this section, these observations about the working of the process are going to be suggestive rather than definitive. Let us begin with a brief history of the U.K. system.

The history of the U.K. scheme has been nicely summarized by Cuthbert, Griffin, and Inman.[64] Although there was an earlier system for controlling certain biologicals, there was no licensing system for drugs until after the thalidomide

Table 3.2 Total Number of Approvals

Year	United States	United Kingdom
1977	17	14
1978	19	17
1979	13	18
1980	12	23
1981	23	25
1982	22	22
1983	12	25
1984	21	11
1985	26	9
1986	20	12
1987	19	10

Source: K. I. Kaitin et al., "The Drug Lag: An Update of New Introductions in the United States and in the United Kingdom, 1977 through 1987," *Clinical Pharmacology and Therapeutics* 46 (1989), p.123.

disaster. As in the United States, that disaster led to a major change in the system for introducing drugs in the United Kingdom. The initial response in 1963 was to set up a Committee on the Safety of Drugs. Although this committee had no legal powers, the major pharmaceutical companies agreed that they would not test new drugs or market them without the prior approval of the committee. This voluntary system functioned from 1964 to 1971. While it was eventually replaced, at least in part because only 600 of 3,600 companies (even if they were the major companies) participated in the scheme, it laid the foundation for the current U.K. scheme. Among its features was an informality of approach, close working relations with the industry, and heavy reliance on postapproval surveillance of adverse effects. The Medicines Act of 1968 called for the replacement of the voluntary scheme by a mandatory scheme, and it came into place in September 1971.

How does that system work?[65] The actual licensing authority is a ministerial committee whose work is carried out by an administrative staff in the Medicines Control Agency (formerly, the Medicines Division of the Department of Health). Applications for approval are submitted to this agency, whose staff then submit the applications for three assessments, pharmaceutical (primarily related to the quality of the production of the product), preclinical (primarily related to safety), and medical (primarily related to efficacy). If these assessments are satisfactory, then a license is issued. If there are doubts, the application is referred to the Committee on the Safety of Medicines, which can recommend approval, ask for changes or further data, or recommend disapproval. If it ultimately recommends disapproval, further appeal can be taken to the Medicines Commission (the senior advisory board to the licensing commission). A similar scheme used to be required for applications from pharmaceutical companies to run clinical trials, but it was replaced in 1981 after considerable complaints about the length of the process. Instead of obtaining a clinical trial certificate, which can be a lengthy process, a company can (and is usually expected to) apply for a clinical trial exemption. Such exemptions had been available from 1968 for doctors who conducted trials under their own initiative and responsibility. Under the 1981 scheme, companies can get the same exemption by submitting an application countersigned by a physician indicating that that physician, serving as the company's medical adviser, thinks the trial is reasonable. The exemption application process cannot take more than 9 weeks.

How well does the final approval system work? We are fortunate to have three good U.K. studies, in addition to the comparative Wardell and Kaitin studies, that guide us in studying this question. Two cover the initial 13 years of the scheme and closely relate to the early comparative U.S.–U.K. data in the Wardell and Kaitin studies.[66] The other provides data on the period 1987–1989 and is thus more recent than the latest Kaitin comparative study.[67] One of the most interesting points to study is the median determination time for new approvals. From 1974 to 1979, the median time in the United Kingdom increased from 7.8 to 14.3 months. It then declined to 9.0 months in 1983. Then came the disaster of 1984, with the median time increasing to 12 months. By 1987–1989, the median time for approval had declined to 31 weeks, which compares extremely favorably with the U.S. median rate for 1987–1989 of 29.8 months.[68] When you combine this with a similar safety record and a better comparative drug lag (at least through the end of 1987, and probably thereafter in light of the 1987–1989 U.K. improvements), you can see why many might conclude that the United States has much to learn from the United Kingdom about an approach to final drug approvals.

Notice that the last claim has been confined to final drug approvals. Analogous data are not available about the U.K. approach to approving clinical trials, and I think that there are real reasons for concern in this area in light of what we saw in Chapter 2 about U.K. practice in connection with clinical trials. So all I am urging here is that the United States look closely at the drug approval process in the United Kingdom to see what it can learn.

It is worth noting before we enter into that analysis that there are some analysts who have argued that even the U.K. system is too cumbersome and imposes excessive costs on British patients. The most notable is David Green, whose positive suggestions will be discussed in the final section of this chapter.[69] All I want to say at this point is that his critique of the U.K. system seems quite unconvincing. In addition to general philosophical observations, Green provides only two sets of data as a basis for his criticism. The first, relating to the delay in approving clinical trials, was rendered obsolete by the development of the exemption scheme. The second, relating to the delay in final approvals in the 1984–1986 period, was rendered obsolete by subsequent improvements which resolved a temporary problem. So I don't think that Green has provided a basis for not continuing to suppose that there are important lessons for the United States to learn from the U.K. drug approval process.

Two possible lessons suggest themselves. One focuses on the claim that the U.K. process is less formal, involves closer cooperation, and has fewer bureaucratic hurdles. The other focuses on the claim that the United Kingdom has a better approach to the trade-off issues and appropriately allows approvals with less data, relying heavily on postapproval surveillance to correct mistakes. The difference between these two possibilities is very great. One would support intensive efforts at procedural reforms in the United States along the lines begun in the pre-AIDS, pre-1987 reforms. The other supports more fundamental changes in the U.S. attitude toward the trade-offs, changes that may even go beyond what has emerged in the United States in the last few years.

How can we determine the correct lesson to be derived from the U.K. experience? As I said at the beginning of this section, we don't yet have a significant number of studies comparing the details of the processes in the two countries and the detailed differences in their answers to the trade-off questions, but I believe that at least one study, which carefully reviews a specific application for approval in both countries, sheds considerable light on this question. If I am right, it is clear that we need more studies of this type.

The illuminating study concerns the use of medroxyprogesterone (Depo-Provera) as a long-term contraceptive agent.[70] Depo-Provera had originally been developed as a treatment for endometriosis, but it has been available in the United States since 1972 primarily as an adjunctive form of therapy for endometrial cancer. It had been approved in the 1960s and the 1970s in many countries for use as a long-term contraceptive, despite concerns about cancer resulting from studies conducted in dogs and monkeys. Applications for approvals were filed in the early 1980s with the FDA in the United States and with the Licensing Authority in the United Kingdom. Approval was granted in the United Kingdom in 1984 after hearings conducted both by the Committee on the Safety of Medicines and by a special panel. As in West Germany and Sweden, approval carried with it the recommendation that other contraceptive measures should be tried before Depo-Provera is used. A similar public board of inquiry in the United States advised against approval, and it was not approved for that use, although some U.S. physicians continued to prescribe it for long-term contraceptive use.[71] In June 1992, an FDA panel once more recommended approval, and it was finally approved in October 1992.[72] In both countries, data were presented to demonstrate efficacy, and data raising safety concerns from animal studies were also presented. In addition, in the United States, the National Women's Health Network played an active role in opposing approval at the hearings.[73]

Why this difference in response? Richard and Lasagna present evidence to support the following conclusion:

> We conclude that the policies concerning the extent of human trials required to gain marketing approval, the acceptability of prescribing drugs for unapproved indications, the evidence required to prove or disprove carcinogenic potential, and, more generally, the threshold of evidence required to prove or disprove causal links all had a profound effect on the decisions made by the two committees.[74]

Most of these points relate directly to our two trade-off issues. So if Richard and Lasagna are right about this case, and if their results are generalizable, then we will have reason to conclude that the lesson to be learned by the United States from the United Kingdom is that procedural reforms are not enough and that substantive changes based upon new responses to the trade-offs are required. But more study of this case and other cases is required before that conclusion can be firmly established.

The original drug lag literature focused on comparisons between the United States and the United Kingdom, simply because Wardell had trained in New Zealand and the United Kingdom before he arrived in the United States, and he was alerted to the issue when he saw that drugs with which he was familiar in the United Kingdom were not available in the United States.[75] But the issue extends beyond those two countries, and important work has been done comparing the outcomes of the drug approval process in many countries. It is important that we examine that literature as well, for that literature can provide us with additional insight into the extent to which comparative drug lags relate to regulatory problems. Moreover, we want to see what we can learn about how to improve the U.S. process by examining the experience of other countries with better records, and it is important that we look at a range of such countries, and not just the United Kingdom.

A significant number of such studies have been undertaken since the early 1980s. Among the most important were an initial multinational study by Grabowski in 1980,[76] an internal study conducted by the FDA in 1982,[77] a study conducted by Ross Cullen from New Zealand in 1983,[78] a series of studies conducted by John Parker, another scholar from New Zealand, in the 1980s,[79] a Swedish study in 1986 by Berlin and Jonsson,[80] and a recently published study by Fredrik Andersson.[81] Unfortunately, even the most recent of these studies, those of Parker and Andersson, employ as their data base drug approvals through 1983. Consequently, they do not shed light upon the issue of the comparative improvement in FDA performance in the period 1984–1987, an issue whose importance we discussed earlier. Nevertheless, they do provide us with some information on the contribution of regulations to comparative drug lags, and they do point us to the countries whose approvals were quicker than those in the United States and from which we might learn something.

Great care must be taken in this process of trying to learn from the experience of other countries. We must be careful to avoid simply assuming that earlier introductions in various countries mean better drug regulation processes while later introductions mean worse drug regulation processes. The rate of diffusion of new drugs into a country, which is what is measured in the drug lag literature, is only partially due to the country's drug regulation process. A drug gets introduced into a country only if a commercial company decides to introduce it and secures approval for introducing it. A drug lag in a given country may mean decisions by companies not to press for introductions into that country because of market factors (cost of marketing, poor reimbursement, size of market, and the like) rather than regulatory delays once the companies apply for permission to market the drugs. Thus relative drug lags may or may not be a sign of inappropriate regulatory delays. Unfortunately, only a few studies have attempted to deal with these issues, and they confine themselves to analyzing the situation in the 1960s and the 1970s.

One of the most systematic of these studies is Cullen's analysis. Cullen begins by pointing out the fundamental failure in the drug lag literature before 1983 to analyze the causes of drug lags:

> To belatedly enter into an arena where all but the FDA appear satisfied with the explanation for times of drug availability may seem foolish. Discussion of these issues has, however, been deficient in scope, myopic in focus and thus inconclusive in result. Consideration suggests that regulations alone may be inadequate explanations for the inter-country pattern of pharmaceuticals diffusion. . . . Absent, too, is any theoretical analysis of the likely determinants of inter-country diffusion of pharmaceuticals. Guilt has been proved by association with little evidence of search for alternatives.[82]

Cullen attempted to meet this problem by analyzing the role of four factors in explaining drug diffusion: market size, ease of marketing, innovativeness of countries, and ease of getting marketing approval. Only the last of these factors is related to the drug regulation process.

Cullen looked at drug introductions between 1961 and 1976 and divided the results into two periods, 1961–1968 and 1969–1976. His hypothesis was that the latter period would show a greater influence of the stringency of drug regulations (as measured by a ranking of drug regulations in 18 countries provided by executives of major drug companies) than the former period. That is, in fact, what he found. The two countries rated as having the most stringent drug regulatory processes—the United States and Japan—suffered the greatest worsening in their relative drug lag, with the United States declining from the best position in the earlier period to the ninth position in the latter period and with Japan declining from the tenth position in the earlier period to the seventeenth position in the latter period. This led him to the following conclusion:

> Two primary conclusions can be drawn from the outcomes of tests of these hypotheses. First, there appears to be considerable evidence that inter-country diffusion of pharmaceutical products first launched during the 1960s was influenced by commercial considerations such as expected sales and costs of marketing in each country. . . . The second conclusion, however, is that these relationships were destroyed by the intervening influence of regulations which changed diffusion from a commercial to an administered process. Despite initial skepticism, the evidence does seem overwhelmingly to indict regulations as the factor which has caused disruption to inter-country diffusion patterns and created a U.S. drug lag.[83]

Similar results were found by Parker, whose data base extended through 1978.[84] We should probably conclude then that the smaller drug lag in such countries as the United Kingdom before the changes in the U.S. regulations was due to the difficulties imposed by the regulations in obtaining approval. This then is the first result that emerges from our examination of multinational studies.

There are many other conclusions that emerge from an examination of these multinational studies. The first is that every one of the countries has some drug lag, in that there are drugs approved in other countries that are not approved in that country and in that there were drugs introduced in other countries before being introduced in that country. The most that one can say is that some countries have less of a drug lag problem than do other countries. The second is that there clearly are countries that had a far greater drug lag problem in the period in question than did the United States. Among those studied by Parker and by Andersson were Japan, Norway, Sweden, Canada, Australia, and New Zealand. The third, and most important conclusion for our purpose, is that while the studies differ in details of methodology and in results, a common ranking emerges from the most recent studies concerning the United States, the United Kingdom, France, and West Germany, as is shown by Table 3.3. This suggests that we should focus our attention now on what can be learned from the drug introduction systems in France and Germany to supplement what we have learned from our examination of the U.K. system, keeping in mind that that was the second purpose of examining the multinational studies.

Great caution must be shown in such an examination. We need to remember that in the case of the United Kingdom, studies of postmarketing withdrawals indicated, even if they did not prove, that British patients were benefiting from the better availability of drugs without paying the price for the premature approval of unsafe drugs. I know of no such studies for France and West Germany, and the lack of such studies should make us very cautious in using their experience to draw any conclusions about how the U.S. system should be modified. Moreover, we need to be very sensitive about cultural differences[85] between Anglo-American, French, and German conceptions of both disease and medications and their impact upon both the drug approval process and the actual utilization of drugs in the dif-

Table 3.3 Relative Drug Lag in Several Studies (years)

	Recent Parker	*Andersson*	*Berlin and Jonsson*
France	2.34	2.6	2.8
Germany	1.76	1.6	1.6
United Kingdom	1.72	1.4	1.3
United States	3.06	3.5	2.8

Note: The Parker data are for drugs introduced in 6 of the 12 countries studied in the period 1970–1983. The Andersson data are for drugs introduced in all 6 countries studied in the period 1960–1983. The Berlin and Jonsson data are for drugs introduced in all 6 countries in the period 1960–1982. Their data for France require further study.

ferent countries. German doctors regularly diagnose latent or actual *Herzinsuf-fizienz* even when Anglo-American doctors would recognize no symptoms of heart failure. French physicians regularly diagnose *crise de foie* even when Anglo-American doctors would point out that the patient has no symptoms of hepatitis or cirrhosis. Over 70 percent of German drugs are combination drugs, in sharp contrast to drug use in other countries. French doctors use drugs in much lower dosages than are used elsewhere. Systems for drug approvals cannot be separated from these broader cultural and institutional settings, and that should make us wary about drawing any firm conclusions from the French and German experience as to how the U.S. system should be modified.

Keeping these cautions in mind, I want to focus on only one difference between those two systems[86] and the U.S. system, a difference that is reflective of a common European approach[87] to the drug approval process. This is the role of experts in the field. Applications for approval are submitted with expert opinions on issues of pharmacology, safety, and efficacy, as opposed to applications being submitted (as they are in the United States) simply with data about those issues. While the regulatory agencies in Europe then review with the help of other experts the original expert's opinions, that original opinion has considerable weight. All of this is not merely a procedural matter, although it has great procedural implications. It also addresses the standards of approval and trade-offs in the approval process.

As noted in the preceding section of this chapter, the 1962 legislation in the United States governing the FDA spoke of approval based upon adequate and well-controlled trials of safety and efficacy and of approval based upon evidence that would enable experts to fairly and reasonably conclude that the drugs are safe and efficacious. As was also noted, the main efforts of the FDA have been to emphasize the former and downplay the latter. The European experience has moved in the opposite direction, and it might well be suggested that this provides greater flexibility to the European drug approval process and explains the better record on the drug lag issue of France and West Germany. But that is at best just a suggestion.

Let us summarize what we have learned in this section from international comparisons to supplement what we learned in the previous section about the U.S. drug approval process. The first lesson, learned from the work of Cullen and Parker, is that regulatory delays have certainly been a very important contributor to the delays in drug approval which constitute the drug lag. The second lesson, learned from the work of Wardell and Kaitin, is that U.S. patients, in comparison with U.K. patients, have paid a serious price in the unavailability of useful drugs without an offsetting gain in greater protection against unsafe drugs. This problem certainly persisted through 1983, and any lessening of the comparative problem in the 1984–1987 period is probably due to problems in the United Kingdom rather

than improvements in the United States. The third lesson, which is the most specu-
lative of the three, is that the advantages of the U.K. system (and perhaps of other
European systems) are reflective of a better substantive response to the trade-off
issues rather than of mere procedural advantages. This reinforces the claims of
the preceding section that the mere procedural reforms in the United States of the
pre-1987 period needed to be supplemented (as they have been in the post-1987,
AIDS-prompted reforms) by explicit modifications in the U.S. approach to the
trade-offs. With the recognition that alternatives to the U.S. approach certainly
deserve a careful examination, we return then to the question of whether these
changes have been sufficient or whether additional fundamental changes are
required.

The Ethical Foundations of
an Appropriate Drug Regulation Scheme

In order to resolve these issues, we need to return to our original trade-off questions and examine a fundamental paradox whose resolution is essential to developing an ethically acceptable drug regulation scheme that can appropriately resolve
these issues. The paradox can be stated in outline form as follows:

1. Any drug regulation scheme necessarily involves an answer to both the
   content question and the epistemic question.
2. Each of these questions calls for a certain balancing of goals, and different
   people will, in light of their different subjective values, balance those goals
   differently.
3. But any drug regulation scheme calls for some society-wide balancing of
   goals, a balancing that will be quite appropriate for some citizens in light of
   their values but very inappropriate for others in light of their values.
4. Therefore, it seems that we will not be able to develop an ethically appropriate society-wide drug regulation scheme, for any scheme will *without justification* embody the values of some and discriminate against the values of
   others. The difficulties and controversies surrounding the standards for drug
   approvals are just a reflection of this lack of a foundation for the drug regulation scheme.

Each step in the statement of the paradox deserves further comment and elabora-
tion.

Throughout this chapter, we have seen that any scheme for regulating the introduction of drugs must involve a process for approval and some standards for
approval. These standards, whether articulated or left implicit, define an appropriate risk–benefit level and an appropriate level of evidence, thereby providing

answers to both our trade-off questions. Moreover, the thrust of our analysis has been that the increasing emphasis in recent discussions is on modifying the standards for approval (especially the standards for the evidence required for approval) at least in those cases where the option of waiting for more data on safety and efficacy comes at great costs given the dismal alternative treatments available. There is no doubt then that any drug regulation scheme involves an answer to both the content question and the epistemic question. So the first claim in the argument for the paradox is surely correct.

What is the appropriate balance between safety and efficacy? To some degree, the answer to this question is a function of the disease being treated. Most people would usually be willing to accept greater risks for an effective treatment of a life-threatening illness than for an equally effective treatment of some cosmetic problem. But to some degree, the answer to this question is also a function of different individual values and goals. People whose goals are intimately connected with their physical appearance and who therefore place great value on that appearance would be willing to accept greater risks for an effective treatment of some cosmetic problem than people who place less value on that appearance because their goals are less intimately connected with it. Similarly, to return to our example of thrombolytic therapy, people who place a great negative value on surviving with the devastating effects of a major stroke would demand a smaller risk of that occurring after use of a thrombolytic agent with substantial efficacy than would people who are more interested in survival even in a substantially disabled condition.

What is the appropriate balance between gathering further evidence of safety and efficacy and approving a drug so that it is available now? To some degree, the answer to this question is a function of the available alternatives. Most people would usually be willing to accept the greater risks involved in an earlier approval if the costs of waiting for more evidence are great because the alternatives available while waiting are very poor. But to some degree the answer to this question is also a function of different individual values and goals. To begin with, how bad the alternatives are depends, for reasons just indicated, on different individual values and goals. Moreover, different people are more or less risk-aversive. That is to say, they have a greater or lesser willingness to take risks, including the risks of trying a new drug that has not been tested as extensively as usual. The more risk-aversive one is, the more evidence one will want of safety and efficacy. The appropriate answer to both the trade-off questions is, then, at least in part a function of the differing goals and values of different people. So the second claim in the argument for the paradox is also correct.

Schemes for the regulation of new drugs are society-wide schemes. In particular, schemes which prohibit the use of (or, at least, the commercial manufacture and distribution of) unapproved drugs limit that use throughout society. Since these society-wide schemes must necessarily involve standards for approval, they must also involve implicit or explicit answers to both the trade-off questions. These standards and answers will match the standards and answers that follow from some citizen's values and goals, and the society-wide scheme will only prohibit drugs that these citizens would not use anyway. But there will be other citizens whose values and goals lead to very different standards and answers, and the society-wide scheme will prohibit drugs that they would use and whose use would be appropriate in light of their values and goals. So the third claim in the argument for the paradox is correct.

We turn to the final claim in the argument for the paradox. How can we justify imposing a scheme that favors the values of some citizens and discriminates against the values of others? One of the fundamental principles of the modern liberal state is, after all, the principle of neutrality between the differing values of different citizens. One possible answer—we need to do so in order to protect nonconsenting third parties from being harmed[88]—is obviously irrelevant here since the use of unapproved drugs is, after all, primarily an activity that imposes risks on the user and not on others. The other possible answer—there is something objectively right about the goals and values lying behind the specific scheme adopted—is implausible; to return to one of our examples, it is unlikely that there is one correct valuation of the importance of one's physical appearance. Even if true, however, it still does not justify the state's intolerance to the values of others. So the final claim in the argument for the paradox is also correct.

Two major resolutions of this paradox seem worthy of exploration. The first accepts the conclusion that current drug regulation schemes, with their emphasis on prohibiting drugs until they are approved by some society-wide approval process, should be dropped. The second rejects that conclusion and attempts to define a rational basis for some society-wide scheme. Let us explore each of these alternatives.

The first alternative has been advocated in the literature from time to time. Grabowski and Vernon put forward such a proposal in 1983, although they conceded that it would have little chance of being adopted. The heart of their proposal was that the role of the government should be to certify the validity of information about safety and efficacy, leaving it for patients and their physicians to decide what drugs to employ in light of that information and in light of their differing values and goals. They summarized that option as follows:

> It is possible to envision an FDA regulatory structure that would operate more as a certifier and disseminator of information for the vast majority of new products introduced. . . . [O]ne could require a premarket review of the evidence carried out under government auspices, using scientific experts within and outside the government. This would provide an independent analysis of the drug's claims of safety and efficacy, which could then lead to required disclosure of information in drug

labeling and advertising. . . . Manufacturers would have the option to market a new drug even if it failed to be certified by the FDA.[89]

A scheme which differs in details but is very similar in basic philosophy was recently advocated for the United Kingdom by David Green:

> Manufacturers would be wholly responsible for the safety of their own products. They would continue to face legal liability for acts of negligence, but would not be required to obtain licenses for new medicines. All new drugs would be launched as trial products and would be submitted to a new regulatory agency for comment. If it objected, the product could still be marketed, so long as the agency's disapproval was printed on the label. All trial products would be required to undergo post-marketing surveillance so that risk levels could be quantified. Once the risk had been thus quantified it would no longer be necessary to use the term "trial product."[90]

Both these proposals are libertarian in spirit, emphasizing the liberty of patients and physicians to use the drugs they wish to and emphasizing their responsibility to make choices in light of the available information. Both these proposals see the government as having an informational, as opposed to a regulatory, role. Finally, both these proposals avoid our paradox since neither involves a society-wide scheme of drug regulation that presupposes society-wide trade-offs based on society-wide values and goals.

These are attractive features. Nevertheless, I don't think we should adopt these proposals as a way out of the paradox. My reasons extend beyond Grabowski and Vernon's worry about these proposals being too radical to be politically viable. They also extend beyond the obvious worries about the capacities of patients and their physicians to assimilate the information that will be provided under these proposals so that they can make choices in light of their values and goals. In the end, I think that we should reject these proposals because of their excessive reliance on the expressed willingness of the patients to take the drugs in question.

One way to see the point I want to make is to think about an analogous issue which we discussed in Chapter 2. We saw there that the regulations governing human research do not accept as legitimate all research in which patients are willing to participate, even if their willingness is fully informed. Some research is so risky that it is judged as inappropriate despite subject consent. To be sure, the rights of the subjects would not be violated if we did the risky research, since they did consent to participate, but that is not sufficient. Similarly, while these proposals for a certification scheme are respectful of the rights of the patients, that is not sufficient to make the resulting use of drugs acceptable; we need to ensure that patients are not being exposed to excessively risky drugs. That is why we need a society-wide drug regulation scheme, one that can be justified despite the paradox.

While suggestive, this analogy is not by itself sufficient to establish our point. To make further progress we need to explore the reasons why it would be wrong both to enroll fully informed consenting subjects in excessively risky research protocols and to provide excessively risky drugs to fully informed consenting patients even though their rights are apparently not being violated in either case because they have provided fully informed consent. Two thoughts come to mind. The first challenges the validity of certain expressed choices and preferences on the grounds that they are so unreasonable that they must represent failures of cognition or pathologies in the values and preferences formation process. The second, extending the first point, challenges the reliance on certain expressed preferences because it is exploitative to use people when the preferences to be so used are so unreasonable as to be invalid. Each of these reasons and the relation between them need amplification.

Even the friends of autonomy have come to recognize that not all preferences and choices can be taken on their face value. Thus John Harsanyi has argued:

> Any sensible ethical theory must make a distinction between rational wants and irrational wants, or between rational preferences and irrational preferences. It would be absurd to assert that we have the same moral obligation to help other people in satisfying their utterly unreasonable wants as we have to help them in satisfying their very reasonable desires. . . . In actual fact, there is no difficulty in maintaining this distinction even without an appeal to any other standard than an individual's own personal preferences. All we have to do is to distinguish between a person's manifest preferences and his true preferences . . . a person's true preferences are the preferences he would have if he had all the relevant factual information, always reasoned with the greatest possible care, and were in a state of mind most conducive to rational choice.[91]

In a somewhat similar fashion, Jon Elster has claimed:

> The criticism I have directed against utilitarian theory is, essentially, that it takes account of wants only as they are given, subject at most to a clause about the need for learning about the alternatives. My objection has been what one might call "backward-looking," arguing the need for an analysis of the genesis of wants.[92]

While Harsanyi's emphasis is more on cognition and Elster's emphasis is more on value formation, both can be seen as supporting the idea that some expressed preferences are not reflections of the true values and preferences of the individual, and are not in that way valid preferences.

Suppose then that the expressed willingness of a subject to participate in a very risky trial or the expressed willingness of a patient to take a very risky drug seems so illogical that we have good reason to suspect that it represents not the subject's true preferences but rather some failure in cognition or some failure in the process of value formation. Even if the subject's rights would not be violated by enrollment in the trial or by administering the drug because of expressed consent, it would still be wrong to proceed because we would be taking advantage of the subject, exploiting his or her failures, to advance our own projects (conducting research, selling drugs). Regulatory schemes are justifiable to protect the vulnerable against exploitation as well as to protect their rights.

This line of thought needs to be supplemented by a theory of true preferences and of exploitation, and this is not the place for the development of such a theory. But enough has been said, I believe, to justify the claim that the Grabowski-Vernon proposal and the Green proposal rely too heavily upon allowing patients to take the drugs that they say that they want to take. We need to look for an alternative solution to the paradox of how we can have a society-wide drug regulation scheme given the differences in people's values.

The alternative resolution of the paradox, the resolution that will provide the theoretical basis for my approach to drug regulation, is based upon the very fact that led us to reject the Grabowski-Vernon–Green drug information proposal, the fact that some preferences to use drugs are sufficiently irrational that we should attribute them to failures in cognition and/or failures in value formation rather than to alternative values.

Suppose a group of patients desire, on the basis of some preliminary information about safety and effectiveness, to use a particular drug. Suppose moreover that the amount of information available and/or the risk-benefit ratio suggested by that information would not under the current drug regulation scheme justify approval of that use. Suppose finally that the patients insist that their values and their answers to the trade-off questions justify their using the drug in question, and that the current regulatory schemes are not respectful of their values. Under what conditions, if any, are we justified in refusing to approve the drug anyway? The answer I would offer is that we are justified only when their desires are sufficiently irrational that we would be justified in saying that their expressed preferences are not their true preferences but are instead the product of cognitive or value formation failure. Put another way, the answer I would offer is that we are justified in denying them access to the drug only when no fully rational agent, whatever their values, would be willing to use the drug. If a fully rational agent, given some set of values, would be willing to use the drug on the basis of the information available, so that we have no basis for saying that the expressed desire of these patients is not their true preference, then we must allow them access to the drug; the most that we can do is make sure that they have available a reliable account of what is known about the drug.

Adopting this approach as the theoretical basis for a morally acceptable drug regulation scheme that is respectful of differences in individual values would obviously lead to a radically different drug regulation scheme. The radical differences between such a scheme and the traditional FDA approach would be substantive, not just procedural. Before turning to the details of the differences, and how they go beyond what the FDA has done in recent years, let me point out three fundamental consequences of adopting this approach.

The first is that this approach calls for new standards that apply to all drugs, and not just drugs for treating life-threatening or severely debilitating or serious illnesses. If some reasonable people, bothered more than most by their allergies, are willing to try a new drug offering better symptomatic relief on the basis of very preliminary evidence that indicates no major health risks and some effectiveness, then our approach would call for the release of the drug (together with reliable information about what little is known about its safety and effectiveness). It would be different, of course, if the preliminary information raised serious safety concerns, for then we might be justified in denying approval on the grounds that their expressed preference for the drug represents a cognitive failure in disregarding the risks or a value formation failure in overemphasizing the unpleasantness of the allergic symptoms. So adopting our approach would modify the approval process for *all* drugs.

The second consequence is that this approach calls for a rejection of the FDA's current near-exclusive reliance on data derived from randomized controlled double-blinded trials. No doubt all reasonable people would agree that information derived from such trials constitutes the paradigm of reliable information. No doubt many reasonable people in many circumstances would insist on relying upon such information exclusively. Still, there is no doubt but that other reasonable people with different values would be willing in certain circumstances to rely upon retrospective data, epidemiological data, clinical impressions of experts, and so on. After all, it is such data that lead to the introduction of many valuable surgical techniques. Given that this is so, the informational standards for drug approval in any scheme based on our approach would have to refer to this wider variety in the sources of information to be used.

The third consequence is that this approach would call for a very different attitude toward risk–benefit assessments in the drug approval process. The FDA, as noted earlier in this chapter, has never been willing to specify a general standard for an acceptable risk-benefit ratio. I am prepared to do so. It is just the standard that at least some reasonable people given their values would be willing to use the drug in question given the ascertained risks and benefits. While hardly precise, this standard at least tells us what question we should be asking.

These three remarks capture the basic differences between my approach and the current drug approval system. Keeping them in mind, let us turn to the details of my approach. I want to focus primarily on the approval process, the standards for approval, and the postapproval process of information dissemination and data monitoring; although my approach has implications for the process by which authorization is given for the commencement of testing (the investigational new drug [IND] process), consideration of those implications lies beyond the scope of this work.

The approval process that I am advocating is meant to be an expedited approval process designed to eliminate any remaining drug lag. It is meant to apply to the approval of all drugs, with special emphasis on drugs of any type that provide meaningful greater therapeutic benefit over existing treatments or offer other advantages over existing treatments. The idea of an improved system covering all drugs, rather than just drugs treating life-threatening or severely debilitating or serious illnesses, is consonant with the proposal of the Council on Competitiveness, is broader than the Accelerated Approval Subpart H proposed regulations, and is justified by our discussion of the drug that offers better symptomatic relief to allergy sufferers. The idea of emphasizing drugs that provide meaningful greater therapeutic benefit over existing treatments is drawn from the accelerated approval regulations and makes sense in light of our basic approach, providing that it is modified by adding the clause about other advantages. After all, reasonable people, whatever their true values, are likely to be willing to use a new drug on an expedited basis after limited evidence about risks and benefits has been gathered only if the new drug offers meaningful greater therapeutic benefit or if it has some other advantage (such as lower price or ease of administration). True "me-too" drugs are drugs for which reasonable people can wait. Finally, drawing upon the European experience and upon the original 1962 statutory standard for evidence of fairly-and-reasonably-concluded-by-experts, it is meant to rely heavily upon the use of expert opinion.

How would such a process work? When a drug company felt that it had accumulated sufficient data about safety and effectiveness drawn from controlled trials, from epidemiological and retrospective studies, or from clinicians' clinical experience, it would present the data to the FDA. The data could be drawn from foreign studies as well as from U.S. studies, could involve surrogate end points, and could include information about foreign approvals. The task of the FDA staff in the approval process would be to review the application to see that it is in the appropriate form, to give it a higher or lower priority for being considered in light of the claimed benefits for the new drug, and to convene a panel of experts to consider the application.

What standard should the panel of experts employ in their deliberations? I have already suggested what it should be: Is there enough evidence at this point of a positive risk-benefit ratio so that some reasonable people with some set of values would be willing to use the drug rather than waiting for further evidence? Adopting this as the standard incorporates both of our trade-offs into the fundamental standard for drug approval. Adopting this as the standard obviously captures the insight of the Lasagna committee that all that is required for approval is substantial evidence (the term used in the 1962 act) rather than definitive evidence (which is what has been required). It also captures the insight of the Council on Competitiveness that the approval process must be sensitive to the costs to patients from delay in the approval process. After all, the answer to the question as to whether reasonable people might be willing to use the drug in question on the basis of the substantial evidence available, rather than waiting for definitive evidence, depends heavily upon the alternatives that are available and the price that would have to be paid by patients who would have to wait if the drug was not approved.

The use of this standard requires a properly constituted committee of experts. A committee composed primarily if not exclusively of academic physicians with substantial research expertise in the area in question is probably the best committee to answer the question as to whether the evidence justifying approval is definitive; it is far from clear, however, that it is the best committee to answer the question as to whether our standard is satisfied. A better committee to answer that question would also contain a substantial number of physicians and other providers, such as nurses, with extensive experience in treating the relevant type of patients in a wide variety of settings and some patient-representatives with sufficient technical knowledge to meaningfully participate in the deliberations. It is only this type of committee that can reasonably be expected to answer the question posed by our standard for approval.

Suppose that the committee of experts recommends approval. On the system I am proposing, that would mean that the drug would, absent special circumstances, be approved. The staff of the FDA would then have two major roles. The first is the development of information for both clinicians and patients. The second is the development of a good system of postapproval monitoring. Let me comment on both these roles.

Under the new system I am proposing, drug approval means only that some reasonable people with certain values would be willing to use the drug on the basis of the information available. For many other patients, use without further evidence would still be inappropriate. This means that this system puts a substantial burden on patients and their clinical advisers to decide whether the drug is appropriate for them. This burden can be met only if there is a central source for reliable information, and the FDA seems ideally suited for that task, although there are other models, such as the Canadian system, where at least part of this role is played by a private coalition of medical and drug industry groups,[93] and the British system, where at least part of this role is played by an industry-sponsored association.[94] Thus the FDA in my approach remains a drug regulation agency as well as a drug information certification agency, but I concur with both Grabowski and Vernon's and Green's emphasis on this drug information certification role.

A recent study reinforces the need for this role.[95] The authors sent to reviewers 109 full-page pharmaceutical advertisements appearing in leading journals. Despite the existence of FDA standards, the reviewers concluded that in 44 percent of the cases the advertisements would lead to improper prescribing if the physician relied on them exclusively. The major problems were not in the claims about safety, but rather in the claims about efficacy and in the balancing of efficacy with side effects and contraindications. Our current system suffers from such misleading claims; a system like the one I am proposing certainly cannot afford them. So the adoption of my system requires a much better approach to checking and certifying the claims made on behalf of drugs.

The role of the FDA does not end on my proposal with the drug approval process. Any scheme for expedited approval of drugs has to place even greater emphasis on postapproval monitoring of data about safety and effectiveness than does the current system. The British, in light of their quicker approval of drugs, have traditionally placed great emphasis on this role, although their success in that process deserves careful study.[96] The Council on Competitiveness emphasized the importance of postapproval monitoring in the context of expedited approval. The Subpart E regulations authorized the FDA to require postmarketing studies on such issues as long-term safety and effectiveness when drugs were approved on the basis of preliminary evidence.[97] They all recognize that changing standards for approval means placing greater emphasis on postapproval activities.

I want to be clear, however, on the proposed FDA role in the postapproval period. The plan is not for the current standards to be reintroduced as the basis for withdrawing approvals. Withdrawals should be based upon the same standard as approvals, so that approvals should be withdrawn only if the additional postapproval data change the available information so that no reasonable people, whatever their values, would be willing to use the drug in question given the new information. But even if the drug is not withdrawn, patients will need guidance about new information as it becomes available, and that informational role should be just as important in the FDA's postapproval activities as in the FDA's initial approval process.

These remarks shed light on the controversy over the FDA's withdrawal of general approval for the use of breast implants filled with silicone gel while allowing access for some patients, for example, postmastectomy patients. An excellent presentation of both sides in this controversy is found in the debate between Dr. Marcia Angell and Dr. David Kessler in the *New England Journal of Medicine*.[98] Both sides agree on the value of additional information but disagree about what should be done in the meantime. Angell, arguing for continued availability, emphasizes the importance of respecting different values and of providing information, themes that are very consonant with my approach. To quote her:

> I believe that the FDA should have permitted women to continue to receive breast implants, regardless of participation in studies and regardless of whether the pur-

pose is augmentation or reconstruction, with the provision that they receive the same information as they would in a trial. . . . It is possible to deplore the pressures that women feel to conform to a stereotyped standard of beauty, while at the same time defending their right to make their own decision.

Kessler presents two arguments on the other side. The first appeals to a social consensus about when implantation is more important:

One can argue that for both groups the benefit is ultimately cosmetic, yet for women with breast cancer who undergo mastectomy, the option of reconstructive surgery is viewed as an integral part of the treatment of the disease. Certainly as a society, we are far from according cosmetic interventions the same importance as a matter of public health that we accord to cancer treatments. The clearest demonstration of this social consensus comes from our policies regarding health insurance.

I find this argument unpersuasive, in part because it links the reconstructive surgery postmastectomy with the rest of the cancer treatment, but primarily because it simply fails to be responsive to social diversity in values. Even if we cannot be responsive to that diversity when designing a health insurance scheme, where we directly or indirectly use the funds of society (thereby involving social values),[99] there is no reason why we cannot respect that diversity by allowing individuals to decide whether they should undergo purely cosmetic surgery in a noncancer case, a purely private decision.

Kessler's second argument does not invoke such public values:

To argue that people ought to be able to choose their own risks, that government should not intervene, even in the face of inadequate information, is to impose an unrealistic burden on people when they are most vulnerable to manufacturers' assertions: when they are desperately ill, when they are hoping against hope for a cure, or when they are seeking to enhance their physical appearance. Those are precisely the situations in which the legal and ethical justification for the FDA's existence is greatest, however. The decision about breast implants reflects that need.

In putting forward this account of why there should be a regulatory scheme enforced by the FDA, Kessler is implicitly appealing to the very distinction between people's explicit preferences and their true preferences that we also invoked. Vulnerable people are entitled to protection from their expressed preferences both on his account and on mine. But I find his lumping together the desperate patient and the patient seeking appearance enhancement most unpersuasive. Moreover, even desperate patients ought to be allowed to follow their choice unless it is totally unreasonable. Kessler has not shown that the women seeking breast augmentation are, in light of the currently available information, choosing something totally unreasonable given the high value they ascribe to the change in appearance. So while he is right about the justification for the existence of the FDA, I think he is wrong about his application of this justification to the case of breast implants.

To summarize, I have argued for a revised drug approval system that emphasizes respecting individual choices and providing information to help people make those choices in a responsible manner, while still allowing for some drugs to be disapproved despite the fact that some patients want to take them. The system incorporates new standards in response to our trade-off questions and new processes for deciding when those standards have been met. While consonant with much of the spirit of recent reforms at the FDA and appreciative of their importance, the proposed system goes beyond them both substantively and procedurally.

We return finally to an analysis of the FDA's handling of tPA and streptokinase at the May 29, 1987, meeting of the Cardio-Renal Drugs Advisory Committee, keeping in mind that we want to focus on the fundamental questions of drug approval and not the special problems encountered that day (the poor timing of the afternoon session, the block on information from NIH studies, and so on). While the committee recommended approval of streptokinase, it did not recommend approval of tPA because it believed the data on efficacy were inadequate and it still had concerns about safety. I offer four observations about that decision.

1. Both streptokinase and tPA appear on the previously discussed internal FDA list of drugs approved in the period January 1, 1980–June 30, 1988, that would have been treated as therapies for life-threatening and severely debilitating illnesses under the Subpart E program if that program had existed when they were approved. It would seem that they would also have been eligible for consideration under the Subpart H program. So it seems that these were valuable drugs whose approval process would have been expedited if the post-AIDS initiatives had been in place a few years earlier. In fact, however, the situation is somewhat more complicated.

2. Given the data on improved survival from GISSI and ISIS-2, streptokinase met the traditional requirements for approval, so the only thing that might have changed is that it might have become available under the Treatment IND program in the period of time between the advisory committee meeting and its final approval. This has happened in other cases (for example, surfactant), and it helped many patients in that interim period.[100] But the period of time in question was relatively short anyway, so that would have been only a limited although nontrivial improvement.

3. With streptokinase approved, tPA might not have been eligible for the Subpart E program since streptokinase is at least a reasonably satisfactory alternative treatment, and the Subpart E program is designed for cases where no satisfactory alternative therapy exists. The situation is less restrictive under the Subpart H program, since it applies so long as the new drug promises to provide a meaningful benefit over existing treatments, and tPA might thus qualify. But the main benefit of falling under that program is that surrogate end points are acceptable as

data of effectiveness. This might not have helped tPA, in part because of the concerns about safety but primarily because many of the skeptics about tPA wanted the end point to be ventricular functioning (about which there were no favorable data) rather than clot lysis (about which there were more favorable data from TIMI). So the admission of data about surrogate end points might still not have led to the approval of tPA in May 1987.

4. TPA would certainly have been approved in May 1987 under the scheme that I am advocating. Given the strongly expressed views of such experts as Braunwald and Topol, it is hard to see how any committee of experts could have avoided the conclusion that tPA ought to be approved because at least some rational people truly wanted to take their chances and use it.

None of this is said by way of providing an argument for my proposal, since those who dislike my proposal will simply challenge the idea that it would have been good for tPA to have been approved in May 1987. I only want to use our example to reinforce my claim that my proposal does go beyond what the FDA has been prepared to do even as a result of the post-AIDS initiatives. The argument for my proposal remains the ethical argument that it seems to be the best way to protect the vulnerable while respecting individual differences. For those of us committed to a public policy based on liberal values, that is a sufficient reason for adopting the proposal.

Notes

1. A good brief history can be found in H. G. Grabowski and J. M. Vernon *The Regulation of Pharmaceuticals* (Washington: American Enterprise Institute, 1983), Chapter 1. A far fuller history can be found in P. Temin, *Taking Your Medicine* (Cambridge, Mass.: Harvard University Press, 1980).

2. An excellent presentation is found in an FDA document entitled "Clinical Testing for Safe and Effective Drugs," an undated document numbered DHEW Publication No. (FDA) 74-3015. While some of the details were modified in recent years in ways that will be described below, the basic account is still accurate and it is a clear exposition of the initial system.

3. 21 USC §355 (b).

4. Ibid., §355 (d).

5. The crucial regulations are found in 21 CFR §312 (governing IND applications) and 21 CFR §314 (governing NDAs).

6. The report in question is the Miles report, a report of a committee appointed by Secretary Gardner which was released on January 17, 1966, the day James Goddard was sworn in as the new FDA commissioner. The quotation comes from p. 1 of this unpublished report.

7. This quotation is cited on p. 56 of the McMahon report, an important report to be analyzed later. The formal reference to that report is Commission on the Federal Drug Approval Process, *Final Report* (Washington: GPO, October 1982).

8. *Federal Register* 35 (May 8, 1970): 7250–53.

9. A detailed account of the first 20 years of the investigations, studies, and reports is found in P. B. Hutt, "Investigations and Reports Respecting FDA Regulation of New Drugs," *Clinical Pharmacology and Therapeutics* 33 (1983): 537–48 and 674–87. The studies have continued, and a similar review article is now needed.

10. In a speech "The FDA Today" delivered before the National Press Club on October 29, 1974, and cited in Grabowski and Vernon, *The Regulation of Pharmaceuticals*, p. 5.

11. He published his results in two main forms, an article entitled "An Evaluation of Consumer Protection Legislation: The 1962 Drug Amendments," *Journal of Political Economy* 81 (1973): 1049–91, and a book entitled *Regulation of Pharmaceutical Innovation* (Washington: American Enterprise Institute, 1974).

12. Wardell published many articles and books on related topics. My initial presentation of his ideas is based upon one of his earliest presentations of them in an article entitled "Introduction of New Therapeutic Drugs in the United States and Great Britain," *Clinical Pharmacology and Therapeutics* 14 (1973): 773–90, and in a follow-up book written by him and Louis Lasagna entitled *Regulation and Drug Development* (Washington: American Enterprise Institute, 1975).

13. *Regulation and Drug Development*, p. 107.

14. D. Kennedy, "A Calm Look at 'Drug Lag'" *JAMA* 239 (1978): 423–26. To get a sense of the level of rhetoric in the debate, one should note the title of Wardell's response in W. Wardell, "A Close Inspection of the 'Calm Look': Rhetorical Amblyopia and Selective Amnesia at the Food and Drug Administration," *JAMA* 239 (1978): 2004–11. It is in this response that Wardell emphasized that the delay in the approval of beta blockers, especially in the post-MI patient, was costing 10,000 lives per year.

15. U.S. General Accounting Office (GAO), *FDA Drug Approval—A Lengthy Process that Delays the Availability of Important New Drugs* (Washington: HRD 80-64, May 28, 1980).

16. Commission on the Federal Drug Approval Process, *Final Report*.

17. U.S. GAO, *FDA Drug Approval*, p. 50.

18. *Federal Register* 44 (October 12, 1979): 58919.

19. *Federal Register* 50 (February 22, 1985): 7452–519; 52 (March 19, 1987): 8798–847.

20. *Federal Register* 50, p. 7455

21. K. Kaitin, N. R. Phelan, D. Raiford, and B. Morris, "Therapeutic Ratings and End-of-Phase II Conferences: Initiatives to Accelerate the Availability of Important New Drugs," *Journal of Clinical Pharmacology* 31 (1991): 17–24.

22. Ibid., p. 22.

23. Grabowski and Vernon, *The Regulation of Pharmaceuticals*.

24. Temin, *Taking Your Medicine*.

25. S. Jenks, "Unclogging the Pipeline: Drug Access," *Medical World News*, October 23, 1989, pp. 28–34.

26. H. Edgar and D. J. Rothman, "New Rules for New Drugs," *Milbank Quarterly* 68, suppl. 1 (1990): 111–41. Quote, p. 138.

27. M. D. Grmek, *History of AIDS* (Princeton: Princeton University Press, 1990), Chapter 16.

28. Ibid., and an article by K. I. Kaitin, "Case Studies of Expedited Review: AZT and L-Dopa," *Law, Medicine, and Health Care* 19 (1991): 242–46 provide useful summaries of that history.

29. F. E. Young et al., "The FDA's New Procedures for the Use of Investigational Drugs in Treatment," *JAMA* 259 (1988): 2267–70.

30. The regulations governing Treatment INDs are found in 21 CFR §312.34. They were issued in the *Federal Register* 52 (May 22, 1987): 19466–77. The regulations governing the Subpart E program are found in 21 CFR §§312.80–88. They were issued in the *Federal Register* 53 (October 21, 1988): 41516–24.

31. The views of the critics, including Representative Waxman and Senator Kennedy, are nicely summarized in M. D. Eaglestein, "Overview of the Reproposed and Final IND Regulations Concerned with the Treatment, Use and Sale of Investigational New Drugs: The Congressional Perspective," *Food Drug Cosmetic Law Journal* 43 (1988): 435–42.

32. *Federal Register* 52 (May 22, 1987): 19468.

33. 21 CFR §312.84.

34. 21 CFR §312.80.

35. The report, obtainable from the FDA, is entitled "Treatment Investigational New Drugs (INDs) Allowed to Proceed." The document is dated June 1993, but it has no other identifying information.

36. For example, cytomegalovirus immune globulin was issued a Treatment IND on October 19, 1987, but was finally approved only in 1990 (see "Year End Review," *Clinical Pharmacology* 10 [1991]: 167). Similarly, pentostatin was issued a Treatment IND on July 28, 1988, but was finally approved only in 1991 (see "Year End Review" *Clinical Pharmacology* 11 [1992]: 208). The latter case is particularly deserving of careful study because the drug received a 1A designation from the FDA, indicating that it is a significant therapeutic gain.

37. The seven 1991–1992 drugs that did not have a Treatment IND, as far as I can tell by comparing the Treatment IND list with the 1990 and 1991 list of approvals, are altretamine, eflornithine, fludarabine, fluconazole, histrelin, idarubicin, and pegademase. Each of the cases would need to be investigated to see whether or not a Treatment IND would have been appropriate, and if so, why it was not issued. Similarly, one would have to see why finasteride, halofantrine hydrochloride, itraconazole, mivacurium chloride, solatol hydrochloride, sumatriptan succinate, and teniposide did not receive Treatment INDs before they were approved in 1992.

38. J. S. Kahan and D. T. Read, "Expedited Availability of New Drugs," *Food Drug Cosmetic Law Journal* 45 (1990): 81–94; the quotation is from footnote 58 of that article.

39. FDA Office of Planning and Evaluation, *A Research Profile of Thirty Recent Therapies for the Treatment of Life-Threatening and Severely-Debilitating Illnesses* (Washington: FDA, OPE Study 79, October 1989).

40. "The AIDS Hoax," *Wall Street Journal* (March 18, 1991).

41. Information about the trials, the parallel Treatment IND program, and the July 18–19 meeting is drawn from a published report in *The Blue Sheet*, July 24, 1991, pp. 2–3, and from a paper presented by Paul Worrall, director of Clinical Research Services at Bristol-Myers Squibb, at the May 6–9, 1990, meeting of the Society for Clinical Trials. A survey of the later data is found in M. S. Hirsch and R. T. D'Aquila, "Therapy for Human Immunodeficiency Virus Infection," *NEJM* 328 (1993): 1686–95.

42. Hirsch and D'Aquila, "Therapy."

43. The preliminary Concorde data were announced in a letter to *Lancet* from Drs. J. R. Aboulker and A. M. Swart published on April 3, 1993 (pp. 889–90). A good account of the resulting controversy, with the quotation from Kessler, is found in L. K. Altman, "AIDS Study Casts Doubt on Value of Hastened Drug Approval in U.S.," *New York Times,* April 6, 1993, p. B6.

44. W. K. Summers et al., "Oral Tetrahydroaminoacridine in Long-Term Treatment of Senile Dementia, Alzheimer Type," *NEJM* 315 (1986): 1241–45.

45. "An Interim Report from the FDA," *NEJM* 324 (1991): 349–52.

46. Ibid.

47. M. Waldholz, "FDA Panel Says More Study Is Needed of Warner-Lambert's Alzheimer Drug," *Wall Street Journal,* July 16, 1991, p. B5.

48. The decision to put tacrine on the Treatment IND program is described in *The Blue Sheet*, December 4, 1991, p. 5. The final decision is described in an unsigned article in the *New York Times* for September 10, 1993, p. A13, entitled "First Drug for Alzheimer's Is Approved by F.D.A."

49. The proposed regulations can be found in *Federal Register* 55 (May 21, 1990): 20856–60.

50. *Federal Register* 57 (April 15, 1992): 13250–59. Following quotes are from pp. 13256, 13257, and 13255.

51. National Committee to Review Current Procedures for Approval of New Drugs for Cancer and AIDS, *Final Report,* August 15, 1990.

52. Ibid., p. 3.

53. Council on Competitiveness, *Improving the Nation's Drug Approval Process* November 13, 1991.

54. G. Annas, "FDA's Compassion for Desperate Drug Companies," *Hastings Center Report* 20 (January, 1990): 35–37.

55. Council on Competitiveness, *Drug Approval Process*, p. 4. Italics added.

56. The letter is described in P. Cotton, "Faster Drug Approval Planned; Safety Questioned," *JAMA* 266 (1991): 2950, and in *The Blue Sheet*, November 20, 1991, p. 8. The text of the hearings is found in Committee on Government Operations, House of Representatives, *Council on Competi-

tiveness and FDA Plans to Alter the Drug Approval Process at FDA (Washington: GPO, March 19, 1992). The report, with dissenting views, was published as *The Quayle Council's Plans for Changing FDA's Drug Approval Process: A Prescription for Harm* (Washington: GPO, October 9, 1992).

57. P. J. Hilts, "Top F.D.A. Staff Members Oppose Looser Drug Approval System," *New York Times*, December 20, 1991, p. A29.

58. The proposed regulations were "New Drug, Antibiotic, and Biological Drug Product Regulations; Accelerated Approval," *Federal Register* 57 (April 15, 1992): 13234–42. The final regulations with important explanations appeared under the same title in the *Federal Register* 57 (December 11, 1992): 58942–60.

59. "DDC Recommended for Approval in Conjunction with AZT by FDA CMTE," *The Blue Sheet*, April 22, 1992, p. 2.

60. K. I. Kaitin et al., "The Drug Lag: An Update of New Introductions in the United States and in the United Kingdom, 1977 through 1987," *Clinical Pharmacology and Therapeutics* 46 (1989): 121–38.

61. O. M. Bakke, W. M. Wardell, and L. Lasagna, "Drug Discontinuations in the United Kingdom and the United States, 1964 to 1983," *Clinical Pharmacology and Therapeutics* 35 (1984): 559–67.

62. P. L. Coppinger, C. C. Peck, and R. J. Temple, "Understanding Comparisons of Drug Introductions between the United States and the United Kingdom," *Clinical Pharmacology and Therapeutics* 46 (1989): 139–45; following excerpt is from pp. 144–45. K. I. Kaitin, "Reply to 'Understanding Comparisons of Drug Introductions between the United States and the United Kingdom,'" *Clinical Pharmacology and Therapeutics* 46 (1989): 146–48; following quote from p. 147.

63. See the discussion in Office of Health Economics, *Crisis in Research* (London: Office of Health Economics, 1986), p. 24.

64. M. F. Cuthbert, J. P. Griffin, and W. H. W. Inman, "The United Kingdom," in W. M. Wardell, ed., *Controlling the Use of Therapeutic Drugs: An International Comparison* (Washington: American Enterprise Institute, 1978), pp. 99–134.

65. Good descriptions of the structure and functioning of the system can be found in Medicines Control Agency, *Guide to the Licensing System* (London: Department of Health, 1988), in the section on the United Kingdom in the *IFPMA Compendium* (Geneva, Switzerland: 1987, with 1989 supplement), and in A. H. Watt, "Medicines Regulation in the United Kingdom," *Health Bulletin* 48 (1990): 219–24.

66. J. P. Griffin, "A Survey of Products Licensed in the United Kingdom from 1971–1981," *British Journal of Clinical Pharmacology* 12 (1981): 453–63, and Office of Health Economics, *Crisis in Research*.

67. M. D. Rawlins and D. B. Jeffreys, "Study of United Kingdom Product Licence Applications Containing New Active Substances, 1987–9," *British Medical Journal* 302 (1991): 223–25. This has been supplemented by M. D. Rawlins and D. B. Jeffreys, "United Kingdom Product Liscence Applications Involving New Active Substances: Their Fate after Appeals," *British Journal of Clinical Pharmacology* 35 (1993): 599–602.

68. This figure is a calculation based upon Table I of K. Kaitin et al., "The New Drug Approvals of 1987, 1988, and 1989," *Journal of Clinical Pharmacology* 31 (1991): 116–22.

69. D. G. Green, *Medicines in the Marketplace* (London: IEA Health Unit, 1987).

70. B. W. Richard and L. Lasagna, "Drug Regulation in the United States and the United Kingdom: The Depo-Provera Story," *Annals of Internal Medicine* 106 (1987): 886–91.

71. "DMPA and Breast Cancer: The Dog Has Had Its Day," *Lancet*, October 5, 1991, pp. 856–57.

72. P. J. Hilts, "Panel Urges Contraceptive's Approval," *New York Times*, June 20, 1992, and W. E. Leary, "U.S. Approves Drug Use by Injection for Birth Control," *New York Times*, October 29, 1992, p. 1.

73. Boston Women's Health Book Collective, *The New Our Bodies, Ourselves* (New York: Simon and Schuster, 1984), pp. 247–48. Much of that opposition was based upon the concern that depo-provera would be prescribed primarily for poor women, women of color, and retarded women, who would agree to being injected without adequate informed consent. One shortcoming of the Richard-

Lasagna study is their failure to consider this additional difference between the United States and the United Kingdom.

74. Richard and Lasagna, "Drug Regulation," p. 890.

75. This is pointed out in an extremely important review of the drug lag literature by Fredrik Andersson, "The Drug Lag Issue: The Debate Seen from an International Perspective," *International Journal of Health Services* 22 (1992): 53–72.

76. H. G. Grabowski, "Regulation and the International Diffusion of Pharmaceuticals" in R. B. Helms, ed., *The International Supply of Medicines* (Washington: American Enterprise Institute, 1980), pp. 5–36.

77. A. E. Hass et al., *A Historical Look at Drug Introductions on a Five-Country Market* (Washington: FDA, OPE Study 60, 1982).

78. R. Cullen, "Pharmaceuticals Inter-Country Diffusion," *Managerial and Decision Economics* 4 (1983): 73–82.

79. The earlier studies were J. Parker, *The International Diffusion of Pharmaceuticals* (New York: St. Martin's Press, 1984), and J. Parker, "Regulatory Stringency and the International Diffusion of Drugs," in B. Lindgren, ed., *Arne Ryde Symposium on Pharmaceutical Economics* (Swedish Institute for Health Economics and Liber Forlag, 1984), pp. 139–58. A more recent study is J. Parker, "Who Has a Drug Lag?" *Managerial and Decision Economics* 10 (1989): 299–309.

80. H. Berlin and B. Jonsson, "International Dissemination of New Drugs: A Comparative Study of Six Countries," *Managerial and Decision Economics* 7 (1986): 235–42.

81. Andersson, "The Drug Lag Issue."

82. Cullen, "Pharmaceuticals," p. 73.

83. Ibid., p. 81.

84. Sources cited in note 79 above.

85. A fascinating and useful, even if somewhat journalistic, account of these differences is presented in L. Payer, *Medicine and Culture: Varieties of Treatments in the United States, England, West Germany, and France* (New York: Henry Holt, 1988). The rest of this paragraph draws heavily on Payer's account.

86. The most recent information about the French system is to be found in the *IFPMA Compendium* for 1987 (with a 1989 supplement) and in E. M. Voisin et al., "New Drug Registration in France," *Food Drug Cosmetic Law Journal* 46 (1991): 707–25. The most recent information about the West German system is also to be found in the *IFPMA Compendium*. A useful history of the beginnings of the German system is H. Kampffmeyer, "West Germany," in W. M. Wardell, ed., *Controlling the Use of Therapeutic Drugs* (Washington: American Enterprise Institute, 1978).

87. The EEC first involved itself in drug approval issues in 1965. Extremely important framework directives were issued in 1975 (75/318/EEC and 75/319/EEC). All of these directives, together with later directives and much detailed regulatory material, are found in the five volumes of *The Rules Governing Medicinal Products in the European Community* (Luxembourg: Office of Official Publications for the European Communities, 1989). The most recent developments are described in L. K. Orzock et al., "Pharmaceutical Regulation in the European Community," *Journal of Health Politics Policy and Law* 17 (1992): 847–68.

88. This classical liberal defense of the use of the state's coercive power to protect nonconsenting third parties has been restated and elaborated most recently in Joel Feinberg's *The Moral Limits of the Criminal Law,* 4 vols. (New York: Oxford University Press, 1984–1988).

89. Grabowski and Vernon, *Regulation of Pharmaceuticals*, p. 71.

90. Green, *Medicines in the Marketplace*, p. 64. A good critique of Green's book, emphasizing the favorable British record on drug approvals, is to be found in M. D. Rawlins, "Drug Regulation: Evolution or Revolution?" *British Medical Journal* 296 (1988): 379–80.

91. J. C. Harsanyi, "Morality and the Theory of Rational Behavior," in A. Sen and B. Williams, eds., *Utilitarianism and Beyond* (Cambridge: Cambridge University Press, 1982), pp. 39–62. Quote, p. 55.

92. J. Elster, "Sour Grapes," in Sen and Williams, *Utilitarianism and Beyond,* pp. 217–38. Quote, p. 237.

93. L. Page, "Canada's Drug Review Panel May Set an Example," *American Medical News,* June 15, 1992, p. 39.

94. A. Herxheimer and J. Collier, "Promotion by the British Pharmaceutical Industry, 1983–8: A Critical Analysis of Self-Regulation," *British Medical Journal* 300 (1990): 307–11.

95. M. S. Wilkes, B. H. Doblin, and M. F. Shapiro, "Pharmaceutical Advertisements in Leading Medical Journals," *Annals of Internal Medicine* 116 (1992): 912–19.

96. See the literature and data discussed in J. L. Bem et al., "25 Years of the Committee on Safety of Medicines," *Drug Safety* 5 (1990): 161–67.

97. *Federal Register* 53 (October 21, 1988): 41524.

98. M. Angell, "Breast Implants—Protection or Paternalism?" *NEJM* 326 (1992): 1695–96, and D. A. Kessler, "The Basis of the FDA's Decision on Breast Implants," *NEJM* 326 (1992): 1713–15. The following excerpts are from pp. 1696, 1714, and 1715.

99. I have argued that we can even in that case. See, for example, B. A. Brody, "The Macro-Allocation of Health Care Resources," in H. M. Sass and R. U. Massey, eds., *Health Care Systems* (Dordrecht: Kluwer, 1988), pp. 213–36.

100. Important data showing the benefits in that period are found in E. M. Zola et al., "Treatment Investigational New Drug Experience with Survanta (Beractant)," *Pediatrics* 91 (1993): 546–51.

4

Troubling Ethical Issues in Drug Adoption

Chapter 1 showed that major ethical issues can arise even after new drugs have been tested and approved. These additional ethical issues all relate in one way or another to the economics of drug adoption and use. In particular, we identified two broad issues that require further discussion:

1. To what extent should clinicians consider costs in deciding which drug to use? To what extent should society consider costs in deciding which treatments will be reimbursed?
2. How should the prices of new drugs be set? Should the price be determined by what the market will pay or should some other mechanism of pricing be used?

These questions are the focus of our attention in this final chapter.

One preliminary observation is in order. Many have said in conversation that ethical reflections are irrelevant to these issues. Matters of economics are real-world problems to be dealt with in a realistic bottom-line fashion without reference to principles and ideals. I believe that this attitude, however prevalent it may be, is fundamentally unacceptable. My hope is that the analysis offered in this chapter, besides shedding light on the specific issues stated above, will also provide positive proof that sound ethical principles and ideals have much to contribute to the discussion of economic issues.

Prices, Clinical Choices, and Reimbursement Policies

Costs and Clinical Choices

In recent years physicians have faced a very difficult question about the choice of thrombolytic agents. On the one hand, tPA costs more than ten times as much as streptokinase, so cost considerations certainly favored the use of SK. On the other hand, there was initially a widespread feeling, supported by data from TIMI about early reperfusion, that tPA was more efficacious, so clinical considerations offered at least some support for the use of tPA. No doubt, the data about mortality from GISSI-2 and ISIS-3 challenged that feeling, but it was reinforced by the favorable findings in the GUSTO trial. Thus between 1987 and 1993 there was to varying degrees a conflict between cost considerations and clinical considerations, and physicians faced the difficult question of which to emphasize. We saw in Chapter 1 that most American physicians initially chose to emphasize clinical considerations over cost considerations, although a significant minority made the opposite choice. We also saw that the number who emphasized costs increased after the appearance of the data from GISSI-2 and ISIS-3. It remains to be seen what will happen now that the data from GUSTO are available. Who was right? More generally, to what extent should doctors consider costs in making clinical decisions? These are the questions we shall now consider. Following the strategy we adopted in previous chapters, we shall first examine the issue in general and then examine it as it applies to the choice of thrombolytic agents in the period 1987–1993.

There is a traditional view that the physician must always emphasize the clinical benefits to the patient regardless of the costs. One well-known articulation of this position is found in the following passage from an article by Marcia Angell, the deputy editor of the *New England Journal of Medicine*:

> As individual physicians, we must do the very best we can for each patient. The patient rightly expects his physician to act single-mindedly in his best interests. If very expensive care is indicated, then the physician should do his utmost to obtain it for the patient. As Levinsky pointed out, the physician cannot serve two masters—his patient and the society's coffers.[1]

An even stronger version of the traditional position is found in the following claim by ethicist Robert Veatch:

> But it should not be the physician's responsibility to eliminate it [a lab test with minimal value] on cost grounds if that physician believes on balance that the procedure is *even infinitesimally beneficial* to the patient. Any campaign to make the clinician more cost-conscious in order to benefit someone other than the patient is a campaign to get the physician to abandon his unequivocal commitment to the patient.[2]

Veatch's claim is so strong precisely because he would require the physician to provide the procedure even when its benefit to the patient is minimal. Advocates of the classical position are not required to uphold their position in this very strong form; they can allow physicians to consider costs when the clinical benefits to the patient are marginal. But if they do that, they will have to provide an account of how marginal the benefits must be before costs can be considered and explain why the justification of their position does not apply to the case of the marginal benefit. The difficulty of doing both explains why some advocates of the classical position are drawn to Veatch's very strong version of it.

There are several points about the classical position that should be noted immediately:

1. Nothing in the classical position prohibits physicians from withholding costly interventions to save money when those interventions are of no benefit to the patient.

2. Nothing in the classical position prohibits physicians from withholding costly interventions to save money for the patient when the patient will have to bear the cost and when the patient judges that the cost that he or she will have to pay is too great a burden when compared to the benefits of the intervention.

3. Nothing in the classical position prohibits society from adopting general policies of withholding costly interventions to save money by not providing physicians with the means to provide those interventions.

Let me elaborate upon each of these points, because an understanding of them is important for a proper understanding and evaluation of the classical position.

In the very same article in which Angell articulates the classical position, she also argues that physicians as individuals and as part of an organized profession can play a major role in cost-containment efforts. As an individual, "the physician should not engage in unnecessary tests and procedures." As members of an organized profession, physicians should advocate fee schedules that do not reward the use of these unnecessary tests and procedures and should press for the adequate funding of technology assessment studies that will enable them to know when interventions are or are not beneficial. Participation in all of these measures, which are part of the process of eliminating waste in the provision of health care, are compatible, according to Angell, with the traditional ethic of the physician's responsibility to the patient. That is the point of claim 1 above.

While the fundamental point of claim 1 is clear, there are important ambiguities within it that I do not find resolved by Angell's treatment. There is, to begin with, the already-noted ambiguity about very minimal benefits. Is claim 1 really confined to legitimizing the withholding of interventions that are of absolutely no benefit to the patient, or does it also allow for the withholding of interventions that are minimally beneficial? The latter version would of course extend the scope of claim 1 considerably. Many of the lab tests that might be thought to fall under claim 1 are actually of some minimal benefit. Angell herself recognizes this when she describes routine chest x-rays on admission, one of the tests she suggests are just wasteful, as being "of almost no benefit."[3] Even more significant is an additional ambiguity about the burden of proof. Is claim 1 really the claim (1a) that the intervention can be withheld only when it is known to be of no additional benefit to the patient, so the burden of proof falls on the doctor who is considering withholding the care? Or is claim 1 better understood as the claim (1b) that the intervention can be withheld as long as it is not known that it will be of additional benefit to the patient, so the burden of proof falls on the advocates of providing the intervention? This ambiguity is particularly important since, as Angell notes, there are at present many interventions whose efficacy has not been adequately studied. We will return to these ambiguities when we apply the classical position to our example of decision making about thrombolytic therapy.

Claim 2 is found in the following statement of the classical position by Pellegrino and Thomasma:

> The physician remains the patient's advocate. As the de facto gatekeeper, the physician is obliged to obtain tests and use treatments that are beneficial to his patient and not to restrict access for purely financial or economic reasons. *The physician may withhold treatment if the patient decides that he does not wish to consume his family's resources.* Thus, limiting access can be part of a legitimate gatekeeper role.[4]

This is a clear and unambiguous statement of claim 2; it emphasizes the legitimacy of withholding care on the basis of the patient's decision about the economic costs compared to the benefits. But there are important issues that remain unaddressed. May the physician make the judgment on behalf of the patient in an emergency situation when the patient cannot reasonably be expected to be able to make an informed decision? May the physician even make that judgment against the expressed wishes of the patient when the physician has good reasons to believe that the patient would agree if there was more time for discussion and less stress? We will return to these unaddressed questions when we apply the classical position to our example of decision making about thrombolytic therapy.

Claim 3 was advocated very early in the discussion of these issues by the lawyer-ethicist Charles Fried in a classic article.[5] Fried pointed out that governments and health-care administrators do not have the same obligations that physicians have to individual patients, and this allows such officials to make decisions about limiting resources for the provision of care. Once such resources are not available to all patients or to certain well-defined classes of patients, their doctors are not of course required to provide them. In this way, Fried argued, cost containment can be realized even within the classical position. To quote him:

> Since the department of health, the legislature, and maybe even the director of the hospital do not have the kind of personal relations with patients that call into being the rights in personal care, respecting these rights is not a constraint upon persons

at that level. . . . Thus, the personal physician must respect the rights of his patients, and the department of health . . . must determine on efficiency and equity grounds how many people, and in what circumstances, will be the beneficiaries of such care. . . . Whatever the patient's right to personal care, and whatever the physician's obligation to his patients, they do not extend to having his doctor engage in political manipulation so that the patient can leapfrog the line or obtain a government benefit that is not properly available to him.

This is an extremely important statement of claim 3 as part of the classical model. However, it was developed to deal with examples such as kidney dialysis where governments can limit the number of machines and can issue mandatory guidelines about who may receive dialysis. But what happens when the government and/or the hospital administration makes a budget available to a service and tells it to use the money as it thinks best? May the physician running such a service and caring for the patients on it withhold some costly but clearly beneficial treatment from one patient in order to have the funds to provide more care to other patients? After all, the single patient may be at the front of the line and there may be no policy that says that the intervention is not available to him. We will return to this unaddressed question when we apply the classical position to our example of decision making about thrombolytic therapy.

We have thus far focused on articulating the classical position. We turn now to an examination of the reasons offered for its adoption. The following are among the most crucial reasons offered in the literature.

First, as Veatch emphasized in his statement of the classical position quoted earlier, the physician has made an unequivocal commitment to the patient, as part of the process of creating the physician–patient relation, to put the patient's interests first. Fulfilling that commitment requires the physician to do what will produce the best clinical outcome for the patient, regardless of the cost borne by society and/or third-party payers. Claim 1 is justified because withholding a nonbeneficial treatment is compatible with (and may even be necessary for) producing the best clinical outcome. Claim 2 is justified because the patient, who must bear the cost in the relevant cases, is waiving the commitment. Claim 3 is justified because the commitment is the commitment of physicians, not of governments or health-care administrators. The legitimacy of claims 1–3, is, however, perfectly compatible with the general validity of the classical position, since both grow out of the same fundamental commitment.

Second, the patient–physician relation must be built upon trust. Patients will trust physicians only if they believe that physicians put the interests of their patients first. If physicians put cost containment first even in a few cases, that trust will disappear. To quote an important recent defense of the classical position: "A policy that makes physicians restrictive gatekeepers disrupts the trust central to the doctor–patient relation. Even . . . the appearance of such a system will further erode the declining sense of trust between doctor and patient."[6] Claim 1 is justified because patients will not stop trusting their physicians if their physicians withhold nonbeneficial treatments; doing that may even increase patient trust. Claim 2 is justified because the patient is requesting that the costly treatment be withheld, and the physician's following the patient's own request is unlikely to lead to patient mistrust of the physician. Claim 3 is justified, especially if the physician makes clear to the patient whose decision it was to make the care unavailable, because the patient will not blame and therefore mistrust the physician. To quote that same recent defense: "It would be less disruptive to the doctor–patient relationship to abandon restrictive gatekeeping in favor of an explicit, public rule. Then . . . at least the doctor could say, 'I'm on your side. I'd like to help you, but I can't.'" The legitimacy of claims 1–3 is, however, perfectly compatible with the general validity of the classical position since they are structured to avoid disrupting the trust which the classical position is trying to build.

Third, when individual physicians withhold care in particular cases on economic grounds, claiming that the costs are too great, there is a tremendous potential introduced for injustices. These decisions, even more than ordinary clinical decisions, can be easily influenced by biases and prejudices that lead the individual clinician to raise these economic concerns only with patients from disadvantaged groups. Adherence to the classical position of putting the interests of the patient first and not considering the costs of the intervention minimizes the potential for this sort of injustice. Claim 1 is justified because it is not an injustice to withhold a nonbeneficial intervention. Claim 2 is justified because it is not an injustice to withhold a treatment that the patient is declining. Claim 3 is justified because the government officials and the hospital administrators will minimize the potential for injustices by drafting general policies about the provision of the intervention in question. The legitimacy of claims 1–3 is, however, compatible with the general validity of the classical position because none of them introduces a potential for prejudicial injustices.

Fourth, it is unfair to put physicians into a position in which they face serious conflicts between their loyalty to their patients and their loyalty to third-party payers, public or private. Adherence to the classical position avoids this problem because loyalty to the individual patient always comes first. Modifying that position by withholding care in some cases to save money is putting other loyalties first, and that, as Angell stressed in the passage quoted above, puts physicians in an intolerable position of dual conflicting loyalties. Claim 1 is justified because one does not put other loyalties first when one withholds nonbeneficial treatments. Claim 2 is justified because one is putting loyalty to the patient first when one respects the patient's request, even if made on economic grounds, to withhold certain treatments. Claim 3 is justified because it is not the physician who is putting other loyalties first. The legitimacy of claims 1–3 is, however, compatible with the general validity of the classical position because none of them creates the conflicting loyalties that the classical position insists must be avoided.

In recent years, a number of authors such as Paul Menzel, Haavi Morreim, and I have begun to challenge the classical position. The reasons offered by these authors, while all beginning with a concern about rising health-care costs, are different, complement each other, and suggest that the classical position requires modification, if not abandonment. We shall now review these reasons and discuss the alternative position which is emerging.

Menzel's point of departure is that the classical position has failed to take into account the possibility that the patient may be willing *in advance* to have his or her clinician withhold some health care on economic grounds in order to keep the costs of health care down, perhaps to make health insurance more affordable to the patient or perhaps for other more altruistic reasons. If that is the case, then the physician is being faithful to the patient in participating in this form of cost control. To quote Menzel's summary of his position:

> I would argue that clinicians may participate actively in the rationing process without diminishing their commitment to individual patients if obvious conflicts of financial interest have been removed, if neither the insurers nor clinicians have claimed that cost is no object . . . and if subscribers and patient representatives have had a significant role in giving at least some general normative guidance for rationing. In all cases the crucial test question for justifying rationing is whether as a subscriber beforehand, the patient would in fact have consented to the limitation on care that the provider is now implementing. To the extent that this question can be answered affirmatively with confidence and justification, the requirement of subscriber-patient involvement in setting rationing guidelines diminishes.[7]

Morreim's point of departure is that limitations of care for economic reasons are inevitable, and that patients have reasons to prefer that their clinicians limit care on economic grounds, rather than having that limitation imposed by administrators using general guidelines. It is only if these decisions are made at the bedside that the needed clinical flexibility will be present. To quote her:

> Only if the physician retains considerable clinical authority is he in a position to offer to each patient the interventions that each most needs. But with this resource control, in turn, comes allocation responsibilities. . . . In sum, clinical authority can only be preserved at some cost to traditional fidelity.[8]

My point of departure is that, like the rest of us, physicians have many different moral commitments that they must balance. As a result, the interests of the patients will often, but not always, take precedence. In some cases the interests of others (other patients, the rest of society) will take precedence and will lead the physicians to withhold certain forms of care on economic grounds. To quote the summary of the argument:

> Like other human beings with many obligations, clinicians must learn to balance these obligations rather than to always give one priority over all others. Rationing that is necessary for cost containment merely extends the set of loyalties that physicians must balance, and there is nothing wrong with that.[9]

These arguments constitute in my opinion a powerful case for the modification of the classical position. In a world that needs to control rapidly increasing health-care costs, clinicians will have to withhold some available and beneficial but costly interventions from their patients even if at the time in question the patients want the interventions to be provided.

How should the classical position be modified? One thing is certain. While these critics are in agreement about the need to modify the classical position, that does not mean that they are in agreement about what modification should be made. For Menzel, clinicians should withhold care for economic reasons only to the extent that rational patients would agree in advance that they do so. For Morreim, clinicians should withhold care for economic reasons only to the extent that economic pressures require that health-care expenditures be limited. For Brody, clinicians should withhold care for economic reasons only to the extent that doing so is required to fulfill their other obligations. There is no reason to believe that these three approaches would lead to exactly the same results.

There is, however, one feature of policies of withholding care to which they might all agree. Consider the contrast between a policy that would withhold care simply on the basis of how expensive it is versus a policy that would withhold care on the basis of a comparison between the costs of the care and the benefits it yields. The former type of policy ranks medical interventions by their costs, withholds the most expensive care first, and continues down the list until enough money has been saved. The latter type of policy ranks medical interventions by comparing their costs and benefits, withholds the intervention which provides the fewest units of benefit per unit of cost first, and continues down the list until enough money has been saved. Although these critics of the classical position might not agree on the extent to which care should be withheld on economic grounds, they appear to agree that clinicians should adopt the second type of policy. If money must be saved, rational citizens would prefer withholding many forms of care that produce the fewest units of benefit per unit of cost to withholding a few expensive forms of care that yield very high benefits. Doing so, moreover, frees the money needed to fulfill the clinician's obligations to others while minimizing the benefits withheld from the patient. So whatever modification is made in the classical position, it should be in the direction of clinicians comparing costs and benefits in decisions to withhold care on economic grounds. As Menzel says very clearly, "Rationing's main target will be high cost-per-benefit care."[10]

With this understanding of both the classical position and recent suggested modifications of it, we turn to the question of the choice of thrombolytic agents in light of the conflict between clinical considerations and cost considerations. We will first examine this question for the period 1987–1989, the period after both tPA and SK had been approved for use but before there were results from comparative trials using mortality as their end point. We will then examine the implications of those comparative trials for this question.

It might seem that the answer to our question during the period 1987–1989 was obvious according to the classical theory. Even though tPA was much more expensive than SK, ethical physicians, following the classical position, should have disregarded the question of cost and used tPA, which had been proven to be more efficacious in terms of early clot lysis in the TIMI-I trial. This presumably was the view of the majority of American physicians in the Brody study[11] who said that they used tPA because it was clinically preferable. On this account, the 40 percent of the responding physicians who chose SK (886 physicians) must have acted wrongly according to the classical position.

I believe that this initial analysis is in error and that the question of which drug should have been used in the period 1987–1989 by adherents of the classical position is far more complex for several reasons. First, claim 3 reminds us that even on the classical position, hospital administrators, using such devices as closed formulary lists, could mandate the use of SK on economic grounds, and ethical physicians practicing in such institutions could then without fault use SK. As pointed out in the Brody study, slightly more than the 5 percent of the responding physicians (114 physicians) used SK for just that reason, and it may well be that more institutions should have adopted that same approach to the choice of thrombolytic agents. Second, claim 1, at least in its version 1b, reminds us that the classical position allows clinicians to withhold on economic grounds the more expensive therapy as long as it has not been proven to be more beneficial to the patient. Given that there were no data in that period showing the greater efficacy of tPA either in terms of survival or in terms of improved ejection fraction, even if there were data showing better clot lysis from tPA, adherents of the use of SK on economic grounds could well argue that their choice was justified even on the classical position. As pointed out in the Brody study, slightly more than 20 percent of the responding physicians (443 physicians) used SK for just that reason, and it may well be that more physicians should have adopted that same approach to the choice of thrombolytic agents. Third, the only physicians using SK whose choice is difficult to justify on the classical position were the slightly more than 11 percent of the responding physicians (248 physicians) who said that they chose SK on economic grounds even though they thought that tPA was the better drug. Even then, however, it may be possible to reconcile their choice with some versions of the classical position. After all, as noted in the Brody study, they were physicians who said that the benefits were insufficient to justify the costs, presumably because they thought that the benefits of the use of tPA over the use of SK were marginal. While their choice was incompatible with Veatch's very strict presentation of the classical position, which demands the use of even infinitesimally better interventions regardless of cost, it may well have been compatible with Angell's less demanding version of the classical position, which allows for the withholding of marginally beneficial interventions on economic grounds. In short, the choices of the physicians who used SK, even if directly or indirectly motivated by economic considerations, can be justified on the classical position.

One other point deserves notice. In another study of choices of thrombolytic agents in the same period, the authors asked users of tPA whether they would change to SK if they knew that the patient had to pay for the treatment because he or she did not have insurance.[12] Thirty-six percent said that they would. This type of economic decision making is also compatible with the classical position because of claim 2, providing that there is some patient input into that decision (an issue not explored by the authors). In this one additional way, then, the classical position turns out to be far more flexible about the choice of thrombolytic agent than was suggested by the initial analysis.

Modifying the classical position makes it easier to justify the decision of even those users of SK in 1987–1989 who believed that tPA was the better drug but that its extra benefits were not sufficient to justify the extra expenditures. As just pointed out, this was the only group of SK users whose decision was difficult, although not impossible to justify on the classical position. Their way of thinking, however, was the very way of thinking about clinicians' withholding care on economic grounds that would be justified if the classical position were to be modified. While the use of tPA rather than SK is not that much of an extra expense in any given case, clinicians would be right in withholding that care if the extra benefits were as marginal as they believed.

All our discussion until now has focused on the ethics of clinicians using SK rather than tPA in the period 1987–1989. But what about that choice in the years that followed? Obviously, the fact that neither GISSI-2 nor ISIS-3 found any benefits in terms of survival from the use of tPA rather than SK provided strong evidence for the idea that the use of SK was justified even by claim 1a of the classical position, the claim that care can be withheld on economic grounds only when there is evidence that it offers no extra benefit to the patient. The use of SK was certainly justified by any of the other versions of the classical position and by the modified position. One might even question the ethics of using a more expensive drug when major trials have not found a compensating extra benefit. In fact, many clinicians switched to SK after the publication of those data.

The publication of the GUSTO results will obviously have a major impact upon these issues. After all, GUSTO showed a reduction in mortality from 7.2–7.4 percent with SK to 6.3 percent with accelerated tPA. Isn't this 15 percent reduction in comparative mortality a sufficiently significant clinical benefit so that clinicians, even on Angell's version of the classical position, ought not to withhold it from their patients? To quote Dr. William Ganz of UCLA, "A doctor does not make his decision based upon price. . . . If we can say that TPA is better, then we have to give it." Even if the classical position is modified, isn't it enough of a benefit to justify the cost? To quote J. Sanford Schwartz of the Institute of Health Economics at the University of Pennsylvania, "Based on the significant life-saving benefit seen in GUSTO, T.P.A.'s cost effectiveness is comparable to that of other widely accepted life-extending standards of care, such as cholesterol-lowering therapy, high blood pressure therapy, mammography, and open heart surgery."[13]

While initially very plausible, this analysis is too superficial. Doubts can be raised both about its account of the results of the GUSTO trial and about the implications it draws from that account. Let us consider each of these doubts separately.

Several doubts have been raised about the claim that GUSTO has shown that tPA saves more lives than SK. Richard Peto has argued that "when the GUSTO-1 results are combined with those of GISSI-2 and ISIS-3, there continues to be no significant difference in the mortality rates between the drugs."[14] But the legitimacy of combining the data from the three trials is questionable. After all, only GUSTO studied the comparative efficacy of the drugs when heparin was begun immediately, thereby helping to preserve tPA's benefit of earlier clot lysis, and the claim that tPA saves more lives than SK is the claim that it does so when heparin is begun immediately. It seems inappropriate then to combine the GUSTO data with the data from the other trials in which heparin was begun later. Others (Ridker and colleagues)[15] have argued that the differences are found only in patients treated during the first 4 hours. Moreover, and more important, they argued that in the GUSTO trial, where bias could have played a role because the trial was an open-label trial, the patients receiving tPA had much more coronary artery bypass surgery on an emergency basis than did the patients receiving SK (9.5 percent compared to 8.5 percent), and this makes it hard to tell whether the benefit in the first 4 hours was due to the tPA or the bypass. Finally, I am troubled by the fact that tPA was administered in an accelerated fashion whereas SK was not, apparently in order to make the SK data comparable to the data from the ISIS-3 trial. Is GUSTO really a proof that tPA is better or is it really a proof that the accelerated provision of thrombolytic therapy saves more lives? Given these doubts, clinicians might well conclude that there is certainly no imperative to use tPA rather than SK for the many patients presenting 4 hours after the onset of symptoms and that even on the classical position, except on the extreme version (1a), there is no moral imperative to provide tPA to patients presenting earlier because GUSTO has not really shown that tPA is better than SK, especially if SK is provided in an accelerated fashion.

Others will see the data differently and will conclude, at least for patients presenting in the first 4 hours, that the GUSTO data do show that the accelerated provision of tPA, when accompanied by the immediate use of heparin, really does save lives. Does this mean that there is then an imperative to provide tPA rather than SK? That does not follow, even on the classical position, in circumstances in which there are formulary restrictions on the use of tPA (as allowed for under claim 3) or where the individual patient must bear a share of the extra costs and would find that too burdensome (as allowed for under claim 2). Otherwise, the classical position does seem to entail, even on Angell's less restrictive version of it, that the physician is required to use tPA. But is that required under the modified position? There are at least two reasons for not immediately concluding, as the preceding analysis did, that it is required because the $200,000 per life saved figure seems comparable to the cost of saving lives with other interventions. First, GUSTO shows, at most, that the expenditure of the extra $200,000 results in one more patient being discharged alive. That does not tell us how long the difference lasts, so we do not know how many years of life (much less quality-adjusted years of life) we are buying with that extra expenditure. That information is needed before any claims of comparability to other interventions can be evaluated. Second, and more important, it is not clear that the modified position would claim that the other interventions are morally required. Their introduction and adoption may reflect the acceptance of the classical position at a time when resource pressures were less critical.

In summary, we have identified two major positions, with several variations of each, on the issue of the extent to which clinicians should consider costs in making clinical decisions. We then applied each of these positions to the choice between tPA and SK in three different periods, the period from the approval of both drugs until the first appearance of the data from the comparative trials (1987–1989), the period in which the relevant data available were the data from GISSI-2 and ISIS-3 (1990–1992), and the period since the data from GUSTO emerged (from 1993). The only unequivocal conclusions were from the middle period, where the use of SK was clearly acceptable and the real issue was the legitimacy of the use of tPA. Most of the variations of both positions would have supported the same conclusions in the earlier period, but some versions of the classical position would have supported, and perhaps even mandated, the use of tPA in that earlier period. The situation is least clear in the post-GUSTO period, in part because of the clinical ambiguities in the GUSTO data and in part because the many versions of the various positions lead in different directions. This is not surprising. We are as a society just beginning to think through the implications of dropping an uncritical acceptance of a poorly defined classical position and of accepting either a more nuanced version of that position or some version of the modified position. The ambiguities of the post-GUSTO period reflect that fact.

Costs and Reimbursement Policies

We have thus far examined the question of the extent to which physicians should consider costs in making clinical decisions such as the choice of thrombolytic agents. But another question needs to be considered: Should third-party payers, governmental or private, consider costs in determining whether they should pay for certain interventions that are admittedly beneficial? This question is obviously very important in and of itself. But it also has an important impact upon our earlier discussion. If third-party payers won't pay for certain interventions because they are trying to control costs, physicians will sometimes find their patients refusing the interventions or will sometimes find their institutions refusing to allow them to provide the interventions, thereby making the question of whether physicians should consider the cost irrelevant.

As we saw in Chapter 1, this question arose in 1988 shortly after the approval of tPA. Medicare decided not to provide extra reimbursement for the use of tPA. We shall return to that decision, but first we shall, following our usual policy, look at the question more generally. We shall focus on public third-party payers, leaving for another occasion the more complex case of private third-party payers.[16]

An excellent point of departure for our discussion is a set of unimplemented regulations that the Health Care Financing Agency (HCFA) proposed in 1989 governing coverage decisions that relate to medical technology.[17] By statute, Medicare covers only services that are reasonable and necessary for diagnosis or treatment. Medicare has traditionally understood this to mean services which are safe and effective, are not experimental, and are provided in appropriate settings by qualified personnel. The main purpose of the unimplemented regulations was to add cost-effectiveness as a consideration in making coverage decisions:

> HCFA is including cost-effectiveness as a proposed criterion because we believe considerations of cost are relevant in deciding whether to expand or continue coverage of technologies, particularly in the context of the current explosion of high-cost medical technologies. We believe the requirement of section 1862(a)(1) that a covered service be "reasonable" encompasses the authority to consider cost as a factor in making Medicare coverage determinations.

To make this work, HCFA would have to be able to define cost-effectiveness and identify procedures for determining whether a given intervention is cost-effective. In the proposed regulations, an intervention is defined as cost-effective if it is:

(i) Very expensive to the program, but provides significant medical benefits not otherwise available;

(ii) Less costly and at least as effective as an alternative covered intervention;

(iii) More effective and more costly than a covered alternative, but the added benefit is significant enough to justify the added cost; and

(iv) Less effective and less costly than an existing alternative, but a viable alternative for some patients.

How will cost-effectiveness be established? The commentary before the proposed regulations identifies the following steps: (1) identify the relevant alternative technologies; (2) identify and quantify the relevant outcomes; (3) identify and quantify the relevant costs whether borne by Medicare or by others; (4) consider nonquantifiable factors. It also adds the following observation which we will find to be very important shortly:

> Consider the case of a service that is closely comparable with respect to the risks associated with its use and its effectiveness to another already covered service, but the new service is substantially more expensive than the one that is already covered. In this situation, we may wish to cover the new service, while providing the results of our cost-effectiveness evaluation to the payment policy staff and/or Medicare contractors for their use in establishing payment levels . . . the amount payable is based on the reasonable cost of the least expensive alternative treatment that appropriately meets the patients' needs.

There are several important points to note about this Medicare proposal. First, it does not exclude coverage simply because a form of treatment is expensive. An intervention is covered as cost-effective under clause (i) even if it is very expensive, providing that it offers significant benefits that would otherwise not be available. Thus the adoption of such a proposal would in no way prevent the coverage of even such expensive modalities of therapy as transplantation, so long as it is used for a class of patients for which it offers significant benefits not otherwise available. In this respect, it is similar to the approach we advocated for clinicians when we discussed modifying the classical position. Second, it defines cost-effectiveness for new technologies only, and it does so by comparing them to technologies already covered by Medicare. This is understandable, because Medicare is usually faced only with decisions about coverage for new technologies. But it is unfortunate, in part because it leaves intact the coverage of already covered interventions which are not cost-effective and in part because it can therefore lead (under [ii]) to the coverage of interventions which are not cost-effective but which are better than already covered interventions which are even less cost-effective.[18] Finally, there are certain crucial ambiguities in the definition. Clause (iii) talks about covering more costly interventions if their additional benefits are significant enough to justify the added costs, but no definition of significant enough is provided. Similarly, clause (iv) covers therapies that are viable alternatives for some patients, even if they are less effective, without clarifying just what is required to make them viable.

This Medicare proposal was only one of a series of proposals put forward in the last few years both in the United States and elsewhere to limit the growth of health-care costs by denying coverage for certain beneficial treatments whose benefits were judged to be insufficient to justify their costs. As is well-known, the state of Oregon engaged for some years in the process of developing a systematic approach to limiting coverage of some forms of insufficiently beneficial care, but there have been setbacks in the actual implementation of that approach.[19] In the United Kingdom, the decision by the North East Thames region of the National Health Service in early 1991 to not cover five common procedures unless there was an "overriding" need[20] led to an extensive public discussion in which many district health authorities made it clear that they were planning to limit the coverage even of life-extending therapies. Among those mentioned were treatment for advanced lung cancer, heart transplants, intensive care for premature (<800 gram) babies, and AIDS treatment. The chief economist at the Department of Health sent a memo to the regional authorities encouraging the systematic making of such decisions. It remains to be seen how these ideas will be incorporated into the British National Health Service. It is clear that the unimplemented Medicare regulations were only one manifestation of a wide-scale international interest, although not success, in limiting social coverage of health-care needs for economic reasons.

Two additional points should be noted. The first is that we are not discussing whether certain interventions that do not meet the proposed definition should be available to those who want them and can afford to pay for them out of their own resources; the question we are discussing is whether those interventions should be provided by public funds. The second, connecting this discussion with our earlier discussion, is that even supporters of the classical position on the commitment of clinicians recognize that clinicians may be limited on economic grounds in what they can do for their patients if that limitation is imposed upon them by social decisions to limit coverage, and it is those decisions that are under discussion now.

Are such policies appropriate social policies? Are they compatible with a social policy of ensuring universal access to beneficial health care? These are some of the obvious questions raised by the policies.

A defense of the Medicare policy of limiting coverage grows out of the widely shared conception of justice in health care as access to an adequate level of health care, the most prominent exposition of which is to be found in a report issued by the President's Commission in 1983.[21] Rejecting the notions of justice and equity as access to what everyone else is getting or even access to everything needed or everything beneficial, the commission defined justice and equity as "access to some level of care: enough care to achieve sufficient welfare, opportunity, information, and evidence of interpersonal concern to facilitate a reasonably full and satisfying life. That level can be termed 'an adequate level of health care.'" Three impressive reasons are offered on behalf of this conception:

> Because an adequate level of care may be less than "all beneficial care" and because it does not require that all needs be satisfied, it acknowledges the need for setting priorities within health care and signals a clear recognition that society's resources are limited and that there are other goods besides health. . . . In addition, since providing an adequate level of care is a limited moral requirement, this definition also avoids the unacceptable restriction on individual liberty entailed by the view that equity requires equality. Provided that an adequate level of care is available to all, those who prefer to use their resources to obtain care that exceeds that level do not offend any ethical principle in doing so. . . . Finally . . . [it] permits the definition of adequacy to be altered as societal resources and expectations change.

Given this plausible, even if incompletely articulated conception of justice in health care, the argument for the policy of limiting coverage is straightforward. Justice requires that everyone have access to an adequate level of health care, not to all health care which is needed or beneficial. Social insurance programs for health care (such as the U.S. Medicare program) are ways of fulfilling that demand of justice. As there are other goods besides health and other commitments besides the commitment to providing access to health care, the amount spent on these programs may legitimately be limited, even if that means that not all beneficial or even needed forms of care are covered. So the unimplemented Medicare policy could be compatible with our commitment to justice in health care by providing universal access to beneficial health care, once that commitment is properly understood.

How can it be just if it reintroduces a multitiered system of health care for the elderly? Some forms of health care which are beneficial but which will not be covered under the proposed policy will be available to those who can pay for them on their own but will not be available to those who must rely upon Medicare, and how can that be just? These objections, while rhetorically powerful, are not that troublesome. As the President's Commission clearly pointed out, the existence of a multitiered system of health care is not inherently objectionable. It is objectionable only if you are committed to the view that justice and equity in the delivery of health care means equality in the delivery of care. A multitiered system in which the basic tier is inadequate, however, is inherently objectionable: justice demands that the basic tier provide adequate care. But the proposed Medicare policy need not threaten the adequacy of the care provided to Medicare recipients who are in the basic tier because they cannot afford to pay for care not covered by Medicare.

As long as the requirement of sufficient benefits to justify the extra cost is not interpreted in an excessively rigorous fashion, the forms of care not covered will be forms of care that offer only modest marginal improvements over care that is covered. The failure to provide these modest marginal benefits hardly challenges the adequacy of the basic tier.

There are no doubt those who understand the commitment to provide universal access in other ways. The Canadian system embodies a different understanding, as has been pointed out by John Iglehart: "In essence, Canadian policy says that simply because people can afford to pay, they should not be able to purchase care that is better or more readily available than that available to the less well off."[22] This different understanding may grow out of a different conception of justice in health care or it may grow out of the idea that we want social solidarity in addition to justice in the provision of health care. In any case, I believe that it is an understanding that should be rejected by all who accept inequalities of wealth. Why should the wealthy be able to buy all sorts of luxuries but not better health care, even when the basic level of health care guaranteed to all is adequate? Health care may be special in that we are all entitled to an adequate level of care, but I see no reason to believe that it is special in that no one should be allowed to purchase at their own expense additional marginally beneficial care. So the proposed Medicare policy, which would result in a situation in which those who have the money get the marginal benefits while those who have to rely on Medicare reimbursement do not, is not a morally inappropriate two-tiered system even if it is a two-tiered system.

There is a harder challenge which must be faced. It raises, quite appropriately, the question of the focus of the limitation of coverage if coverage must be limited to save money. Should the focus be on limiting the coverage of certain forms of care, as Medicare had proposed, making them available only to the more affluent, who can pay for them out of their own funds, or should the focus be on more stringent limitations on the coverage of more affluent individuals, leaving them to rely even more upon their own resources, so that all beneficial forms of care can be provided to the less affluent?

A full response to this challenge would require developing a complete theory of justice in the allocation of health-care resources, and this is not the place to do so.[23] Instead, I will defuse this challenge by relying upon a useful distinction recently introduced by Norman Daniels, whose work represents one of the main sources of the view that justice in health care requires special attention to the health-care needs of the least well off.[24] Daniels distinguishes three versions of that view in allocation decisions:

> How stringent is the priority owed the poorest groups when we seek to improve aggregate well-being? Three positions are possible: (1) help the poor as much as

possible (strict priority); (2) make sure the poor get some benefit (modified priority); (3) allow only modest harms to the poor in return for significant gains to others who are not well off (weak priority).[25]

Actually, still a fourth version allows modest harms to the poor in return for significant enough gains to others, regardless of their wealth (weaker priority position). By not covering some forms of care that provide only marginal benefits, the proposed Medicare policy does harm the least well-off, who cannot pay for these forms of care by themselves. But the harm is at most very modest because the benefits of these forms of care are very marginal. The money saved can be used to ensure coverage of much more beneficial forms of care for all Medicare beneficiaries, many of whom are not that well-off, even if they are not the least well-off. So theories of justice which assign a weak or a weaker priority to the needs of the least well-off can accept the proposed Medicare policy. Only theories of justice that insist that all allocational inequalities must benefit the least well-off (the strict or the modified priority) can object to the proposed Medicare policies, and such a requirement seems excessive.[26]

It seems reasonable to conclude therefore that while there are many ambiguities in the proposed Medicare policy on limiting reimbursement, the judicious use of such a policy, once the ambiguities are properly resolved, could, in a world of limited resources, improve the outcomes from the medical care which is covered without doing an injustice to anyone. However, I do want to issue an important caution about the use of this approach. We must ensure that we consider all the benefits to the patient, including benefits that are not easily quantifiable, in making these decisions. In fact, the proposed Medicare policy insisted on the need to do this. An example will help illustrate the need for this caution.

In an important recent article, Friedman and Katt discuss how clinicians can help control costs without significantly compromising care by making cost-conscious choices among the drugs they use.[27] While they do not extend their discussion to reimbursement policy, such an extension seems quite reasonable. One example they give is from the management of hypertension:

> Regarding differences among each of these agents, ACE [angiotensin-converting enzyme] inhibitors and calcium channel blockers in general are significantly more expensive than diuretics and beta blockers, especially if the less expensive atenolol, propranolol, furosemide, or hydrochlorothiazide is used. Certainly, in an otherwise healthy patient with hypertension unresponsive to dietary changes and weight loss, it would be reasonable to begin treatment with these less expensive choices, especially since no one of the above agents has been proved to be more effective.

The main exceptions they offer to these recommendations are for patients with diabetes (for whom ACE inhibitors are recommended) and patients with chronic obstructive pulmonary disease (COPD) or severe occlusive vascular disease (for whom calcium channel blockers are indicated). While sympathetic with the philosophy they are expounding, I do feel that this is a good example of a case in which the philosophy must be applied with caution.

Friedman and Katt's discussion does not attend to some important side-effect issues, especially issues about side effects that are of concern to patients. Consider the question of sexual functioning after taking antihypertensive medications. In one very important recent study, S. H. Croog and his colleagues reported that patients taking an ACE inhibitor showed less worsening of sexual functioning that patients taking the beta blocker propranolol.[28] The implications of that study have been complicated by the more recent findings of the TAIM study[29] and of a study comparing sexual functioning after the use of different ACE inhibitors;[30] the question obviously deserves much further investigation, as do questions relating to other side effects that trouble patients. The point that I want to make now is that the extra costs of calcium channel blockers and ACE inhibitors may well be justified if they have fewer of these side effects, either because patients are more willing to take them and they are therefore more effective in controlling hypertension or because the avoidance of those side effects by itself justifies the extra costs of those drugs. The Friedman and Katt study suffers from a failure to even consider these issues. My point simply is that the proposed regulations were right in insisting that these patient-experienced side effects must be considered in deciding whether the more expensive drug is worth the extra cost.

We turn finally to an analysis of how the proposed policy, and other reasonable reimbursement policies of the same type, should have dealt with the reimbursement for the extra cost of tPA over SK. Two points need to be kept in mind. The first is that this decision would not have fallen directly under the proposed policy for technical reasons (in part because both were approved for myocardial infarctions at the same time, and in part because thrombolytic therapy was not covered directly, but only as part of the reimbursement for the treatment of myocardial infarctions, under Medicare's DRG policy). But for the sake of analyzing the policy issue, let us disregard these technical matters. The second point that is worth noting is that there was a close connection in time between the actual decision by Medicare at the beginning of 1988 to not increase the DRG reimbursement for myocardial infarctions in light of the cost of tPA and the issuance of the proposed regulations in 1989. While I do not want to overstate the connection between these two events, it seems plausible to hypothesize that the conflict over increasing reimbursements in the case of tPA reinforced interest that may already have existed in formulating such a policy.

Given the evidence available at the time of the initial approval of SK and tPA, it seems clear that it would have been hard to justify covering tPA, with its much greater cost. Its best chance would be the claim that it fell under clause (iii) of the proposed definition of a cost-effective new therapy in that its added benefits were significant enough to justify its added costs. But such a claim would have to confront the fact that no added benefits had been demonstrated either in terms of improved left ejection fraction or in terms of survival. This does not mean that Medicare under the proposed policy should have refused to cover tPA. It does mean that Medicare under the proposed policy should have been willing to pay only the same amount that it was willing to pay for SK. This would be an implementation of its announced policy, cited previously, that reimbursement in such cases should be "based on the reasonable cost of the least expensive alternative treatment that appropriately meets the patients' needs." And if this was true in that earlier period, it seems even more true for the period after the results of GISSI-2 and ISIS-3 were in and showed no difference in mortality.

The much more complicated issue is whether or not the results of GUSTO lead to the conclusion that the extra costs of tPA should be reimbursed. First, it is far from clear, for reasons already given, that GUSTO showed that tPA offers benefits that are considerably greater than those offered by SK. Second, for reasons also given previously, it is far from clear that the additional benefits, if any, are sufficient to justify the additional costs. The comparisons that some have drawn with other life-saving therapies which are covered are, as we showed above, not necessarily appropriate, and in any case they may at most show that we should question the coverage of those other interventions. As in the case of the clinical question, the ambiguities in the GUSTO data combined with our inexperience in thinking through these issues lead to lack of clarity in the post-GUSTO period about the appropriateness of paying for the extra costs of tPA.

We have argued in this section for a number of very controversial claims. Our understanding of the patient–physician relation should be transformed to allow for a fuller consideration of the economic implications of clinical decisions. Our understanding of justice in health care should be transformed to accept the appropriateness of certain types of two-tiered systems. Such transformations would have supported the clinical decision to use SK and the policy decision to offer no extra reimbursement for the use of tPA until the results of GUSTO became available. Because of the ambiguities in the GUSTO data and our need to better understand these transformations, there is great uncertainty about the appropriate clinical and reimbursement decisions in the post-GUSTO period.

The Prices of Drugs

Throughout the discussion in the last section, the price differential between tPA and SK was taken for granted and we discussed the issue of how clinicians and reimbursement policies should deal with it. But should it really be taken for granted? Should tPA cost so much more? As we saw in Chapter 1, these questions were raised by several people during the debates in 1988. In this section, we will examine them.

Any serious examination of these questions needs to begin with a broader discussion of the basis for the pricing of drugs. At the beginning of this chapter, I indicated two fundamental questions that need to be discussed: Should the prices of drugs be set by whatever the market will pay? If not, what other pricing mechanism should be used? We turn first to an examination of these fundamental questions.

Concerns and Responses in the United States

The prices of prescription drugs have attracted considerable attention in the United States in the last few years. It might seem surprising that this is so, since the total cost of these drugs used outside institutions in 1991 was $36.4 billion, which was less than 5 percent of the total national health care expenditures of $751.8 billion. Moreover, the percentage of health care expenditures devoted to prescription drugs has dropped in half since 1965.[31] I suspect that one of the reasons why so much attention has been paid to the prices of drugs is that consumers pay a comparatively high percentage of those costs directly out of pocket. In 1991, consumers paid directly out of their own pockets $20 billion for out-of-institution use of prescription drugs, 55 percent of their total cost. This is very high when compared to the 19 percent of total health-care expenditures paid by consumers directly out of their own pockets. When Americans are not reimbursed for expenditures, they become very aware of them. But this is not the whole story; the rest, I suspect, is related to a growing recognition that other health-care bills (especially hospital bills) reflect the high cost of drugs paid for by those institutions, and that any attempt to control these other health-care bills must also address the cost of the drugs used.

The first focus of attention has been on the unusually high prices of individual new drugs. One of the most recent controversies has been over the price of Taxol, the drug derived from the bark of the Pacific yew tree, which has recently been approved for use by women with advanced ovarian cancer. The initially announced price was in the $3,000–$4,000 range per person treated.[32] Another controversy has been over the price of Betaseron, a new drug for the treatment of multiple sclerosis, whose initial price will be about $10,000 per year.[33] Other new drugs whose prices have attracted considerable attention in recent years include AZT (initially $8,000 per year) for HIV-positive patients, cyclosporine ($5,000–$7,000 per year) for the suppression of the rejection of transplanted organs, Ceredase (initially $250,000 per year) for treating Gaucher's disease, growth hormone ($8,000–$30,000 per year) for stimulating growth in children, and clozapine (initially $8,944 per year). The last three cases are particularly interesting. Ceredase and growth hormone are protected against competition under the Orphan Drug Act of 1983, which was designed to encourage the development of drugs to treat rare diseases. Moreover, growth hormone therapy is one of the few very expensive treatments used electively, even if it is conceded that extreme shortness can be psychologically devastating in certain cases.[34] Clozapine's high cost included a mandatory licensed weekly program of drug tests. That requirement was dropped in response to considerable pressures, resulting in a 30–40 percent lowering of the annual cost.[35]

In response to criticisms of these costs, many of the pharmaceutical companies have introduced programs of assistance for uninsured or underinsured individuals in need of these drugs.[36] These programs can sometimes aid people with considerable means who are nevertheless underinsured for the high cost of some of these drugs. Critics remain dissatisfied. To quote one report, "In Congress, the industry's voluntary actions are generally seen as public relations efforts meant to ward off further government moves to curb drug prices."[37]

The second focus of attention has been on the high general price increases for prescription drugs in recent years. One recent study which attracted considerable attention was performed at the request of Representatives Byron Dorgan and Fortney (Pete) Stark. At their request, the General Accounting Office prepared a report on price increases between 1985 and 1991 of 29 drugs selected by the congressmen. The reasons for picking those drugs and the possible biases involved in the selection were not disclosed. In any case, the study found that in a period in which the general Consumer Price Index rose 26.2 percent and the medical-care Consumer Price Index rose 56.3 percent, only 3 of the 29 drugs showed a smaller increase. The median maximum percentage price increase was 124.8 percent.[38] Similar results of a broader nature were found by the Congressional Research Service and announced by a congressional committee in a report on drug prices. According to that finding, prescription drug price inflation in the period 1980–1990 was 152 percent, almost three times the general inflation rate for that period of 58 percent. The report noted that the difference continued through the first half of 1991.[39]

All such studies suffer from substantial methodological issues related to such questions as the variable pricing of drugs to different purchasers, changes in manufacturing processes and quality, and the introduction of new drugs.[40] Moreover, one might question whether the increase in drug prices should be compared to the general increase in prices or to the general increase in health-care prices, since the latter is often far greater than the former. The most recent study shows, in fact, that prescription drug inflation in the period 1980–1992 (188 percent) was only moderately greater than medical price inflation (151 percent), although it was much greater than the general inflation rate (68 percent).[41] Nevertheless, in response to these studies, segments of the drug industry held down price increases in 1992 to the general rate of consumer price increases:

> Heightened public sensitivity to hyperinflationary price trends coupled with fears of greater government intervention has led leading drug makers to voluntarily cut back on price increases. After price run-ups at triple the rate of inflation for over a decade, many leading firms, including Merck, Marion Merrell Dow, ICI, and Roche, are limiting 1992 price increases to the general inflation rate as measured by the consumer price index (CPI). The Pharmaceutical Manufacturers Association (PMA) recently estimated that drug companies representing one-third of the total market are holding price increases to the CPI.[42]

The extent to which this has actually happened is, however, a matter of some controversy.[43] In any case, there is a tension between this development in the industry and possible developments relating to the cost of new drugs. The more price increases on existing drugs are controlled, the greater will be the pressure to price new drugs as high as possible. We shall return to this theme.

A third focus of attention has been on studies of the prices of the same drugs in different countries. A number of studies have appeared which indicate that American consumers pay much more for the same drugs than do their counterparts in other countries. Two of these studies were done in Europe, one by the Italian pharmaceutical manufacturers association (Farmindustria) and one by the Belgian Consumer Association (BEUC), and were reported in the United States in a series of congressional reports.[44] To quote a summary of these studies:

> Average drug prices paid by American consumers are 54% higher than the average for all EEC nations, and are higher than drug prices even in the EEC nations with "free markets" for prescription drug prices. . . . These data provided by the Belgian Consumer Association confirm the relationship between U.S. and EEC prices found in a methodologically different analysis performed in 1988 by the Italian pharmaceutical manufacturers' association, Farmindustria.

Another report, produced by the General Accounting Office, compared drug prices in the United States and Canada.[45] The general finding of that study was that Americans pay 32 percent more for a carefully selected basket of 121 frequently dispensed drugs than do Canadians unless the Americans are institutional buyers getting special discounts.

These types of studies have provoked different responses by different observers. Richard Zeckhauser, a Harvard economist, interpreted them as follows: "Obviously, we subsidize the world." On the other hand, Gordon Binder, CEO of Amgen, a biotechnology company, saw those higher prices as crucial to the success of the American pharmaceutical industry and its development of new drugs:

"The U.S. drug industry is one of the strongest in the world. . . . If the Government meddles with the free market, it could well destroy the industry."[46]

Given these sources of concern about the prices of drugs, it is not surprising that some members of Congress have turned their attention to this issue—hardly a new concern.[47] As early as 1959, Senator Estes Kefauver held hearings on the price of drugs, focusing both on the enormous gap between production costs and prices and on the contribution to costs of a patent system without compulsory licensing. No legislation on drug prices was actually passed, however, as attention turned to the need to revise the laws governing the FDA in light of the thalidomide problem. Almost 30 years later, the drafters of the 1988 Medicare Catastrophic Coverage Act, responding to studies showing the high out-of-pocket cost of drugs for the elderly, incorporated into that ill-fated act coverage for outpatient prescription drugs, coverage that was later repealed because of financing problems. But congressional attention to this issue in the last few years has been particularly intense.

The leading congressman addressing this issue has been Senator David Pryor of Arkansas, chairman of the Senate Special Committee on Aging. That committee published between August 1989 and September 1991 three reports on the price of drugs.[48] Moreover, Senator Pryor has introduced crucial legislation on the price of drugs.

Senator Pryor's first legislative proposal in this area was an attempt to aid the state Medicaid programs, which were struggling with the burdens of the high cost of outpatient drugs covered under those programs. Its basic goal was to ensure that the state Medicaid programs would get the benefits of the pricing discounts that manufacturers were offering to large-scale purchasers such as the VA system, hospital chains, and HMOs. A modified version of this proposal was passed in the Omnibus Budget Reconciliation Act (OBRA) of 1990.[49] Manufacturers who agreed to this pricing change for Medicaid patients were guaranteed that all their prescription drugs would be covered under Medicaid for all indicated uses. Almost immediately, many drug companies began to increase their discounted prices, especially to the VA hospitals, to avoid having to give similar rebates to Medicaid. Ultimately Congress was forced to change the law so that discounts to VA hospitals did not count in determining Medicaid prices.[50] It remains to be seen whether OBRA of 1990 will actually help control Medicaid drug expenditures.

This proposal was a very partial measure, since it addressed only Medicaid expenditures on drugs, and not drug prices in general. In an attempt to deal with that broader issue, Senator Pryor introduced legislation designed to encourage drug companies to limit their increases in the prices of drugs to the general rate of inflation. Drug companies benefit significantly from tax credits they receive for locating production facilities in Puerto Rico. The Pryor proposal was designed to limit those benefits to companies whose price increases did not exceed the rate of inflation. It was, however, defeated in March 1992,[51] perhaps because senators, learning from the experience of OBRA of 1990, were hesitant to pass measures that might lead to unanticipated effects (such as drug companies moving production facilities to other countries). Even if it had passed, however, it would not have dealt with the issue of the prices of new drugs, one of the issues that has attracted so much attention in recent years.

Senator Pryor is not the only legislator who has devoted attention to the prices of drugs. Representative Henry Waxman and Senator Howard Metzenbaum have called attention to the high price of a few drugs (for example, growth hormone and Ceredase) which were protected against competition under the Orphan Drug Act. They proposed a bill that would limit such protection once sales reached $200 million. Although they were successful in having their bill passed, it was vetoed by President Bush, who argued that the bill would undercut the incentives required to encourage the development of such drugs.[52]

These congressional developments have led to very few firm results. Medicaid is paying less for drugs, but in light of the changes in pricing policy developed by many manufacturers, the extent of those savings is unclear. Nothing has been done legislatively to control the increase in drug prices or limit the initial high prices on breakthrough drugs, although some companies did begin to limit price increases in 1991.

Attention to the prices of drugs has switched from Congress to the new presidency. The 1993 Clinton health-care reform proposal, as initially presented, while increasing both Medicare and private third-party coverage for prescription drugs, contains a provision for a form of price control on the prices of drugs by a new National Health Board and by the secretary of the Department of Health and Human Services. In testimony before Congress, both Hillary Rodham Clinton and Secretary Donna Shalala have made it clear that they are committed to this provision. What will happen to it in the legislative process remains to be seen.[53]

In the meantime, the pricing of drugs, for better or worse, is the province of the drug companies. We shall shortly be examining whether the three factors cited earlier indicate that this needs to be changed or whether the current system of pricing can be defended. But before doing so, we turn to the experience of other countries to see what their drug pricing policies can teach us.

International Comparisons and Lessons

In looking at drug prices from a comparative perspective, two points emerge very clearly. The first is that the United States is not alone in struggling with the question of the pricing of drugs. Many of the most developed countries, especially those with advanced health-care systems and important pharmaceutical industries, are struggling with this issue of how drugs should be priced. To quote a recent German commentary in *The Economist*:

> In theory, drug companies and governments should work in partnership to raise health standards: the companies by creating revolutionary new treatments, governments by deftly allocating tax revenues so that their health services can afford them. In practice, that relationship is rapidly going wrong, because of the astronomical prices drug firms are charging for their innovations. Governments accuse the industry of profiteering and causing havoc in their health services, and want to cut back the rising drugs bill. The industry retorts that this would not only hit its profits but also impede medical progress.[54]

The second point is that the United States differs from the rest of these countries in that it alone lets the prices of drugs be determined by market forces, with the exception of the recent legislation about the prices paid by Medicaid. It also differs from the rest of these countries in that it has the largest drug industry responsible for the introduction of the largest number of new medicines. The relation between these two facts will be very important for our analysis in the section on profits and costs that follows.

To see why and how other countries regulate the initial prices of new drugs and increases in the prices of old drugs, we will examine the United Kingdom, Germany, France, and Canada, and we will pay some attention to other countries as well. We are fortunate that three comprehensive studies have recently appeared which provide extensive information about these matters.[55]

The drug industry in the United Kingdom is extremely important, both in terms of its prominence in the world drug industry and in terms of its contribution to the economy of the United Kingdom. Twelve percent of worldwide pharmaceutical research and development takes place in the United Kingdom. The British drug industry is responsible for the discovery and/or development of the cephalosporins for treating infections, the beta blockers for treating cardiovascular disease, the H2 antagonists for treating ulcers, acyclovir for treating certain viruses, and AZT for treating HIV-positive patients. It is the second largest contributor to the United Kingdom positive balance of payments for manufactured goods and it has been the fastest growing manufacturing sector in the United Kingdom in recent years. For all of these reasons, there is considerable interest in ensuring the success of the drug industry by allowing it to make an adequate profit to support research and development.[56]

At the same time, the government of the United Kingdom pays for most prescription drugs under the National Health Service and is therefore concerned about its costs. The NHS expenditure on drugs (currently in excess of £3 billion) is the second highest item after staff costs in the NHS budget, and it is currently viewed as a matter of concern.[57]

The U.K. system of price controls is based upon an attempt to control total profits rather than the price of individual drugs. Under the Pharmaceutical Price Regulation Scheme, the large drug companies are expected to charge prices that yield them a return on capital employed for serving the U.K. market of 17–21 percent. As costs before profit companies are allowed the costs of production, a sales promotion allowance, and a research and development allowance to cover the cost of developing new drugs. In recent years, the R&D allowance has been around 20 percent. Companies whose prices lead to profits beyond a certain acceptable excess must reduce future prices or pay a rebate to the NHS.[58]

How well has this system worked to control costs? The annual rate for the increase in drug expenditures has run around 10 percent (2 percent due to a volume increase, 6 percent to the substitution of newer products for older products, and 2 percent for price increases on older products). This has produced some of the current concern, which is reinforced by the BEUC study showing that for 125 commonly used drugs used in 12 European countries, the United Kingdom paid the fifth highest amount for the drugs in question.[59] In any case, the system has worked to control costs as compared to the cost of drugs in some other European countries (the Netherlands, Denmark, and Germany), and it has certainly produced lower prices than those found in the United States. Table 4.1 shows how U.K. prices compare to other European prices. The 1989 Farmindustria (Italian Pharmaceutical Manufacturers Association) study showed that U.K. prices were less than half U.S. prices. The data are summarized in Table 4.2.[60]

Table 4.1 Relative Drug Prices, Various Countries, from BEUC Study

Country	Price level of 125 drugs
Portugal	100
France	111
Spain	112
Greece	115
Italy	127
Belgium	139
Luxembourg	155
United Kingdom	**180**
Ireland	193
The Netherlands	214
Denmark	231
Germany	239

Table 4.2 Relative Drug Prices, Various Countries,
from Farmindustria Study

Country	Weighted average retail price
Spain	100
France	104
Italy	152
Belgium	159
United Kingdom	**205**
Germany	271
Holland	291
United States	**427**

What can be learned from an examination of drug pricing in the United Kingdom? The first lesson is that it is technically feasible to have a system of price controls based on the concept of limiting profits. It should be noted, however, that while a system of price controls based on limiting profits is possible in many health-care systems, it is both easier to administer in and particularly well-suited for systems with single payers that don't have to worry about who pays for what drugs. The second lesson is that such a system of price controls could significantly reduce the cost of drugs for U.S. consumers. In fact, the beauty of the U.K. system is that different price levels, all below the current U.S. price levels, are attainable by modifying the allowance for promotion costs and for research costs and/or by adjusting the acceptable profit level. The third lesson is that such a system is compatible with a substantial research effort. As we have seen, the U.K. system is designed to promote research and development as well as to control costs, and it has an explicit mechanism for doing so: the research and development allowance. We will return to a further discussion of these features of the U.K. system.

The German drug pricing system operates very differently from the U.K. system, largely because of the difference in the history of the two systems. While the United Kingdom has had a drug pricing system in place for many years, the German system is just emerging in response to the Health Care Reform Act of 1989.[61]

Germany's health-care system has attracted much attention because it managed during the 1980s to control the growth of heath-care costs so that they did not grow more rapidly than the general economy. Nevertheless, pressure was felt to more stringently control the cost of health care since the cost of health insurance was perceived as rising too rapidly. These pressures led to the Health Care Reform Act of 1989, with its special approach to the pricing of drugs.

Traditionally, Germany has had a very strong pharmaceutical industry, one that has spent 15 percent of sales on research and development and has the highest export rate among all drug-exporting countries in the world. Prices were not controlled before 1989, and the government's main effort to control drug expenditures focused on the development of a list of drugs that would not be covered under health insurance.[62] As a result, German drug prices, as shown in the previously discussed BEUC and Farmindustria studies, were among the highest in Europe.

The basic philosophy behind the new German approach to the pricing of drugs is found in the following statement by Norbert Blum, minister of labor and social affairs:

> One medicine cost DM30 and another, equally good with the same active substance, costs DM90. Why should the health insurance scheme pay for the most expensive, why shouldn't it buy the DM30 product? The health insurance system has always been based on the principle that the services financed must represent value for money.[63]

This philosophy is being carried out by a system of reference pricing. A fixed price is set for drugs with the same active ingredient, for drugs with therapeutically equivalent ingredients, and for drugs with comparable pharmacological profiles. That fixed price is based on the lowest available price for that class of drugs. Any manufacturer of another member of the class can charge more for its product, but the patient then has to pay the difference. The expectation is that all prices will drop close to the reference price because consumers will resist paying for the difference.

Iglehart reports that in the first stage of setting reference prices, the stage that focused on classes of drugs with the same active ingredients, reference prices were set at 30–66 percent below the previous market prices. Setting reference prices is more complicated in the other stages, as Macarthur has shown.[64] Moreover, there is at least some evidence that the German industry found ways to circumvent the intentions of the program, in part by marketing products in such a way that they fell outside of the system. Total German drug bills rose by 9 percent in 1990 and by 10 percent in 1991.[65] As a result, a new law adopted in late 1992 imposed a new global budget on payments for prescription drugs. This led to a 20 percent decline in drug expenditures in the first half of 1993.[66]

A crucial issue is the impact of this pricing scheme on research and on the development of new drugs. Unlike the U.K. system, which attempts to both control costs and promote research and development, the new German system is simply a price-control system. No provision is made to ensure that the prices paid provide a revenue stream sufficient to fund research and development. Concern about the implications of this feature was expressed as early as 1988 in the following private memo prepared for the U.S. Pharmaceutical Manufacturers Association:

> To the extent that pharmaceutical prices are forced down in Germany through the reference price system, the funds to support research, development, and promotion will have to come from somewhere else. . . . Only in another large and open market, such as the United States, could pharmaceutical manufacturers hope to recoup at least a portion of the funds that will be needed for self-sustaining future innovation.[67]

A full discussion of this issue is reserved for our later analysis; it is sufficient to note for now that this is certainly a matter that requires serious concern and thought.

What can be learned from an examination of this recent German experience? There are several lessons that deserve to be noted. The first is that it is possible for a system that has previously imposed no controls on the cost of drugs to reverse itself in this practice. The second is that a system of price controls must cover all (or at least most) drugs if it is to be effective. The third is that systems that consider only prices and not profits may in the long run fail to promote adequate drug development.

Some of these issues also arise when one looks at the French system for the pricing of drugs. The French system is of particular interest because of the very low prices that the French pay for drugs. As seen in Tables 4.1 and 4.2, the French prices for drugs are near the lowest in all of western Europe. How does this come about?

The French system is based upon strict price controls for drugs whose costs are to be reimbursed to patients under the Social Security System.[68] The price is set at the time the drug is approved for reimbursement; the price of nonreimbursable drugs is not controlled. Among the factors considered at that time are the cost of similar drugs in France, the cost of the drug being considered in other European countries, and the place of the new drug and the company in the French economy (more on this last factor below). Drugs that are very similar to already-approved drugs are likely to be approved for reimbursement only if they are priced considerably below those already-approved drugs. Price increases have been granted over the years, but data suggest that these price increases have been considerably below general price increases. Thus, with 1970 taken as the base year and the base prices set at 100, the price index for pharmaceuticals in 1987 was 198.4 compared to the general cost-of-living index of 420.2. A similar calculation taking 1980 as the base year shows the index price for pharmaceuticals in 1988 as 125.4 as compared to the general price index of 171.8 and the price index of nonreimbursable drugs as 193.4. This suggests that the limit on price increases is central to the French system for controlling drug prices.

What impact has this had on the development of new drugs in France? Without drawing any firm conclusions about causality at this point, we can at least point to data which suggest that the French pharmaceutical industry has fallen behind the industry in other countries. A King's Fund Institute study of 66 global, innovative drugs introduced from 1975 to 1989, presented in Table 4.3, is illustrative of the basis for the concern.[69] Brudon and Viala add the following observation: "Recent studies have shown that France fell behind during the period 1975–86. It was second in world drug research and has now dropped to fourth in the total number of drugs representing both a clinical advance and a new chemical structure."[70]

The French have not been unaware of this problem. In the early 1980s, better initial prices and better price increases could be obtained by companies that agreed to increase investments in research and development in France. The formal system for allowing these higher prices disappeared in the mid-1980s, but there is some evidence that it continues to operate on an informal basis.[71]

One important lesson emerging from this examination of the French system is that it is possible to use a system of price controls to keep the prices of drugs very low in comparison to the prices in other countries. A second lesson is that doing this may result in a low level of pharmaceutical research and development unless special attention is paid in the pricing system to encouraging such research.

Before we turn from these three European approaches to a look at approaches adopted elsewhere, we need to remember that developments in Europe in terms of integrating national economies may mean that these national differences may not persist in the years to come. The same sort of phenomenon may also lessen the differences between U.S. and Canadian prices as free trade increases between those countries. To see why, let us look at the Canadian system.

Interest in the Canadian scheme for controlling drug prices is part of the general U.S. interest in the Canadian health-care system, but it was certainly increased after the appearance in September 1992 of the GAO report which indicated that Canadians were paying much less for prescription drugs.[72] How were these savings produced? The GAO felt that there were two mechanisms that produced these savings. (1) Since 1987, Canada has had in place a price monitoring body, the Patented Medicine Prices Review Board, which examines both introductory prices

Table 4.3 Drug Introductions, by Country

Country	Percentage of global, innovative drugs
United States	45
United Kingdom	17
Germany	12
Switzerland	6
France	5
Japan	5

and price increases. If these are deemed to be excessive, and if the manufacturer refuses to lower prices, then market exclusivity under the patent system can be removed. (2) Provincial health-care plans, such as the Ontario Drug Benefit Plan, include a drug in their formulary (list of drugs for which it will reimburse those patients, mostly elderly and low income, covered under the plan) only if the price proposed by the manufacturer as the best available price is found acceptable.

These recent measures have not had a deleterious effect on Canadian pharmaceutical research and development, primarily because there has traditionally been very little of this research and development anyway. Until 1986, Canadian patent law called for compulsory licensing of patented drugs, so that competitors could undercut the sales of new patented drugs by introducing cheaper generic equivalents. As a result, pharmaceutical research amounted to only 5–6 percent of sales. The creation of the Price Review Board was part of a package plan by which a company's patents were protected from compulsory licensing for additional years if the company's research and development expenditures were at least 10 percent of sales. This is why the Price Review Board's major mechanism for enforcing price controls is the removal of patent protection by the removal of market exclusivity.[73]

The North American Free Trade Agreement, recently signed by the United States, Canada, and Mexico, requires, in one of its provisions, the unification of patent protection in the pharmaceutical industry. As a result, Canada's parliament must now repeal the compulsory licensing provisions of Canadian patent law, thereby destroying the enforcement mechanisms of the Price Review Board. It is anticipated that this will lead to a significant increase in Canadian prices.[74] As in the case of Europe, the greater integration of national economies in North America may limit the differences in the prices of drugs.

This brief look at the Canadian system adds one more dimension to the lessons we can learn by comparing drug pricing. The crucial Canadian lesson is that the system of patent protection is an important component of the process by which drugs are priced and the process by which research and development is encouraged or discouraged. This lesson will be crucial for our own analysis to follow.

The schemes for price controls which we have examined are not the only ones attracting attention. Australia recently proposed making future drug approvals conditional on a satisfactory cost-effectiveness analysis.[75] This measure is in addition to other earlier Australian initiatives that have kept its prices far below international averages. Since this approach is consonant with other initiatives throughout the world to submit medical interventions to careful economic analysis, it can be expected that the Australian approach will be carefully examined and widely imitated in the years to come.

Several lessons emerge from these international comparisons. The first is that it is possible to control the price of drugs. The second is that this can be accomplished in a variety of ways, ranging all the way from profit controls to strict price controls. The third is that support for research and development can be built into price-control systems, but this is likely to occur only when there are explicit mechanisms for ensuring this support. The final lesson is that one needs to consider issues of patent protection when one is trying to develop an adequate system. None of these lessons settles the question of whether any system of price controls is desirable; that question will be examined in the next section. But these lessons will be very important if we decide that such a system is desirable.

Profit Levels, Cost of R&D, and Suggested Policies

In a world increasingly relying on market mechanisms to set the price of consumer goods, it seems appropriate to ask whether there are any good reasons for not allowing drug companies to charge what they want and for not relying on competitive forces in the marketplace to control the price of drugs. None of the data we have examined thus far provides reasons. Even if drug prices in the United States, which relies on such a system, are higher than drug prices elsewhere and have been rising more rapidly than other prices, that may be a reflection of the rapidly increasing costs of developing new drugs. Perhaps other developed countries should free up the prices of drugs and pay their share of the costs of research and development. This was the viewpoint expressed by Dr. P. Roy Vagelos, the CEO of Merck and Co., in a well-known and frequently cited article:

> The basic principle governing the free enterprise system is that free and unrestrained competition should force fair prices. The more segmented the industry, the truer that is, and the pharmaceutical industry . . . is highly competitive. Research and development costs are a major consideration in setting the price of a new medicine. . . . [O]n an industry-wide basis, counting all of the investments in the failed and successful projects, it costs $231 million, on average, to bring one new prescription medicine to market in the United States. . . . So in countries where we believe prices for innovative medicines are set unfairly low, we try to market our medicines at those prices while lobbying for a change in the government's pricing policy.[76]

Two reasons might be offered to explain why competitive pricing cannot be relied upon to produce fair prices. The first refers to patents and the monopolies they create. The second refers to the lack of a connection between prices paid by consumers (who are sometimes, but not always, reimbursed) and choices about drugs made by clinicians. Let us examine each reason separately.

The first reason focuses on the fact that the market in pharmaceuticals is not totally free. As long as newly developed drugs are under patent protection, they are protected from competition and the manufacturer can charge higher prices than would be sustainable in a competitive marketplace. While pharmaceuticals do not get the standard 17-year patent protection in the United States because of the years lost while approval is sought from the FDA, the Drug Price Competition and Patent Term Restoration Act of 1984 has resulted in a greater than 10-year effective patent protection for new drugs.[77] Patent protection and the resulting monopolies are required to protect innovation and cannot therefore be eliminated. Consequently, drug prices need to be set by some nonmarket mechanism to produce fair prices. A recent analysis summarizes this argument:

> The monopoly provided a prescription drug by the patent is not accidental. Congress established that monopoly in the form of a patent because, in a market economy, capital invested in creating a product must be returned to the investor with a profit. . . . Economic theory has long recognized that a monopoly seller sets his price at what he estimates is the highest price he can sustain without stimulating excessive buyer resistance, i.e., declining demand. In the case of medications, viewed by many as necessities, this price may be the highest price the buyer can pay.[78]

As it stands, this argument is inadequate. First, it overemphasizes the lack of competitiveness produced by the patent system. Even during the period of patent protection, competitors can often produce drugs which are sufficiently different so that they are not covered by the patent but which are sufficiently similar so that they compete for the same uses. These are the "me-too" drugs. So the extent to which there truly are monopolies in the drug industry is not equivalent to the extent to which drugs are covered by patents. Second, and even more important, this account cannot explain what actually happens to drug prices after drugs are no longer covered by patents. It would seem, on this account, that drug prices should decline rapidly after that point as manufacturers meet the newly emerging price competition from the newly permitted generic drugs. Two studies showed that this does not happen. The first examined the effect of patent expiration on 30 drugs that lost their protection in the period 1976–1987.[79] The authors found that prices actually increased until a generic competitor entered the market and then decreased only marginally, and that generics captured only 25.2 percent of the market even though their cost was less than half that of branded drugs. The second study examined 35 drugs that lost their patent protection in the years 1984–1987.[80] The trends found were even more surprising. The average price of the drugs which lost their patent protection increased 69 percent in constant dollars in the 6 years after that protection was lost. While this resulted in an even greater discrepancy between generic prices and branded prices (with the generic price being just 20 percent of the branded price), the formerly patented products still had a 40 percent market share.

There is no doubt that the existence of patents means that a reliance on the market to set drug prices cannot be justified by a simple appeal to the virtues of pricing in free markets. But there is also no doubt that there are other factors that are even more important in understanding why the drug market is not appropriately viewed as a free competitive market. This leads us to an examination of our second answer.

It has long been recognized that the market for the purchase of health-care services, including the market for the purchase of pharmaceuticals, is very different from the market for the purchase of most consumer goods. Because of the asymmetry of information between the physician and the patient, the person who makes the decision as to which drugs will be purchased is the physician, while the person who purchases the drug is the patient. To be sure, the problem of noncompliance shows that patients are not purely passive followers of physicians' orders; nevertheless, the physician still is the primary decision maker. But since that primary decision maker is neither the purchaser of the pharmaceutical nor the person who pays for that purchase, there is little incentive for that decision maker to consider the cost of the pharmaceutical. This means that price competition cannot be counted on to produce fair prices. These reflections are strengthened by the observation that even in the United States, the majority of patients are reimbursed to varying degrees for the money they spend on pharmaceuticals. The most recent study showed that 70 to 74 percent of the noninstitutionalized civilian population had some outpatient prescription drug coverage, although only 3 percent had full coverage that covered the entire cost of all pharmaceuticals.[81] Consequently, manufacturers know that patients will not be that sensitive to the price of drugs, and this means that price competition will not be as effective in this market as it is in other markets.

This account helps explain the failure of price competition to modify the prices of branded products after generics enter the market; physicians continue to order the branded products because of inertia and because they have no incentive to change. To quote Peter Temin:

> In the absence of information generated by consumers, behavior appears to exhibit hysteresis. Even trained professionals act very conservatively in the presence of new suppliers. As Senator Kefauver said thirty years ago, their incentives to save other people's moneys are not strong.[82]

Thus we have good reasons for rejecting Vagelos's suggestion that we rely upon the free market and unrestrained competition to set the price of drugs. Some system of price control seems justified. At the same time, it would be foolish to disregard Vagelos's observations about the high cost of the development of new drugs and the need for adequate pricing to cover those costs.

A recent study by DiMasi and his colleagues emphasized the extent of those costs and the need to consider them in deciding about the pricing of new drugs.[83] The study examined the cost of developing new drugs that were first tested in humans in the period 1970–1982. In 1987 dollars, the cost of developing a newly approved drug was $231 million. Of that sum, $114 million represented out-of-pocket expenditures, while the rest represented interest costs on money spent over the years before approval (assuming a 9 percent discount rate). The authors reported that this represented a 230 percent increase in total costs in real terms over the previous period. They attributed the bulk of it to increased out-of-pocket costs required to generate the data needed to secure FDA approval, although some of it was also due to a longer development period and to a higher discount rate. In any case, those expenses must be paid for and drug costs must cover them.

This study can be criticized on a number of grounds.[84] On the one hand, it does not seem to have taken into account the tax savings companies obtain when they spend money on research and development. During the period in question, these would have reduced the cost of developing new drugs, at least for companies with taxable income, by more than 45 percent. This reduction would be different in recent years, in part because of lower tax rates and in part because of new tax credits. On the other hand, it may have underestimated interest rates on money used for research and development, so that a 9 percent discount rate would be too low. This means that they may have underestimated the cost of developing new drugs. In any case, none of this changes the basic fact that the cost of research and development for new drugs has increased and must be paid for by the purchasers of the resulting drugs.

This observation needs to be correlated with our thesis in Chapter 3. We argued there for modifications in the standards of evidence required for drug approval. The main argument we offered was based upon philosophical reflection about individual freedoms and about constraints on government interferences with them. It is reasonable to expect, however, that the modifications we proposed will reduce expenditures for research and development, both directly and by shortening the development period and the resulting interest costs. That could result in lower drug costs. This is another argument for our proposals.

Returning to the issue of the pricing of drugs, what emerges from our discussion is that we have good reasons for not allowing the market to set the price of drugs but we also have good reasons for ensuring that the pricing which emerges is sensitive to the need to cover the costs of the continuing research on, and development of, new drugs. All of this means to me that we need to consider systems which, like the British system, incorporate both these features. The British system has, moreover, another feature that seems very worthwhile: it imposes limitations on the money spent on promotion and advertising. Let me explain why this is a desirable feature.

In the recent debate in the United States about the pricing of drugs, spokespersons for the pharmaceutical industry, such as Vagelos, have emphasized the high costs of research and development. Critics have responded by challenging the heavy expenditures on promotion and advertising. For example, Dr. Barry Bleidt claimed that "the industry spends more on promotion than on research and development, so when they say they don't have enough money to develop new drugs, I don't believe them."[85] While data on this matter are hard to come by, the *Pink Sheet*, an industry newsletter, reported that in 1991 companies spent $10 billion on promotion while spending only $9 billion on research and development. Dr. Stephen Schondelmeyer calculated that this is an underestimate, and that the industry spends up to 20 percent of its budget on promotion while only spending 16 percent of its budget on research and development. We do not at this point need to agree on an appropriate level to spend on promotion; it is sufficient to conclude that any system of setting prices needs to settle that question, and another desirable feature of the British system is that it attempts to control such expenditures in the course of setting prices. Consumers should not be required to subsidize excessive promotional expenses.

In short, our analysis suggests that drug prices should be set so that there is adequate coverage for production costs and for limited promotional activities and adequate support for research and development (either directly or through an appropriate rate of return). It also suggests that the market cannot be relied upon to set drug prices. To be sure, adopting such an approach, as evidenced by the British experience, will produce prices that are relatively high compared to most European prices even if not compared to present U.S. prices. But the goal is not to produce the lowest prices; it is to produce a set of prices that are supportive of appropriate research and development while not being excessive. I am not arguing for adopting the exact British system for setting the prices of drugs; we shouldn't do that because of the many differences between the American and the British health-care systems. But none of those differences prevent us from incorporating the basic philosophy behind the British system of drug pricing into a system that is more appropriate for the U.S. context.

Are current American drug prices too high? Nothing that we have seen so far settles this question. We have seen that they are much higher than anyone else's prices. We have argued that we cannot be certain that the market ensures that they are not too high, and we have provided an outline of a theory as to what the prices should be. But none of this settles the question. For all that we have seen so far, the high American prices may be appropriate, especially in light of the fact that other countries have so controlled prices that they may not be paying for their fair share of the costs of research and development.

There are considerable data available on the profitability of the American pharmaceutical industry, data that indicate that the industry has done extremely well in recent years. Typical is one recent analysis in which the pharmaceutical industry was shown to have a return on stockholders' equity which was at least 50 percent higher than the median rate of return on stockholders' equity for the Fortune

500 industrial companies, with the gap widening.[86] The return on stockholders' equity in the pharmaceutical industry climbed to 26 percent in 1990. This has been taken as evidence that drug prices as currently set are too high. But such a conclusion is premature for two different reasons. First, as a matter of accounting convention, expenditures on research and development and on promotion are treated as expenditures in the year in which they occur rather than as investments in future earnings, which is what they really are. Consequently, corporate balance sheets in industries with extensive expenditures on research and development and on promotion, such as the pharmaceutical industry, understate the value of the company's assets and artificially inflate its rate of return.[87] Second, the cost of capital must be higher in riskier industries than in safer industries, to compensate for the risk of the investment. Consequently, a higher rate of return might be justified for industries such as the pharmaceutical industry in which investments in research and development often yield no return because the research project fails.

Since these defects in the standard analysis are well known, considerable interest was generated by a number of studies commissioned by the congressional Office of Technology Assessment (OTA) and reported on in its recent study on pharmaceutical research and development.[88]

The first study examined the revenues to companies from new chemical entities approved for sale in the United States in the period 1981–1983 and compared them to the cost for developing those entities (including the cost of capital and the cost of failed projects) as adapted by the OTA from the previously cited DiMasi study. The conclusion of the study was that there was $36 million in excess revenues. As the OTA pointed out, this excess would have been eliminated by a 4.3 percent price reduction. This means that excess profits were not the major source of the price differential between the United States and other developed countries, which was much more than 4.3 percent; it was due to some combination of other excessive U.S. expenditures (perhaps on promotion) and underpricing by the other countries.

The second study attempted to correct for the defects in the standard comparisons between the profits of pharmaceutical companies and the profits on other companies. Estimates by outside consultants of the rates of return for pharmaceutical companies compared to matched nonpharmaceutical firms, making various assumptions about the investment life of research and development expenditures, suggested a higher rate of return of 2–3 percent per year in the pharmaceutical industry. Further OTA analysis suggested that this difference could not be explained on the grounds that pharmaceutical investments were riskier, thereby requiring a higher rate of return. The OTA reached the following conclusion:

> Evidence on the economic rate of return to the pharmaceutical industry as a whole
> over a relatively long period (1976–87) shows returns that were higher than returns

on nonpharmaceutical firms by about 2 to 3 percentage points per year after adjustment for differences in risk among firms. This is a much lower differential than is suggested by conventional comparisons of profit ratios, but it is still high enough to have made the industry a relatively lucrative investment.[89]

The OTA report did not translate this second finding into any conclusions about the prices of drugs, so I will attempt to do so. The excess rate of return from that period was about 20 percent of the actual rate of return for the pharmaceutical industry, which means that pharmaceutical company profits would have had to decline by 20 percent to eliminate the unjustified differential. A recent study by the Prime Institute reported that company profits represented 13 percent of the average wholesale price of drugs in 1992 ($2.31 out of $17.96).[90] Projecting that back to the earlier period, the average wholesale price would have to drop 2.6 percent, or 46 cents, to abolish the unjustified excessive profits as calculated by the OTA.[91] While not trivial, this is much smaller than the differential between U.S. prices and the prices in other countries noted earlier. There may be other explanations of the price differential which justify the claim that U.S. prices are too high. One possibility is that U.S. marketing costs, averaging 20 percent of wholesale sales in the Prime Institute study as opposed to the allowed 9 percent in the British pricing scheme,[92] are too high. Alternatively, the prices in the other countries may be too low and the United States may be bearing an unfair percentage of the cost of research and development.

Let me summarize what we have learned, add a few observations in connection with these lessons, and then apply these lessons to the case of tPA:

1. There are good reasons for not allowing the market to set the prices of drugs, including the monopoly aspect of patents but primarily the isolation of decisions to order drugs from economic considerations.

2. A good nonmarket system for pricing drugs is not a system that produces the lowest prices. Instead, it is one that covers all costs of production, allows for an appropriate level of promotion, and provides an adequate rate of return to encourage research and development.

3. There will be very hard decisions that need to be made in developing such a nonmarket system. One issue involves an adequate rate of return. The OTA analysis shows that it is possible to develop an approach to that question based on adjusting for the timing of investments and on comparing rates of return with rates of return on investments with comparable risks, but this is obviously an approach whose details will generate much controversy. An even more controversial question is what constitutes an appropriate level of promotion, an issue whose importance has emerged in the course of our analysis.

4. While American prices are much higher than European prices, this is not primarily due to excessive American profits. Factors that seem more relevant are very high promotional costs in America and inadequate support for research and development in many other countries.

5. One very hard problem in implementing our approach is that pricing decisions will have to be made on the basis of estimates about sales over time, since it is the estimate of the sales over time multiplied by the allowed price (which may change over time) that must cover all of the items listed in 2 above. What will be the basis for such estimates? What will happen if the estimate turns out to be too low (depriving the company of part of the revenue to which it is entitled) or too high (giving the company a windfall)?

6. Another difficult problem in implementing this approach is its international dimensions. Unless all countries agree on a similar approach to pricing, those whose pricing policies keep the prices too low will have a free ride on the support of research and development provided by countries who have more appropriate pricing.

7. TPA is an excellent example of why the market cannot be trusted to set the price of drugs. As we saw in Chapter 1, the success of Genentech in getting a broad interpretation of its patent in the United States led Burroughs Wellcome to abandon its development of a competitor drug, so patent monopolies were particularly efficacious in limiting competition in this case. Moreover, the setting of an emergency such as a myocardial infarction is one in which there is little chance that a concern about price on the part of the patient will check the physician's desire to order the most efficacious drug, even if it is only a little more efficacious and much more expensive.

8. The actual high price of tPA is not by itself evidence of overpricing. We could decide whether or not tPA was properly priced only if society had settled the questions raised in 3 above, only if we had complete data about research and development costs for tPA and about their timing, and only if we had good projections about its total sales over time. This latter requirement is particularly difficult to satisfy in light of the conflicting results from the major trials and in light of the ambiguous meaning of the GUSTO results.

One final observation is in order. It would obviously be a complicated task to implement the approach advocated here. But a failure to do so means an inappropriate reliance on the market to set prices. As long as we do that, clinicians and policymakers, struggling with the issue of whether the high extra cost of a new drug is justified by the benefits to the patients, will also have to be concerned with the legitimacy of the extra cost. Patients and professionals deserve better. Let them at least be sure that the price they are considering is an appropriate price.

Notes

1. M. Angell, "Cost Containment and the Physician" *JAMA* 254 (1985): 1203–7. Quote, p. 1206.

2. R. M. Veatch, *A Theory of Medical Ethics* (New York: Basic Books, 1981). Quote, p. 285; italics added.

3. Ibid., p. 1204. This is her assessment of the findings of a well-known study of this topic. The study is F. A. Hubbell et al., "The Impact of Routine Admission Chest X-Ray Films on Patient Care," *NEJM* 312 (1985): 209–13. That assessment is shared by the authors. I do not myself share that assessment since the routine studies led to quicker treatment of real problems in at least three (maybe as many as 11) cases and to one diagnosis of a sometimes successfully treatable (but not in this case) lethal condition. But the point in the text stands, even if the example needs to be changed.

4. E. D. Pellegrino and D. C. Thomasma, *For the Patient's Good* (New York: Oxford University Press, 1988). Quote, p. 175; italics added.

5. C. Fried, "Rights and Health Care—Beyond Equity and Efficiency," *NEJM* 295 (1975): 241–45. Following excerpt is from p. 244.

6. D. P. Sulmasy, "Physicians, Cost Control, and Ethics," *Annals of Internal Medicine* 116 (1992): 920–26. This quote and the following quote, p. 922.

7. P. Menzel, *Strong Medicine* (New York: Oxford University Press, 1990), and P. Menzel, "Some Ethical Costs of Rationing," *Law, Medicine, and Health Care* 20 (1992): 57–66. Quote, p. 59.

8. The most recent and fullest version of her views is to be found in E. H. Morreim, *Balancing Act: The New Medical Ethics of Medicine's New Economics* (Dordrecht: Kluwer, 1991). Quote, p. 62.

9. B. A. Brody, *Life and Death Decision Making* (New York: Oxford University Press, 1988), and B. A. Brody, "Physicians and Rationing," *Texas Medicine* 87 (1991): 86–90. Quote, "Physicians and Rationing," p. 89.

10. Menzel, "Some Ethical Costs of Rationing," p. 59.

11. B. A. Brody et al., "The Impact of Economic Considerations on Clinical Decision Making," *Medical Care* 29 (1991): 899–910.

12. D. S. Lessler and A. L. Avins, "Cost, Uncertainty, and Doctors' Decisions," *Archives of Internal Medicine* 152 (1992): 1665–72.

13. The first quotation is from "Costly Clot-Dissolving Drug Has Slight Advantage, Research Finds," *The Houston Chronicle,* May 1, 1993, p. A17. The second quotation is from L. M. Fisher, "Drug Maker's Key Product Gets a Lift," *New York Times,* May 1, 1993, p. 6.

14. Quoted in an undated document (from late spring 1993) distributed by Astra, USA, a distributor of SK, under the signature of William Dwyer, product manager.

15. P. M. Ridker, C. O'Donnell, V. J. Marder, and C. H. Hennekens, "Large Scale Trials of Thrombolytic Therapy for Acute Myocardial Infarction," *Annals of Internal Medicine* 119 (1993): 530–32.

16. This case is more complex for two reasons. Consider, on the one hand, the claim that what should be covered by private insurance should be settled by private negotiations between insurers and purchasers of their policies and not by social policies and, on the other hand, the claim that private insurance in the United States is partially paid for out of public funds because of favorable tax treatment, and is therefore really disguised public insurance.

17. "Medicare Program: Criteria and Procedures for Making Medical Services Coverage Decisions that Relate to Health Care Technology" (BERC-432-P) *Federal Register* 54 (January 30, 1989): 4302–18. The following excerpts are from pp. 4308–9, 4317, and 4309.

18. This problem is a common, although not inevitable, problem for programs designed to use cost considerations in deciding about coverage. A good discussion of it, and of related problems, is found in S. Birch and A. Gafni, "Cost Effectiveness/ Utility Analyses," *Journal of Health Economics* 11 (1992): 279–96.

19. A tremendous amount has been written about that effort. An excellent summary and evaluation are found in a report from the Office of Technology Assessment, *Evaluation of the Oregon Medicaid Proposal* (Washington: Office of Technology Assessment, May 1992). An up-to-date ac-

count of the latest implementation setbacks is found in C. Campbell, "Gridlock on the Oregon Trail," *Hastings Center Report* 23 (July–August 1993): 6–7. See also Donald L. Patrick and Pennifer Erickson, *Health Status and Health Policy* (New York: Oxford University Press, 1993).

20. Information about these U.K. developments are found in two reports by Malcolm Dean in the *Lancet*: "End of a Comprehensive NHS" (February 9, 1991, pp. 351–52) and "Is Your Treatment Economic, Effective, Efficient?" (February 23, 1991, pp. 480–81).

21. President's Commission for the Study of Ethical Problems in Medicine and Biomedical and Behavioral Research, *Securing Access to Health Care,* vol. 1 (Washington: GPO, 1983). Following quotes from p. 20.

22. J. K. Iglehart, "Canada's Health Care System Faces Its Problems," *NEJM* 322 (1990): 562–68. Quote, p. 562.

23. I have attempted to develop such a theory in a series of recent articles, the most important of which are B. A. Brody, "The Macro-Allocation of Health Care Resources" in H. M. Sass and R. U. Massey, eds., *Health Care Systems* (Dordrecht: Kluwer, 1988), pp. 211–36, and "Ethical Reflections on International Health Care Expenditures," in E. Matthews and M. Menlowe, eds., *Philosophy and Health Care* (Aldershot, England: Avebury, 1992).

24. N. Daniels, *Just Health Care* (New York: Cambridge University Press, 1985), and N. Daniels, *Am I My Parents' Keeper?* (New York: Oxford University Press, 1988).

25. N. Daniels, "Is the Oregon Rationing Plan Fair?" *JAMA* 265 (1991): 2232–35. Quote, p. 2233.

26. This point is the familiar point that Rawlsian theories of justice, such as the theory proposed by Daniels, impose an excessively stringent requirement on inequalities, one that would not be chosen by rational individuals operating under the veil of ignorance. Even strong egalitarians, such as Thomas Nagel in *Equality and Partiality* (New York: Oxford University Press, 1991), allow (p. 73) for the legitimacy of the weak and the weaker priority.

27. R. B. Friedman and J. A. Katt, "Cost–Benefit Issues in the Practice of Internal Medicine," *Archives of Internal Medicine* 151 (1991): 1165–68. The following excerpt is from p. 1166.

28. S. H. Croog et al., "Sexual Symptoms in Hypertensive Patients," *Archives of Internal Medicine* 148 (1988): 788–94.

29. S. Wassertheil-Smoller et al., "Effect of Antihypertensives on Sexual Function and Quality of Life," *Annals of Internal Medicine* 114 (1991): 613–20.

30. M. A. Testa et al., "Quality of Life and Antihypertensive Therapy in Men," *NEJM* 328 (1993): 907–13.

31. S. W. Letsch et al., "National Health Expenditures, 1991," *Health Care Financing Review* 14 (1992): 1–30. For the analysis of the percentage of health-care expenditures devoted to prescription drugs, see the Boston Consulting Group, *The Contribution of Pharmaceutical Companies* (September 1993), p. 53.

32. T. Noah and E. Tanouye, "FDA Approves Taxol to Treat Ovarian Cancer," *Wall Street Journal,* December 30, 1992, p. B1.

33. "Betaseron Price Decisions Appear to Employ Cost Shifting," *The Blue Sheet,* September 8, 1993, pp. 9–10.

34. A whole literature has grown up surrounding the treatment of short stature. See, for example, the review of the issues in D. B. Allen and N. C. Fost, "Growth Hormone Therapy for Short Stature," *Journal of Pediatrics* 117 (1990): 16–21.

35. M. Freudenheim, "Method of Pricing Drug Is Assailed," *New York Times*, August 28, 1990, p. C2, and M. Freudenheim, "Cost Cut on Drug for Schizophrenia," *New York Times*, December 6, 1992, p. 1.

36. Pharmaceutical Manufacturers Association, *1992 Directory of Prescription Drug Indigent Programs* (Washington, D.C.). As noted in the article about betaseron, (note 33), these programs may actually result in higher prices for those who pay for the drugs.

37. L. Jones, "Industry's Charity Won't Stop Federal Push to Curb Drug Prices," *American Medical News*, February 10, 1992, p. 1.

38. General Accounting Office, *Prescription Drugs: Changes in Prices for Selected Drugs* (August 1992, GAO/HRD-92-128).

39. Special Committee on Aging, United States Senate, *The Drug Manufacturing Industry: A Prescription for Profits* (September 1991, Serial No. 102-F), p. 1.

40. Recent studies exploring some of these issues include D. L. Cleeton et al., "What Does the Consumer Price Index for Prescription Drugs Really Measure?" *Health Care Financing Review* 13 (1992): 45–51, and P. A. Ensor, "Projecting Future Drug Expenditures—1992," *American Journal of Hospital Pharmacy* 49 (1992): 140–45. A good summary of these problems, and of the most recent attempts to correct them, is found in a recent *Wall Street Journal* editorial, "Drug Price Rise May Be Exaggerated," October 8, 1993.

41. Staff Report to the U.S. Senate, Special Committee on Aging, *Earning a Failing Grade: A Report Card on 1992 Drug Manufacturer Price Inflation* (February 1993).

42. *Standard & Poor's Industry Surveys* (August 20, 1992), Health Care, p. H19.

43. Staff Report, *Earning a Failing Grade*, pp. 12–16.

44. The most important of these are Special Committee on Aging, United States Senate, *Prescription Drug Prices* (August 1989, Serial No. 101-D), Appendix F, and Special Committee on Aging, United States Senate, *Skyrocketing Prescription Drug Prices* (January 1990, Serial No. 101F), pp. 1–28. Quote from p. 14 of latter.

45. GAO, *Prescription Drugs: Companies Typically Charge More in the United States than in Canada* (September 30, 1992, HRD-92-110).

46. Both quotations from G. Kolata, "Why Drugs Cost More in the U.S.," *New York Times*, May 24, 1991, p. C1.

47. P. Temin, *Taking Your Medicine* (Cambridge, Mass.: Harvard University Press, 1980), Chapter 6.

48. Reports cited in notes 39 and 44 above.

49. The history and immediate impact of OBRA of 1990 is carefully analyzed in M. R. Pollard and J. M. Coster, "Savings for Medicaid Drug Spending," *Health Affairs* 10 (1991): 196–206. Senator Pryor's perspective on these issues is to be found in D. Pryor, "A Prescription for High Drug Prices," *Health Affairs* 9 (1990): 101–9.

50. J. Rovner, "The Senate Hones Its Revision of Drug Discounts; Bill Clears," *Congressional Quarterly* 50 (October 10, 1992): 3170.

51. J. Rovner, "Drug Manufacturers Win Round in Senate Debate on Prices," *Congressional Quarterly* 50 (March 14, 1992): 622.

52. The text of the Bush veto message is to be found in "Bush Vetoes Amendments to Orphan Drug Act," *Congressional Quarterly* 50 (November 17, 1992): 3893.

53. M. Freudenheim, "Drug Companies Feeling Pressure of Clinton's Plan to Keep Their Prices Down," *New York Times*, September 30, 1993, p. A12, and "Clinton, Shalala Testify to Future of Bioscience Research Pharmaceutical R&D under Health Care Reform," *Washington Fax: Life Science,* October 13, 1993.

54. "The Cost of Drugs: Hard to Swallow," *The Economist*, April 18, 1992, p. 76.

55. The first two are D. Macarthur, *Pricing and Reimbursement of Pharmaceuticals in the European Community* (Richmond, Surrey: PJB Publications, 1989), and G. Sermeus and G. Adriaenssens, *Drug Prices and Drug Legislation in Europe* (Brussels: BEUC, 1989). The most recent is R. N. Spivey, A. I. Wertheimer, and T. D. Rucker, eds., *International Pharmaceutical Services* (New York: Pharmaceutical Products Press, 1992).

56. The information in this paragraph is derived from Spivey et al., *International Pharmaceutical Services*, pp. 575–80.

57. M. Dean, "Curbing the Drugs Bill," *Lancet*, December 19–26, 1992, pp. 1531–32.

58. Further details are found in Macarthur, *Pricing and Reimbursement*, pp. 67–75.

59. Sermeus and Adriaenssens, *Drug Prices*.

60. This study is cited in the Special Committee on Aging, *The Drug Manufacturing Industry*, p. 28.

61. This act, and the background to it, is described in J. W. Hurst, "Reform of Health Care in Germany," *Health Care Financing Review* 12 (1991): 73–101, and in J. K. Iglehart, "Germany's Health Care System," *NEJM* 324 (1991): 503–8, 1750–56.

62. Details about the German pharmaceutical industry can be found in H. Sitzius- Zehender et al.,

"Federal Republic of Germany," in Spivey et al., *International Pharmaceutical Services*, Chapter 9.

63. Cited in Iglehart, "Germany's Health Care System," p. 1754.

64. Macarthur, *Pricing and Reimbursement*, pp. 36–41.

65. "Hard to Swallow," *The Economist*, April 18, 1992, p. 76.

66. H. Meyer, "New Health Cost Controls Are Approved in Germany,"*American Medical News*, February 15, 1993, p. 9, and GAO, *1993 German Health Reforms* (July 1993, GAO/HRD-93-103). The figures on the 1993 expenditures are from C. Whitney, "German Health Plan Cuts Prescription Costs," *New York Times*, September 15, 1993, p. 5.

67. Cited in Iglehart, "Germany's Health Care System," p. 1755.

68. The French system is described in detail in J. Brudon and G. Viala, "France," in Spivey et al., *International Pharmaceutical Services*, in Macarthur, *Pricing and Reimbursement*, pp. 45–56, and in Sermeus and Adriaenssens, *Drug Prices*, pp. 62–103.

69. Cited in Institute for Pharmaceutical Economics, *Government Influence in Pharmaceutical Pricing* (Philadelphia: Institute, 1991), p. 41.

70. Brudon and Viala, "France," p. 211.

71. The fullest discussion of this is to be found in Macarthur, *Pricing and Reimbursement*, pp. 53–55.

72. GAO, *Prescription Drugs*.

73. A good analysis of these issues is to be found in J. A. Bachynsky, "Canada," in Spivey et al., *International Pharmaceutical Services*, pp. 63–91.

74. M. Freudenheim, "For Canada, Free Trade Accord Includes Higher Prices for Drugs," *New York Times*, November 16, 1992, p. 1.

75. The Australian proposal is discussed in a series of articles in *Health Affairs* 11 (Winter 1992).

76. P. Roy Vagelos, "Are Prescription Drug Prices High?" *Science* 252 (1991): 1080–84. Quote, p. 1081.

77. P.L. 98-417.

78. S. Morrison, "Pharmaceutical Pricing and Patent Law," *CRS Report for Congress* 91-748E (November 22, 1991), p. 2.

79. R. E. Caves, M. D. Whinston, and M. A. Hurwitz, "Patent Expiration, Entry, and Competition in the U.S. Pharmaceutical Industry," *Brookings Papers: Microeconomics* (1991).

80. Performed by Stephen W. Schondelmeyer of the University of Minnesota and reported in OTA, *Pharmaceutical R&D* (Washington: GOP, OTA-H-522, February 1993), Appendix F.

81. Ibid., p. 241.

82. Quoted in Caves, Whinston, and Hurwitz, "Patent Expiration," p. 61.

83. J. A. DiMasi et al., "Cost of Innovation in the Pharmaceutical Industry," *Journal of Health Economics* 10 (1991): 107–42.

84. These are presented in OTA, *Pharmaceutical R&D*, pp. 66–72.

85. This remark is quoted by Elisabeth Rosenthal, "Drug Companies' Profits Finance More Promotion than Research," *New York Times*, February 21, 1993, p. 1. The article contains an extensive discussion of this issue and is the source of the remaining statistics in this paragraph.

86. B. O'Reilly, "Drugmakers under Attack," *Fortune*, July 29, 1991, pp. 48–63.

87. An important study which examines this issue is P. Megna and D. C. Mueller, "Profit Rates and Intangible Capital," *Review of Economics and Statistics* 73 (1991): 632–42.

88. OTA, *Pharmaceutical R&D*.

89. Ibid., p. 104.

90. This information is presented in chart 6, appended to a February 1993 staff report to the United States Senate Special Committee on Aging entitled *Earning a Failing Grade: A Report Card on 1992 Drug Manufacturer Price Inflation*. This staff report has not been formally published, but is obtainable from the committee.

91. This assumes no increase in sales through a lowering of price. That assumption seems reasonable in light of the very small price decrease.

92. Spivey et al., *International Pharmaceutical Services*, p. 582.

Conclusions

This book has traveled down many paths. We have studied aspects of the development of cardiology from Herrick to GUSTO. We have looked at a wide variety of theoretical issues, ranging all the way from informed consent in emergency research, to accelerated approval for life-saving drugs, to the right profit level for drug companies. It seems appropriate, therefore, to retrace our steps and to summarize what we have learned.

The following conclusions have emerged about the development of thrombolytic therapy:

1. The rapid progress in the 1980s, from improved knowledge about the cause of myocardial infarctions and about the benefits of various thrombolytic agents to the approved clinical use of several such agents to save many lives, is eloquent testimony to the innovative capacity of modern medicine.

2. This innovative capacity has progressed far more rapidly than has our understanding of how drugs should be tested, approved, and adopted. As a result, many problems were encountered during this period of rapid scientific innovation.

3. In the process of testing the thrombolytic agents, the most tragic of the problems was the continued use of placebo-controlled trials that were no longer appropriate rather than using active-controlled trials. Placebo-controlled trials of intravenous thrombolytic agents may well have been inappropriate after the results of the Western Washington trial confirmed the validity of the approval of intracoronary SK; they were certainly inappropriate by the time the TIMI investigators decided not to run any placebo-controlled trials because of the results of the GISSI trial and the Yusuf analysis. The decisions by other investigators to continue to run placebo-controlled trials were tragic as well as inappropriate because of the extra deaths in the placebo control groups.

4. In addition, none of the trials properly dealt with the issue of informed consent in emergency research. Some inappropriately disregarded informed consent because of the emergency situation while others inappropriately used the normal informed-consent process despite the special features of the emergency situation. The fundamental problem was their failure to recognize the existence of partially

valid consent in the emergency situation and to fashion techniques for dealing with partially valid consent.

5. Some of the clinical trials were structured by people who had financial conflicts of interest during the trials. This was a problem not because of the potential for fraud but because of the potential for inappropriate decisions about the structure and conduct of the trials.

6. The initial refusal of the FDA's advisory committee to recommend the approval of tPA was unfortunate. In part it was due to easily remediable factors such as the poor scheduling of the meeting and the lack of coordination between the NIH and the FDA. The more fundamental problem, however, was the failure of the approval process to properly reflect the appropriate trade-offs between safety and efficacy and between better proof and quicker approval when dealing with potentially significant therapeutic advances in the treatment of life-threatening illnesses.

7. Until the results of GUSTO became available, but especially after the results of GISSI-2 and ISIS-3 were known, it was perfectly appropriate for clinicians to use SK because it was cheaper and for reimbursement schemes to refuse to pay the extra cost of tPA. The situation is much more complicated now that the results of GUSTO have been published, in part because of substantial questions about the results of that trial and in part because we have not yet developed a proper ethic for a health-care world which must be cost-conscious to replace the classical ethic that costs should be disregarded if patients can benefit from more costly interventions.

8. Although the price of tPA is high in comparison to the price of SK, we cannot say at this point that it is inappropriately high. This is because we lack enough knowledge both about the capital investments in its development and about its sales potential, but it is also because we have not yet decided as a society how we want to price drugs, given that we have good reasons for not depending on the market to set drug prices.

It should be remembered that all of these conclusions emerged as a result of our theoretical analyses of a wide variety of issues. These theoretical analyses led us to a series of far broader conclusions, the most important of which are the following:

9. The current regulations governing research on human subjects have not adequately dealt with the limits on the use of placebo control groups in clinical trials and with the process of obtaining informed consent in emergency research.

10. The proposed federal rules for dealing with conflicts of interest in clinical trials need to be expanded to deal with the conflicts produced by grant income as well as the conflicts resulting from financial relations (for example, equity ownership) with commercial sponsors of clinical trials.

11. Despite the growing recognition that the FDA's rules need to be modified to better reflect the need for more appropriate trade-offs in the drug approval pro-

cess, not enough has been done to change those rules to accommodate the different values of different citizens with different perspectives.

12. The classical position on the relation between clinical decisions and cost considerations is not as inflexible as sometimes portrayed, but it is still inadequate for a health-care world in which cost control is a vital need. Better alternatives are now available, although more work needs to be done on them.

13. We have good reason to reject the market as the mechanism for setting the prices of drugs. We also have good reason to reject many of the European mechanisms used for setting drug prices, including those of France and Germany, which inadequately support needed research and development. While the details of the British approach are probably inappropriate for the American setting, its basic philosophy of controlling prices while allowing for an adequate return to encourage research and development seems right. Special attention will need to be paid to the appropriate level of drug promotion and to the problem of other countries that try to take advantage of the U.S. support of research and development through higher drug prices in the United States.

These are, no doubt, controversial conclusions. I welcome controversy about them because it may stimulate more people to reflect on these important issues. If it can achieve this, I will consider this book a success.

Index